MEDICAL RADIOLOGY

Diagnostic Imaging

A. H. Freeman · E. Sala (Eds.)

Radiology of the Stomach and Duodenum

With Contributions by

K. Balan · A. Ba-Ssalamah · N. R. Carroll · C. Cousins · M. Dux · T. Fork · A. H. Freeman
K. M. Harris · H.-U. Laasch · D. Martin · M. Memarsadeghi · P. Pokieser · M. Prokop
J. W. A. J. Reeders · E. Sala · T.C. See · P. J. Shorvon · M. Uffmann · R. Zissin

Foreword by

A. L. Baert

With 322 Figures in 588 Separate Illustrations, 129 in Color and 9 Tables

Springer

Alan H. Freeman, MB, BS, FRCR
Consultant Radiologist
Department of Radiology
Addenbrooke's Hospital
Box 219, Hills Road
Cambridge, CB2 2QQ
UK

Evis Sala, MD, PhD
University Lecturer/Honorary Consultant Radiologist
University Department of Radiology
Addenbrooke's Hospital
Box 219, Hills Road
Cambridge CB2 2QQ
UK

Medical Radiology · Diagnostic Imaging and Radiation Oncology
Series Editors:
A. L. Baert · L. W. Brady · H.-P. Heilmann · M. Knauth · M. Molls · C. Nieder · K. Sartor

Continuation of Handbuch der medizinischen Radiologie
Encyclopedia of Medical Radiology

ISBN 978-3-662-49605-3 Springer Berlin Heidelberg New York
DOI 10.1007/978-3-540-49897-1

Springer is part of Springer Science+Business Media

http//www.springer.com

Softcover re-print of the Hardcover 1st edition 2008

Medical Editor: Dr. Ute Heilmann, Heidelberg
Desk Editor: Ursula N. Davis, Heidelberg
Production Editor: Kurt Teichmann, Mauer
Cover-Design and Typesetting: Verlagsservice Teichmann, Mauer

Printed on acid-free paper – 21/3180xq – 5 4 3 2 1 0

To my wife

Jackie
for all her patience
during the preparation of this book

Alan H. Freeman

To my son

Pier

and my husband

Gezim

Evis Sala

Foreword

Notwithstanding the major contributions of endoscopy in the diagnosis and management of disorders of the stomach and the duodenum, radiology still has an important role in specific disease settings.

This volume provides up to date information on multimodality imaging of this anatomic section of the upper gastrointestinal tract within the framework of a multidisciplinary approach.

The editors, A.H. Freeman and E. Sala, judiciously selected the topics and were very successful in engaging the help of several other internationally recognised experts in gastrointestinal radiological imaging. The book comprehensively covers all main areas of interest, is superbly illustrated and the references include the most important recent publications in the field.

I am confident that this outstanding volume will find a great interest from general as well as specialised gastrointestinal radiologists but also from gastroenterologists and abdominal surgeons, who want to update their knowledge and abilities on the actual value of radiological imaging for patients with stomach or duodenal disorders. I hope that it will meet the same success as the previous volumes in our series.

Leuven — Albert L. Baert

Preface

Following Roentgen's discovery of X-rays, early experimenters quickly realised that this new technology held promise for investigating the hitherto unknown area of the gastrointestinal tract. Only 1 year after the publication of Roentgen's paper, W. Becher fed lead subacetate to a guinea pig and thus performed probably the first contrast study of a living stomach. Studies on humans soon followed, with Roux and Balthazard reporting their findings using bismuth subnitrate as a contrast agent in 1897. Herman Rieder in 1904 was the first to standardise the gastric examination, using as a contrast agent a mixture of 40 g of bismuth subnitrate mixed with gruel – henceforth known as the "Rieder meal". However, it was realised that bismuth subnitrate had toxic side effects so investigators had to search for another form of contrast agent. They soon realised that barium sulphate, a naturally occurring mineral, possessed the ideal parameters of inertness, non-absorption from the gastrointestinal tract and excellent X-ray diffraction properties, which made it a perfect contrast agent for opacifying the upper GI tract. Its potential use had been suggested by Walter Cannon but it was Bachem and Gunter in 1910 that first described the use of barium sulphate in the stomach, and thus was borne the barium meal. Modifications occurred over the years, particularly with the introduction of double contrast, in an attempt to provide better delineation of the mucosal surface. Although the principle of double contrast in the colon had been first advocated by Fischer in 1923, its use in the stomach was slow to catch on in the Western world. The major stimulus for double contrast studies came from Japan in the 1960s, when a population screening programme was started to detect early gastric cancer – a condition with a very high prevalence in Japan. Hikoo Shirakabe, in particular, popularised the technique which requires the adherence of a thin film of high density barium sulphate to the gastric mucosa whilst the stomach is inflated with gas – usually CO_2. Improvements in barium preparations, including the addition of numerous gums and anti-flocculating agents, meant that by the late 1970s excellent mucosal detail could be demonstrated of the entire stomach and duodenum. And then along came flexible endoscopy, with its ability not only to see all the mucosa in glorious technicolour, but also to take biopsies of any suspicious or doubtful lesion. Here was a simple outpatient procedure requiring minimal sedation and within a decade the barium meal virtually died. However, conventional examination of the upper GI tract is still performed, although now the indications are different – often for function as well as morphological detail. New indications, such as studying the stomach after surgery for morbid obesity, have come into vogue and are likely to increase with the obesity epidemic in the Western world. It should also be remembered that endoscopy is not infallible – a point addressed in Chapter 4 – and that there are still occasions when a patient cannot or will not tolerate an endoscopy.

Whilst demand for conventional radiology of the stomach has substantially dropped, aided by the discovery of *Helicobacter pylori* and its relationship to peptic ulcer disease, new technology has introduced a host of indications for radiological imaging of the stomach and duodenum. This particularly applies to CT with the subsequent development of multidetector CT (MDCT). Early CT rapidly proved its worth in staging gastric carcinoma, particularly in the sphere of distant spread to nodes and the liver. Delineation of the wall of the stomach, however, proved difficult both because of duration of scan time as well as lack of fine detail. These problems have been largely overcome with MDCT, which can now offer exquisite detail of the gastric wall acquired in the space of a few seconds. Very fine detail of the distinction between the mucosa and submucosa can still only be achieved by the use of endoscopic US as is outlined in Chap. 8. It is interesting to speculate as to whether or not CT will eventually have this capability or will MRI possibly supersede both, aided by its real time capabilities. The latter clearly takes the radiologist into the role of functional studies, a sphere up to now dominated by Nuclear Medicine examinations. Radiological intervention in the stomach and duodenum is also growing in importance and whilst it is helpful to have endoscopic expertise, this is not essential, as is shown in Chapter 11.

Finally, it goes without saying that accurate interpretation of radiological images (however they are acquired) requires a full knowledge of pathological processes and the way that they affect the organ. The principle of radiologic/pathologic correlation is now well established, but it is always helpful to remind ourselves of the macroscopic changes and how they come about from different disease processes. This we have attempted to do in Chaptre 2.

In conclusion, we would like to thank Prof. A. Baert for entrusting us with the preparation of this project in the Medical Radiology series, and our particular thanks go to all our authors for contributing to this volume. We hope that it will provide useful and informative reading for any radiologist with an interest in the stomach and duodenum. Finally we wish to thank Ms Ursula Davis, Mr Kurt Teichmann and all the production team at Springer, whose tremendous help and expertise brought the project to fruition.

Cambridge

Alan H. Freeman
Evis Sala

Contents

Introduction and Clinical Overview

1

Alan H. Freeman

CONTENTS

Diseases of the stomach and duodenum are immensely common, accounting for 4% of family doctor visits per year. The generic title "indigestion" encompasses a collection of symptoms including heartburn, nausea, bloating, belching and sometimes vomiting. All of these may arise from disorders of the lower oesophagus, stomach or duodenum. In addition, disorders of the biliary tree may also cause such symptoms, resulting in diagnostic and treatment dilemmas

In many instances there may not be an underlying physical abnormality, so-called functional dyspepsia which is probably related to motor disturbances of the stomach and duodenum (Hammer and Talley 2000). In particular, this may be related to personal habits such as smoking, eating too much and too quickly or drinking too much alcohol.

When organic causes are present, they most commonly relate to gastro-oesophageal reflux disease (GORD), gastritis and duodenitis, as well as frank ulceration. Occasionally, ominous symptoms such as loss of appetite, increased satiety and loss of weight suggest a more sinister cause such as a carcinoma.

Understandably, most patients are aware of an association between indigestion and excess gastric acid and are therefore likely to self medicate – as witness the large number of proprietary antacids available across pharmacy counters. If simple measures fail then the patient is likely to consult his family doctor. Here, a brief history is essential, if only to rule out ominous symptoms as indicated above. Physical examination is largely unrewarding, unless there are obvious signs such as a gastric mass, lymphadenopathy, etc. Again in the first instance treatment is likely to be symptomatic; for example, if GORD is suspected then simple measures such as the avoidance of large meals late at night, elevating the head of the bed and weight reduction are indicated. If symptoms persist, then consideration has to be given to the prescription of a proton pump inhibitor (PPI). This is usually administered first thing in the morning over a 4- to 8-week trial period. Failure to respond to this regime is common, probably in the order of a quarter of the patients, and therefore the dose has to be increased. Usually this is doubled so the medication is taken before breakfast and before dinner. Alternatively a trial of another manufacturer's PPI is often advocated and it has to be noted that there are different genetic responses to the various PPIs. It is also worth remembering that there are other causes of oesophagitis apart from GORD. Medications such as doxycycline, tetracycline, aledronate, potassium chloride, non steroidal anti-inflammatory agents (NSAIDs) and quinidine are all well recognised causes of oesophagitis. If the patient remains symptomatic after these manoeuvres, and a confounding drug history has been excluded, then it is time to consider endoscopy (see below) and probably ph testing. Endoscopy is also necessary to exclude rarer causes of oesophagitis such as eosinophilic oesophagitis in which the oesophageal wall becomes infiltrated with eosinophils; usually without a peripheral eosinophilia. This condition typically responds to steroids.

Diseases of the stomach and duodenum account for about 50% of cases of dyspepsia, in the form of gastritis, duodenitis and duodenal ulcer. Most of these conditions are linked to infection with *Helicobacter pylori* (HP); for example it is shown to be present in 95% of cases of duodenal ulcer. Therefore, the goal here is the detection and eradication of this

A. H. Freeman, MB, BS, FRCR
Consultant Radiologist, Department of Radiology, Addenbrooke's Hospital, Box 219, Hills Road, Cambridge, CB2 2QQ, UK

organism. How should this be done? The urea breath test is the most accurate method of HP detection. This test relies on the fact that HP in the stomach produces urease. If the patient ingests 13C labelled urea, this will react with urease in the stomach and thus release 13C labelled CO2. In turn this is absorbed and then exhaled in the patient's breath, whence it can be quantified by mass spectrometry. Alternatively, radioactive C14 may be used as the labelling agent and will require a scintillation counter to measure the resultant C14CO2. The test has sensitivity and specificity of around 96% and is simple to perform. Patients need to stop taking PPIs for at least 2 weeks prior to the test and Histamine H2 receptor antagonists for 3 days before. In addition, antibiotics should cease at least 4 weeks before the test.

There are two other non-invasive tests for HP and these include serology and the stool antigen test. Serology is less specific than either of the other tests because it will remain positive long after the infection has been eradicated, but it is simple to perform and requires no preparation on the part of the patient. With a sensitivity of 92% and a specificity of 91% the stool antigen test is almost as accurate as the breath test. However, it requires the same patient preparation as the breath test and so cannot be conducted instantly.

The final and invasive test to ascertain the presence of HP is endoscopy and biopsy. The biopsies should be taken from the antrum of the stomach which is the area most frequented by the organism, although there is evidence that it colonises the more proximal body in patients who are taking PPIs. Histological examination reveals the organism. Apart from formal histology the biopsy specimens can be instantly examined for the presence of HP by the rapid urease test. This again utilises the fact that the organism secretes urease, but in this instance it is the conversion of urea to ammonia and bicarbonate which is the key. The specimen is placed in a medium containing phenol red. Subsequent production of ammonia raises the pH and changes the colour of the specimen, thus providing a useful instant diagnosis.

1.1 Which Patients Should Undergo Endoscopy?

This will be determined by local and national guidelines (National Institute for Health and Clinical Excellence 2004). As a general rule it is imperative to endoscope patients over the age of 50 who have persisting symptoms despite the use of PPIs, or whose dyspepsia is unexplained by other factors such as NSAID ingestion. In addition, there are a number of alarm features which should always lead to urgent endoscopy. These include the following: difficulty in swallowing, vomiting, sudden and unintentional weight loss, chronic gastrointestinal bleeding, epigastric mass, abnormal barium meal and iron deficiency anaemia. With the last mentioned not only can endoscopy exclude serious disease of the stomach and duodenum, but by obtaining biopsy material from the second part of the duodenum will also exclude celiac disease. All gastric ulcers must be biopsied even if they exhibit characteristic benign appearances; though it should be noted that only about 2% of gastric ulcers will be malignant. The usual technique involves biopsies from all four quadrants plus or minus brushing for cytology. If the biopsies are negative then repeat endoscopy is indicated to confirm complete healing, though even that may not be infallible as sometimes malignant ulcers can heal over on treatment. Immediate prepyloric and duodenal ulcers may be regarded as benign.

If HP is present what treatment regimes are recommended? The recommended treatment is that of triple therapy comprising of a full dose PPI together with metronidazole and clarithromycin or amoxicillin and clarithromycin. This course is for a 7-day period though will need to be extended to 1 month if a gastric ulcer has been demonstrated. In some circumstances it may be appropriate to consider such a course of treatment in patients who are asymptomatic but harbour HP. This group includes patients who are on other drugs, particularly NSAIDS, as it is known that about 10%–20% of patients taking these drugs will develop peptic ulcer disease, sometimes with serious complications(Hippisley-Cox et al. 2005) This issue particularly applies to elderly patients who are taking NSAIDs and who may have extensive other co-morbidity factors.

1.2 Is There Ever a Role for the Upper Gastrointestinal Series (Barium Meal)?

Whilst there has been a huge decline in the numbers performed, this procedure, unlike the oral cholecystogram, has not passed into history. Perhaps the commonest indication is the failed endoscopy. Despite sedation and/or local anaesthetic throat spray, there are still patients who are unable to tolerate the procedure and still require evaluation of the stomach and duodenum. It also has to be remembered that endoscopy is not infallible (see Chapter 4).There are several situations where endoscopic interpretation may be problematic or downright erroneous. The first concerns alteration in anatomy which may preclude full endoscopic interrogation. Typically this results from large hiatal hernias, an intrathoracic stomach or frank gastric volvulus. All of these may prevent the passage of the endoscope or obscure large areas of the stomach. For this reason spatial relationships of the stomach may be better appreciated at a barium meal. Secondly, endoscopic demonstration is largely that of the mucosal surface and submucosal lesions may be overlooked. Most typical of these is linitis plastica or leather bottle stomach, which may completely escape notice because failure to distend the stomach is attributed to the patient belching. Finally, it must not be forgotten that successful endoscopies inspect the duodenum down to the level of the inferior duodenal flexure and disease in the third and fourth parts may not be noted. The common endoscopic report of "no abnormality seen in the oesophagus, stomach or duodenum" must on occasion be treated with caution, particularly if it does not fit with the clinical picture.

Dyspeptic symptoms may of course arise from structures other than the stomach and duodenum. The commonest of these is disease of the gall bladder and biliary tract, with tumours of the pancreas a less frequent consideration. Many of these conditions are well ascertained by trans-abdominal ultrasound; particularly diseases of the gall bladder. As the symptomatology often overlaps it may be prudent in many cases to perform this simple test, in the knowledge that more sophisticated cross section imaging, i.e. CT, may be required if there is excess fat, gas, etc.

The advent of multi-detector CT (MDCT) has unquestionably enhanced its role in the diagnosis of diseases of the stomach and duodenum, (see Chaps. 6.1, 6.2), but it also still retains a major role in the staging of tumours. Whilst the overall incidence of carcinoma of the stomach may be going down, there is good evidence of the increase of tumours of the gastro-oesophageal junction – so-called junctional tumours. Thus a history of dysphagia, particularly if allied to dyspepsia and weight loss has to be taken with extreme seriousness. Initial diagnosis is made by endoscopy and biopsy, but subsequent management then requires accurate staging. The following questions need to be answered: Is the tumour amenable to surgical resection? If not, can it be down-staged by chemotherapy? If still unresectable is it suitable for palliative treatment such as stenting and/or laser treatment? Is there extensive metastatic disease or are there other co-morbidity factors that prevent intervention? Many of these questions can be answered by MDCT which, of course, is particularly good at demonstrating loco-regional nodes as well as local invasion into adjacent structures. Naturally, it excels at demonstrating more distant metastatic disease, particularly in the liver. However, the emerging role of PET/CT will challenge it in several of these areas (lymph nodes and the liver in particular), and this will have to be incorporated into management protocols when important clinical decisions have to be made. It must also be remembered that CT cannot as yet compete with endoscopic ultrasound for T1/2 staging.

Naturally, CT plays a major role in the follow-up of these patients, whether they have had formal surgery or palliation in the form of a stent. Tumour recurrence and/or more distant spread always will remain a possibility and the role of radiology in the post-operative situation is reviewed in Chapter 13. The biggest practical issues following stent insertion is local recurrence, which may be through the mesh if it is uncovered, or over the top of the stent if covered. However, covered stents are more prone to distal migration than uncovered, which also presents its own problem. Tumour recurrence through the wall can be dealt with by laser therapy or, on occasion, by the insertion of a second stent through the lumen of the original.

The prevalence of pancreatic cancer is also increasing and its presenting features often overlap with those of gastro-duodenal origin. Of course, if the tumour is situated in the head of the pancreas then obstructive jaundice is likely to be the first sign. However, tumours arising from the neck or body of the gland often have a more insidious and occult mode of presentation, usually with vague epigastric discomfort, together with loss of appetite and weight. Urgent CT examination will usually reveal the diagnosis and should be performed at the slightest suggestion, as it is the mainstay of diagnosis.

In summary, it can be seen that the role of radiology in investigating diseases of the stomach and duodenum has changed. Endoscopy and endoscopic techniques are now pre-eminent in the initial diagnosis, but radiology, particularly in the various forms of cross sectional imaging, has a major and increasing role to play.

References

Hammer J, Talley NJ (2000) Non-ulcer dyspepsia. Curr Opin Gastroenterol 16:503–507

National Institute for Health and Clinical Excellence (2004) Managing dyspepsia in adults in primary care. NICE, London (www.nice.org.uk)

Hippisley-Cox J, Coupland C, Logan R (2005) Risk of adverse gastrointestinal outcomes in patients taking cyclo-oxygenase-2 inhibitors or conventional non-steroidal anti-inflammatory drugs: population based nested case-control analysis. BMJ 331:1310–1316

Additional Reading

British Society of Gastroenterology (2002) Guidelines for the management of oesophageal and gastric cancer. BSG, London (www.bsg.org.uk)

Radiological–Pathological Correlation

2

Jacques W. A. J. Reeders, Alan H. Freeman, and Evis Sala

Radiology as a discipline is one which is dominated by images. Nowhere is this truer than imaging of the upper gastrointestinal tract, which was the first area to experience the correlation of images produced by indirect radiological techniques with those produced by direct endoscopic methods. Knowledge of the macroscopic appearances as shown either by endoscopy or from pathological specimens is the key to interpreting radiological images. The following chapter attempts to bring these facets together so that the reader is able to understand better the pathological base of the common and not so common conditions affecting the stomach and duodenum, and how these processes manifest themselves on radiological images.

a

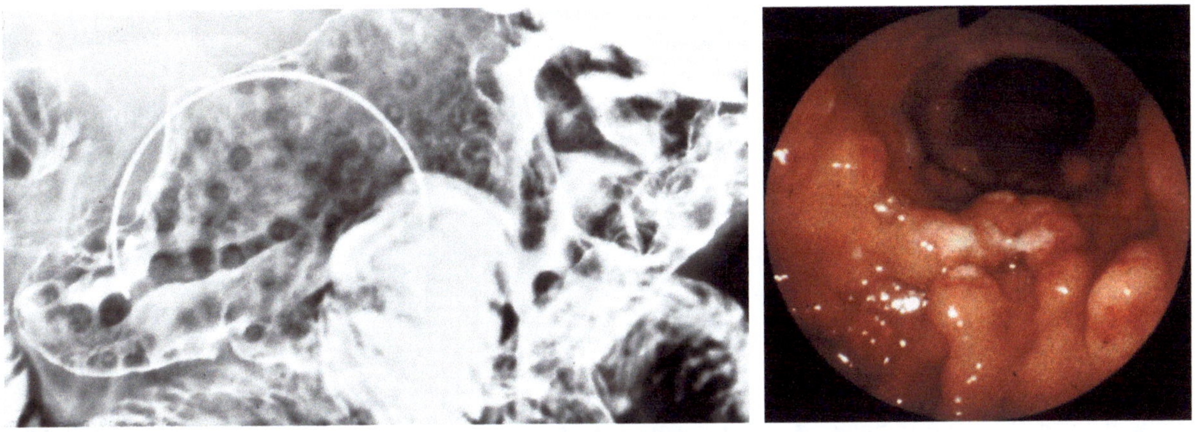

b

Fig. 2.1a,b. Erosive Gastritis. Double Contrast barium study (**a**) showing multiple erosions in the body and antrum of the stomach. Note the typical round lucencies with a central pit of barium. Endoscopy (**b**) confirms the small bulbous elevations with central ulcerations

J. W. A. J. Reeders, MD, PhD
Consultant Radiologist, Department of Radiology, St. Elisabeth Hospital Willemstad, Breedestraat 193(O), Curaçao, Netherlands Antilles
A. H. Freeman, MB, BS, FRCR
Consultant Radiologist, Department of Radiology, Addenbrooke's Hospital, Box 219, Hills Road, Cambridge, CB2 2QQ, UK
E. Sala, MD, PhD, FRCR
Univerity Lecturer/Honorary Consultant Radiologist, Department of Radiology, Addenbrooke's Hospital, Box 219, Hills Road, Cambridge, CB2 2QQ, UK

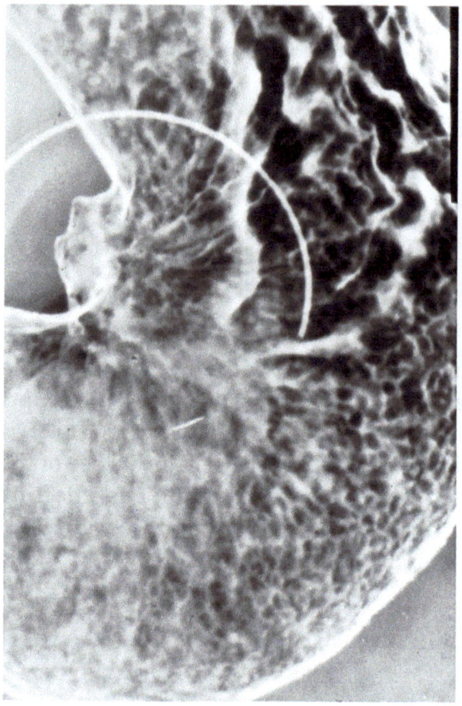

a

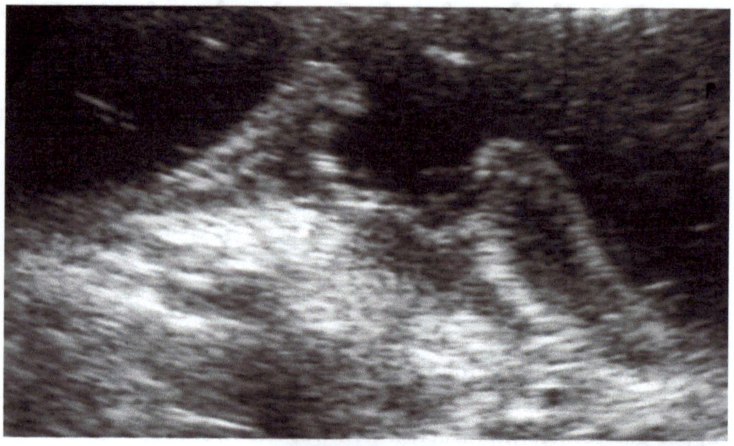

b

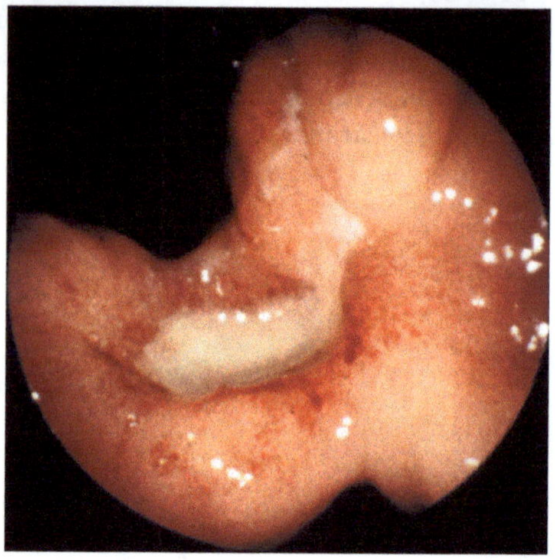

c

Fig. 2.2a–c. Benign gastric ulcer. Double contrast barium study (a) showing a large deep penetrating ulcer at the incisura angularis. Ultrasound of the water-filled stomach (b) illustrates the oedematous border of the ulcer. Endoscopy (c) confirms deep ulceration with thickening of the surrounding margin. Biopsy proved this to be a benign ulcer

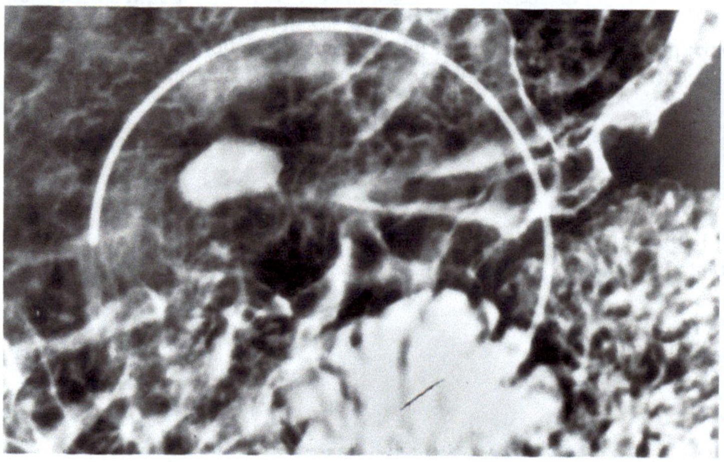

a

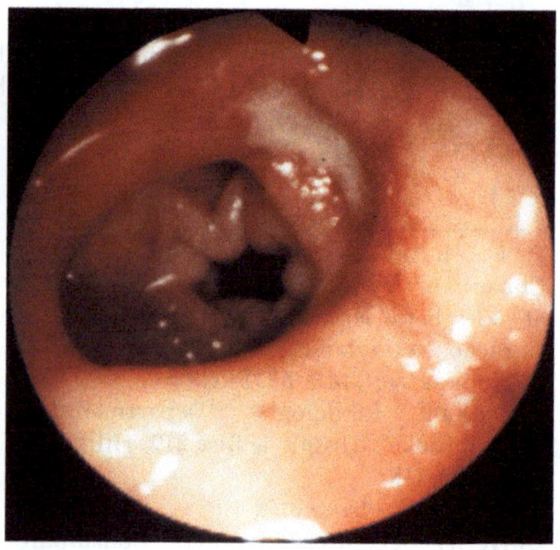

b

Fig. 2.3a,b. Benign gastric ulcer. Double Contrast barium study (a) shows a small benign ulcer niche on the greater curve of the body of the stomach, with folds radiating to the ulcer crater. Endoscopy (b) confirmed a benign ulcer

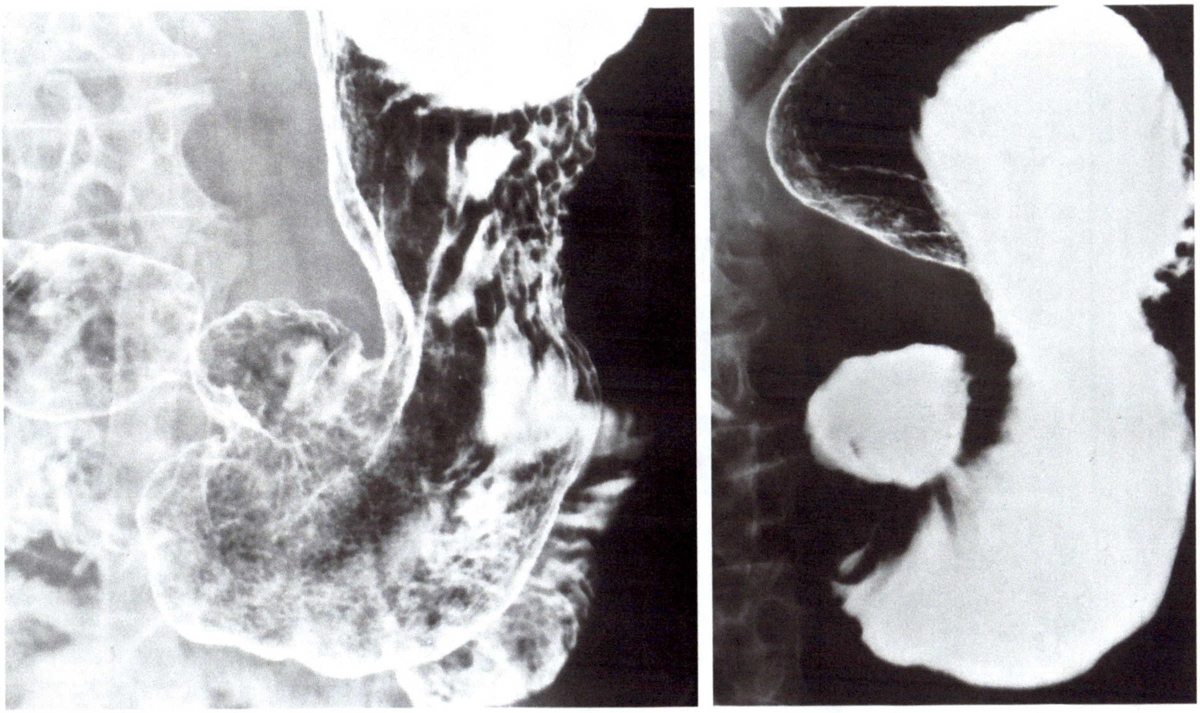

a b

Fig. 2.4a,b. Malignant gastric ulcer. Double Contrast barium study (**a**) and a single contrast study (**b**) show a large deep penetrating malignant ulcer on the lesser curve of the body of the stomach. Note the prominent tumour collar around the margin of the ulcer

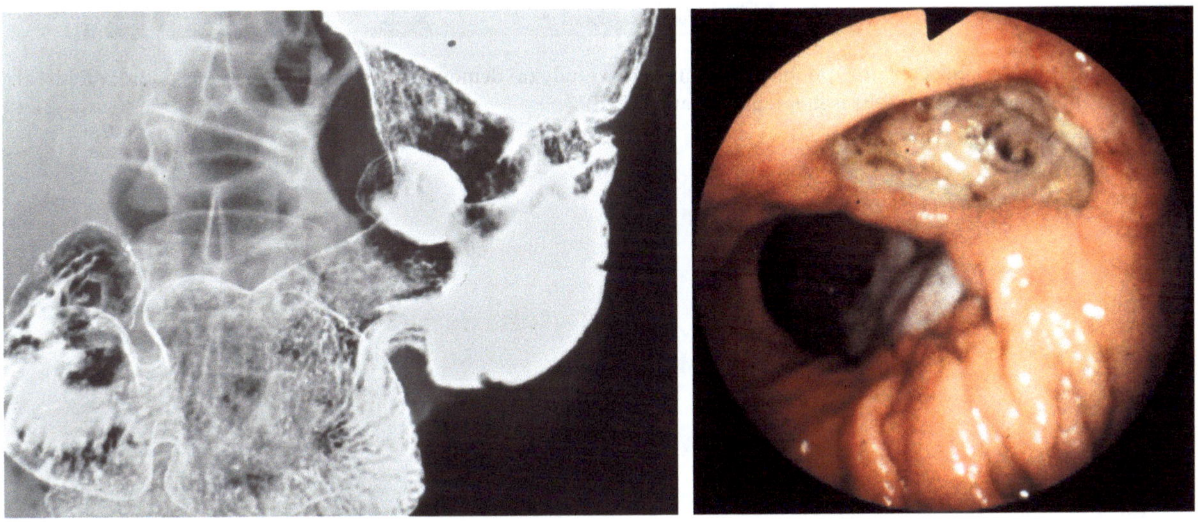

a b

Fig. 2.5a,b. Ischaemic gastric ulcer (iatrogenic). Double Contrast barium study (**a**) showing a deep penetrating ulcer affecting the greater curve of the body of the stomach, mimicking a malignant ulcer. Three months prior to this investigation, the patient had undergone a coeliac axis plexus blockade with the injection of 96% alcohol partly within the gastric wall. Endoscopy (**b**) demonstrates the deep ulcer with well defined margins

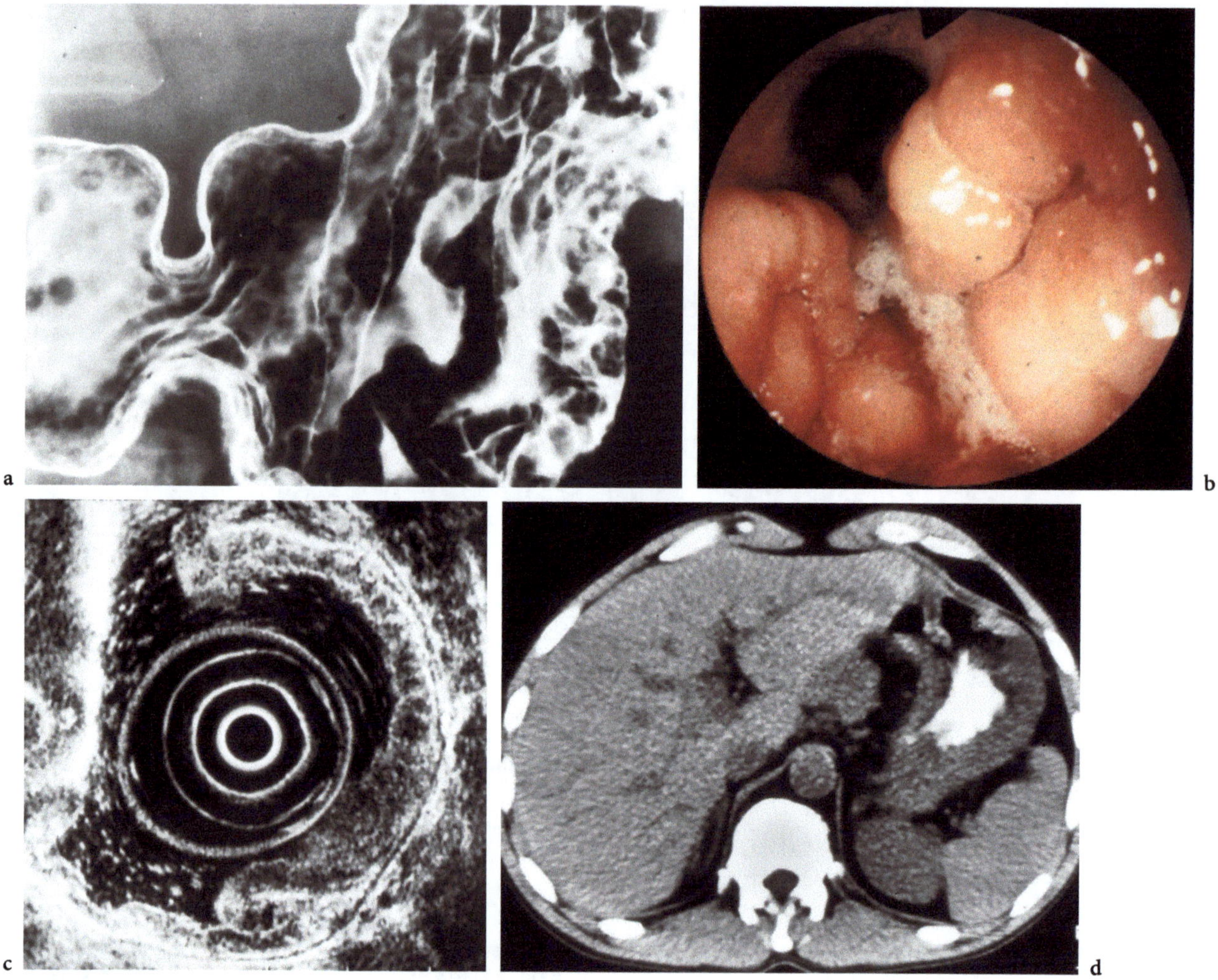

Fig. 2.6a–d. Hypertrophic Gastritis. Double Contrast barium study (a) demonstrating enlarged tortuous nodular folds, also shown at endoscopy (b), endo-ultrasonography (c) and CT (d)

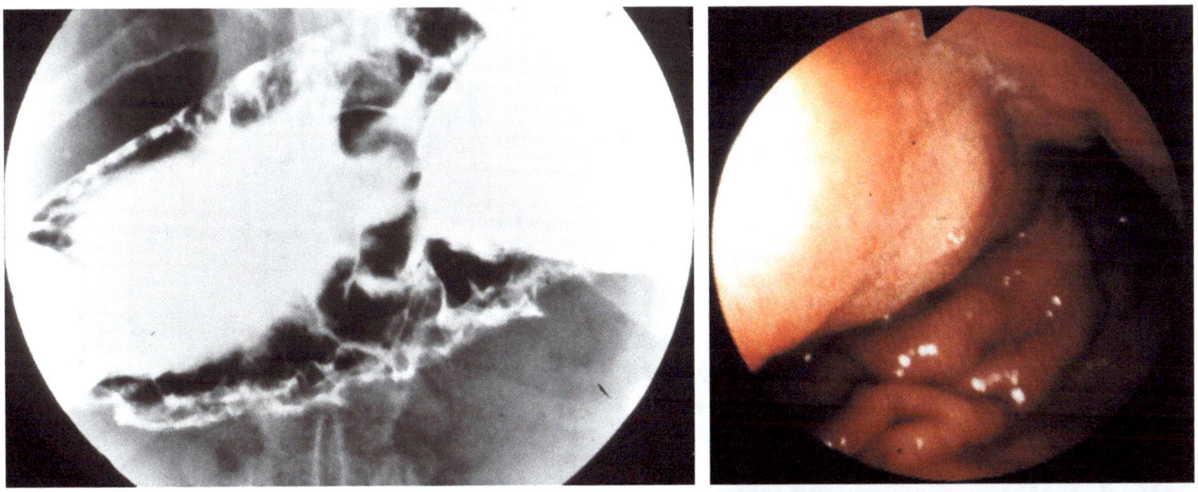

a b

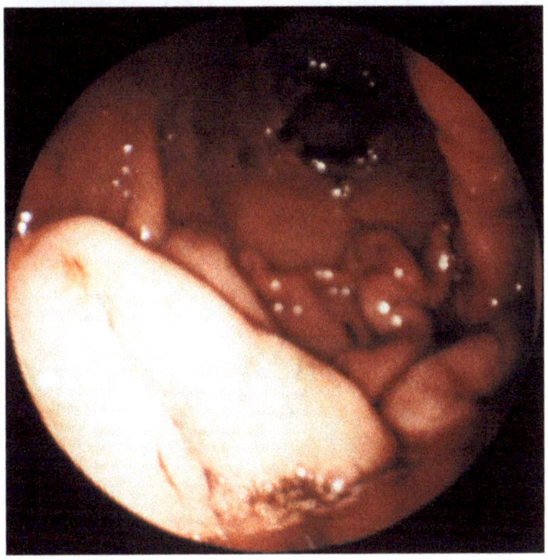

c

Fig. 2.7a–c. Zollinger-Ellison Syndrome. Double Contrast barium study (**a**) showing enlarged thickened tortuous folds in the body of the stomach, also well demonstrated at endoscopy (**b,c**)

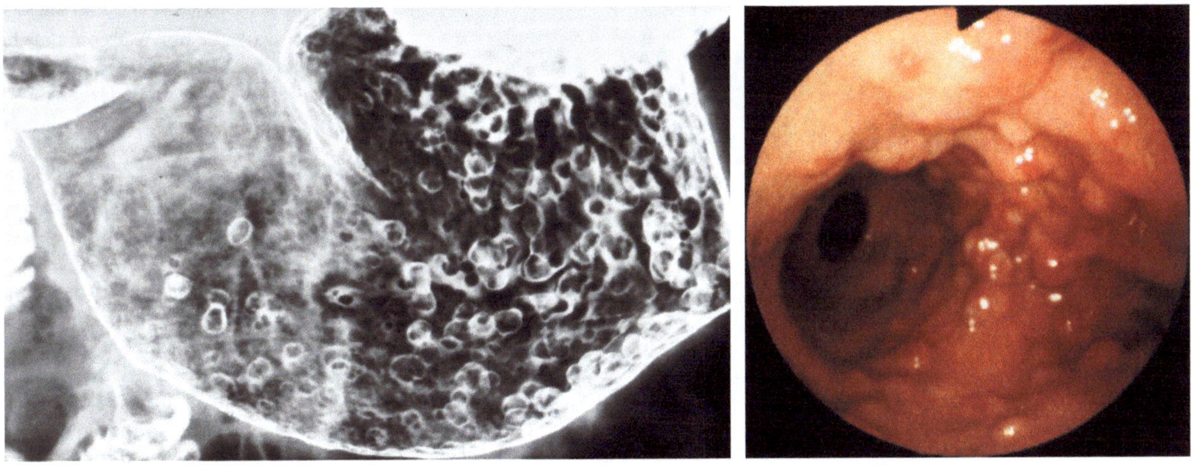

a b

Fig. 2.8a,b. Gastric Polyps. Double Contrast barium study (**a**) and Endoscopy (**b**) demonstrating innumerable benign hyperplastic polyps in the body and antrum of the stomach

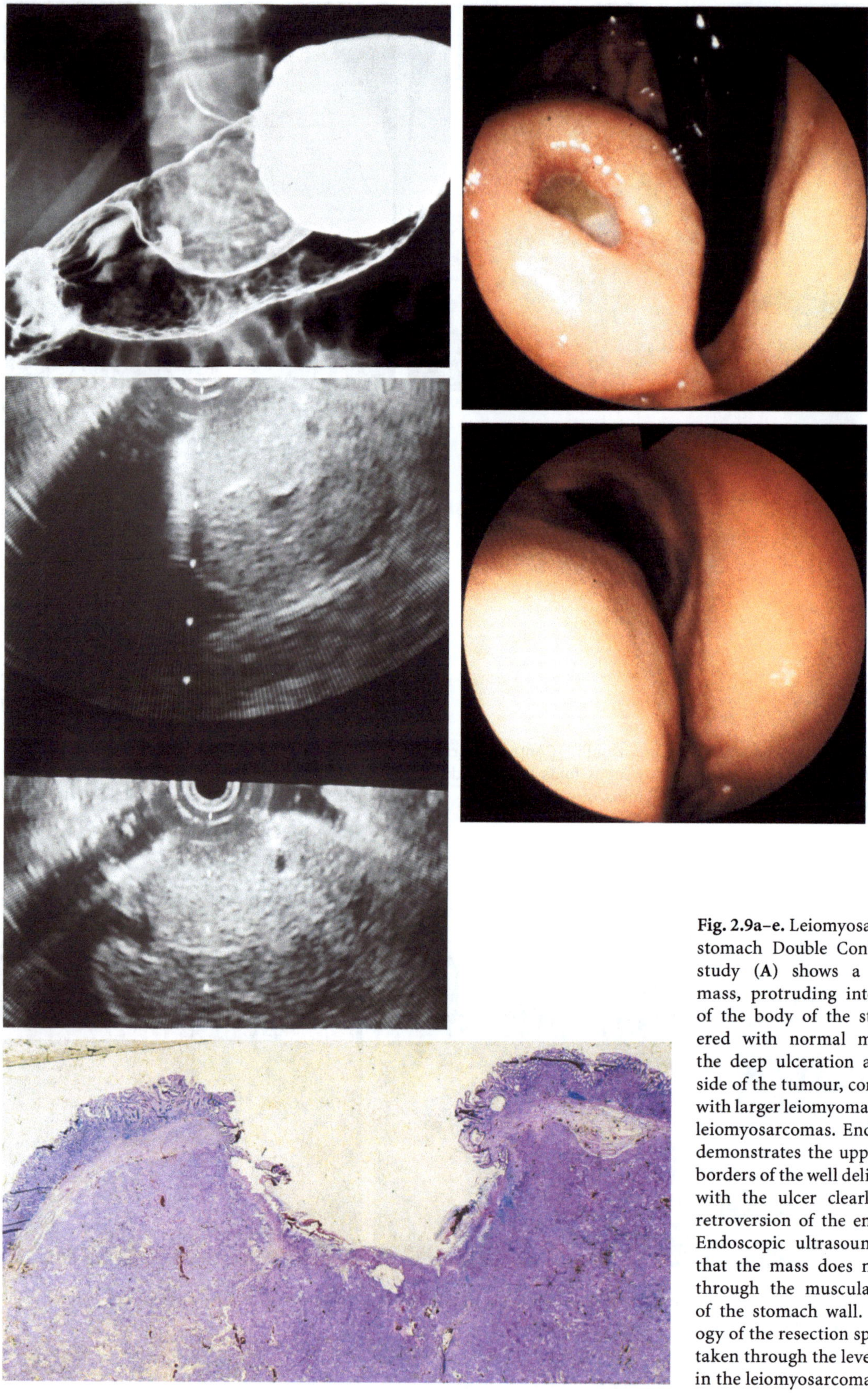

a b c d e

Fig. 2.9a–e. Leiomyosarcoma of the stomach Double Contrast barium study (**A**) shows a large bulky mass, protruding into the lumen of the body of the stomach, covered with normal mucosa. Note the deep ulceration at the caudal side of the tumour, commonly seen with larger leiomyomas (GISTs) and leiomyosarcomas. Endoscopy (**b,c**) demonstrates the upper and lower borders of the well delineated mass, with the ulcer clearly seen with retroversion of the endoscope (**b**). Endoscopic ultrasound (**d**) shows that the mass does not penetrate through the muscularis mucosae of the stomach wall. Histopathology of the resection specimen (**e**) is taken through the level of the ulcer in the leiomyosarcoma

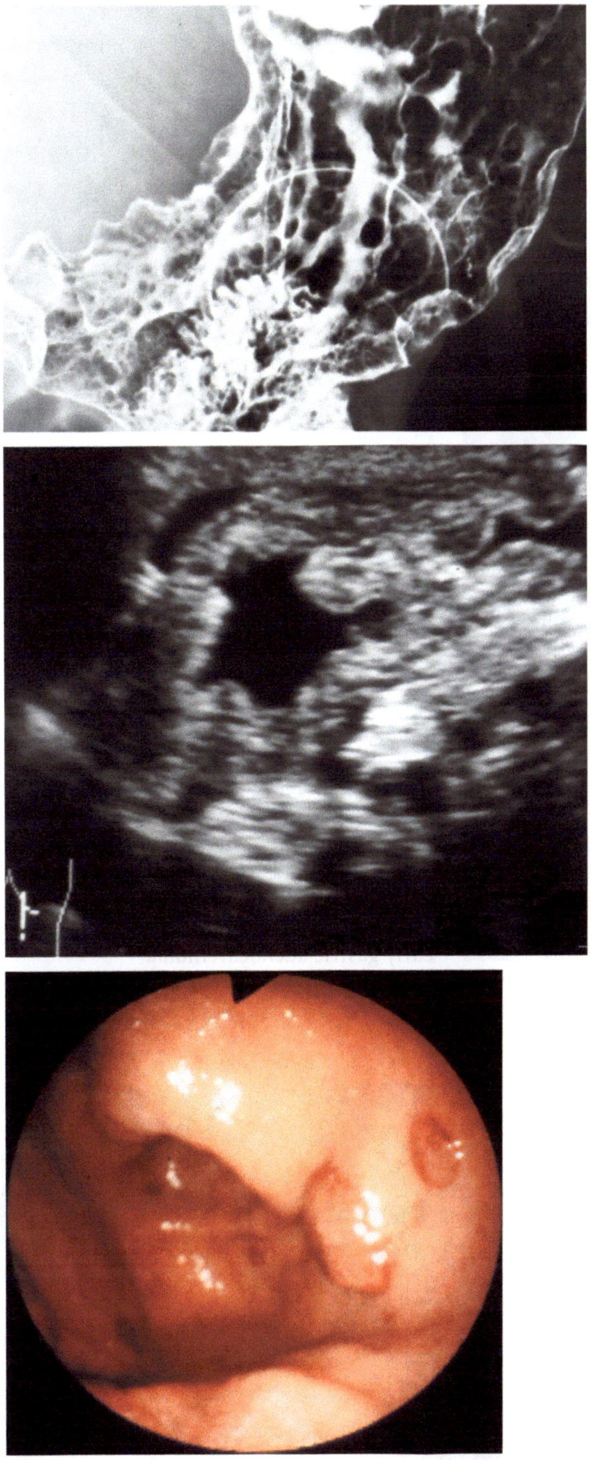

Fig. 2.10a–c. Kaposi's sarcoma of the stomach. Double Contrast barium study (a) shows multiple well delineated small bullous protrusions into the lumen of the body and antrum of the stomach. Ultrasound (b) shows multiple protrusions into the water-filled lumen. Endoscopy (c) demonstrates purple coloured round sharply delineated lesions, on a background of normal mucosa, typical of Kaposi's sarcoma

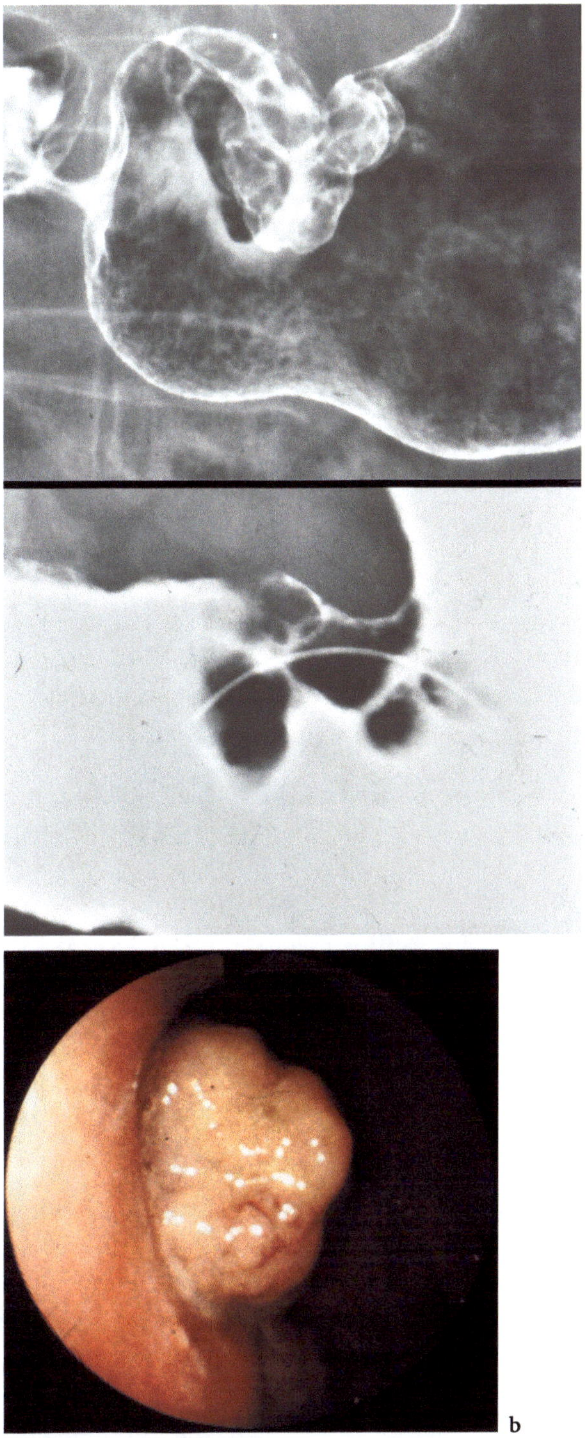

Fig. 2.11a,b. Metastasis to the stomach. Double Contrast and Single Contrast barium studies (a) demonstrate a villous type tumour arising from the lesser curve aspect of the antrum, confirmed at endoscopy (b). Biopsy revealed a metastasis from breast cancer

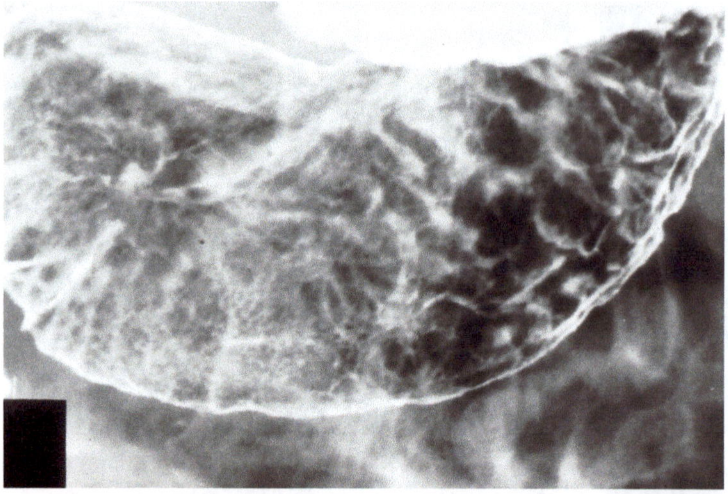

a

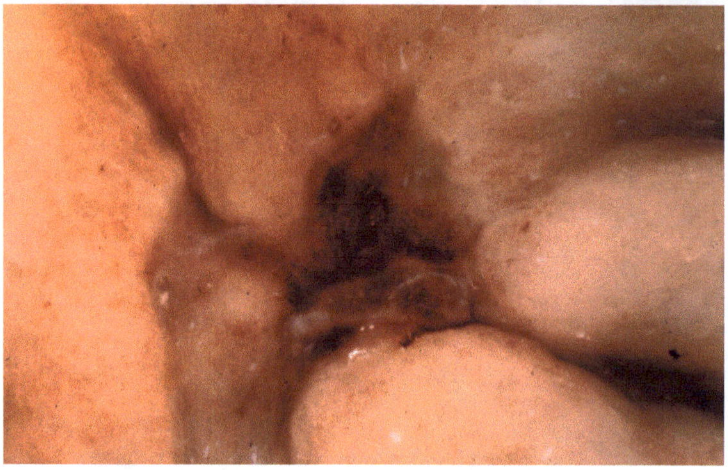

b

Fig. 2.12a,b. Early Gastric Cancer. Double Contrast barium study (a) shows a flat ulcerated lesion on a background of normal mucosa. The folds are distorted and truncated at the level of the flat lesion. Histopathology of the resection specimen (b) confirmed an early gastric adenocarcinoma

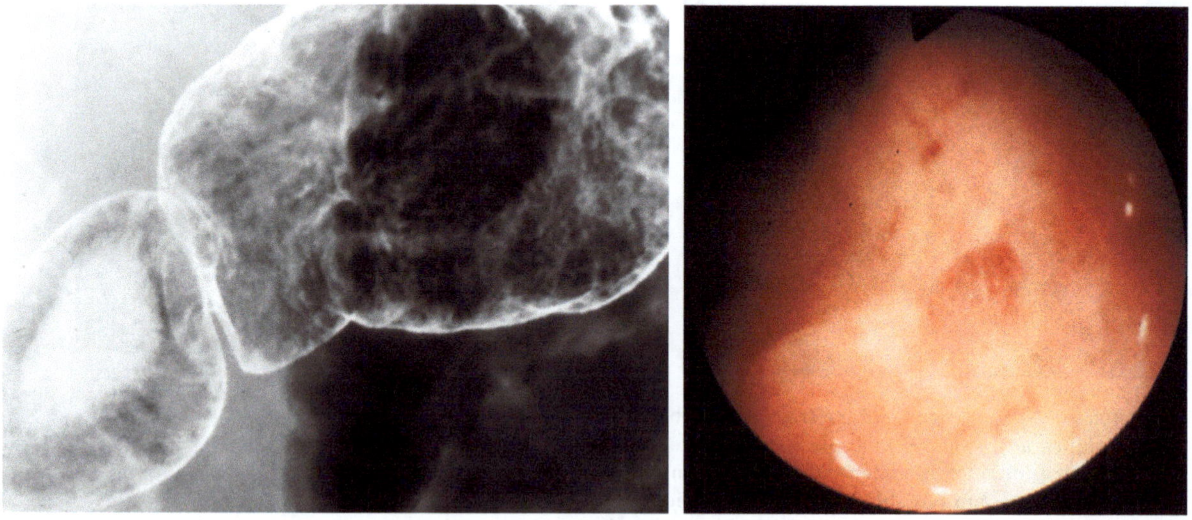

a b

Fig. 2.13a,b. Early Gastric Cancer. Double Contrast barium study (a) shows slight distortion of normal mucosal folds on the posterior wall of the antrum of the stomach. Endoscopy (b) demonstrates the non-depressed lesion, with distortion of the normal gastric mucosal pattern. Histopathology confirmed early gastric cancer

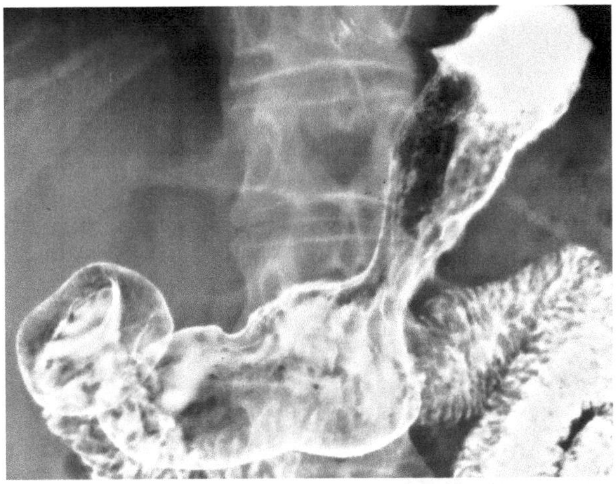

a

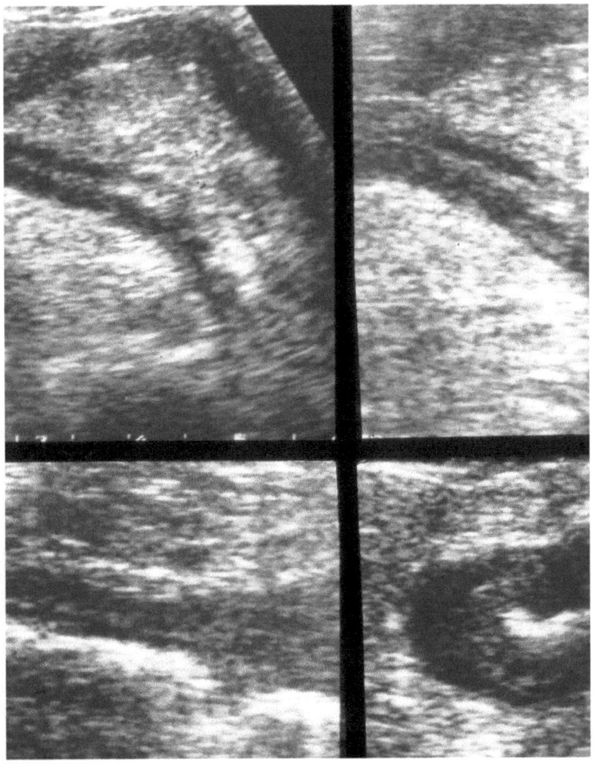

b

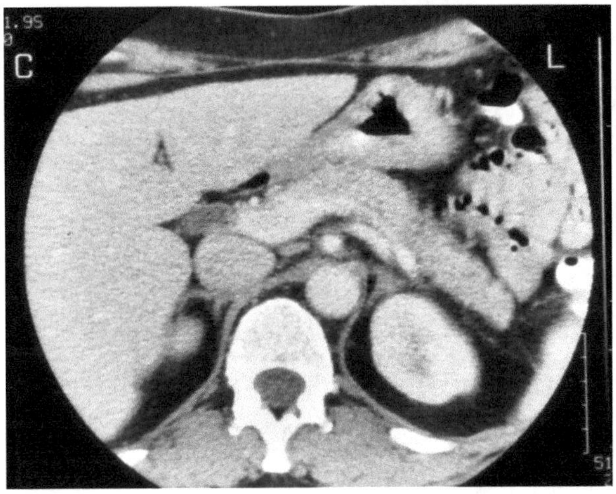

c

Fig. 2.14a–c. Linitis Plastica of the stomach. Double Contrast barium study (**a**) shows a marked circumferential narrowing of the fundus and proximal body of the stomach. Ultrasound (**b**) and CT (**c**) confirm extensive thickening of the gastric wall. Multiple biopsies confirmed the presence of linitis plastica

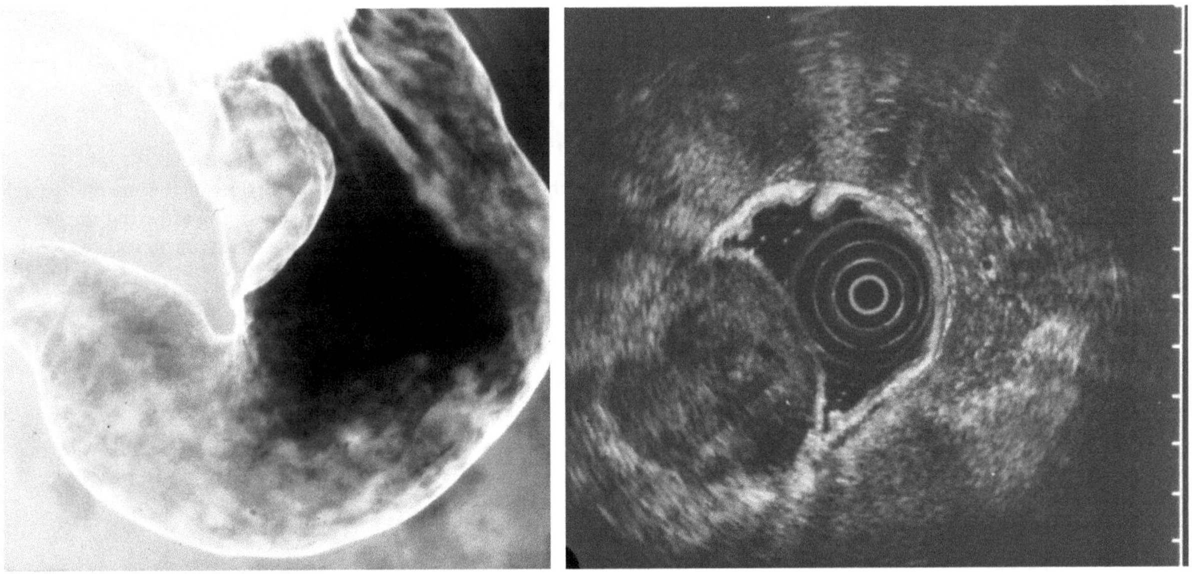

a b

Fig. 2.15a,b. Leiomyoma of the stomach. Double Contrast barium study (**a**) shows a well delineated smooth mass arising from the lesser curve of the stomach. Endoscopic-ultrasound (**b**) demonstrates a massive lesion which does not penetrate through the gastric wall. Biopsy revealed a benign leiomyoma

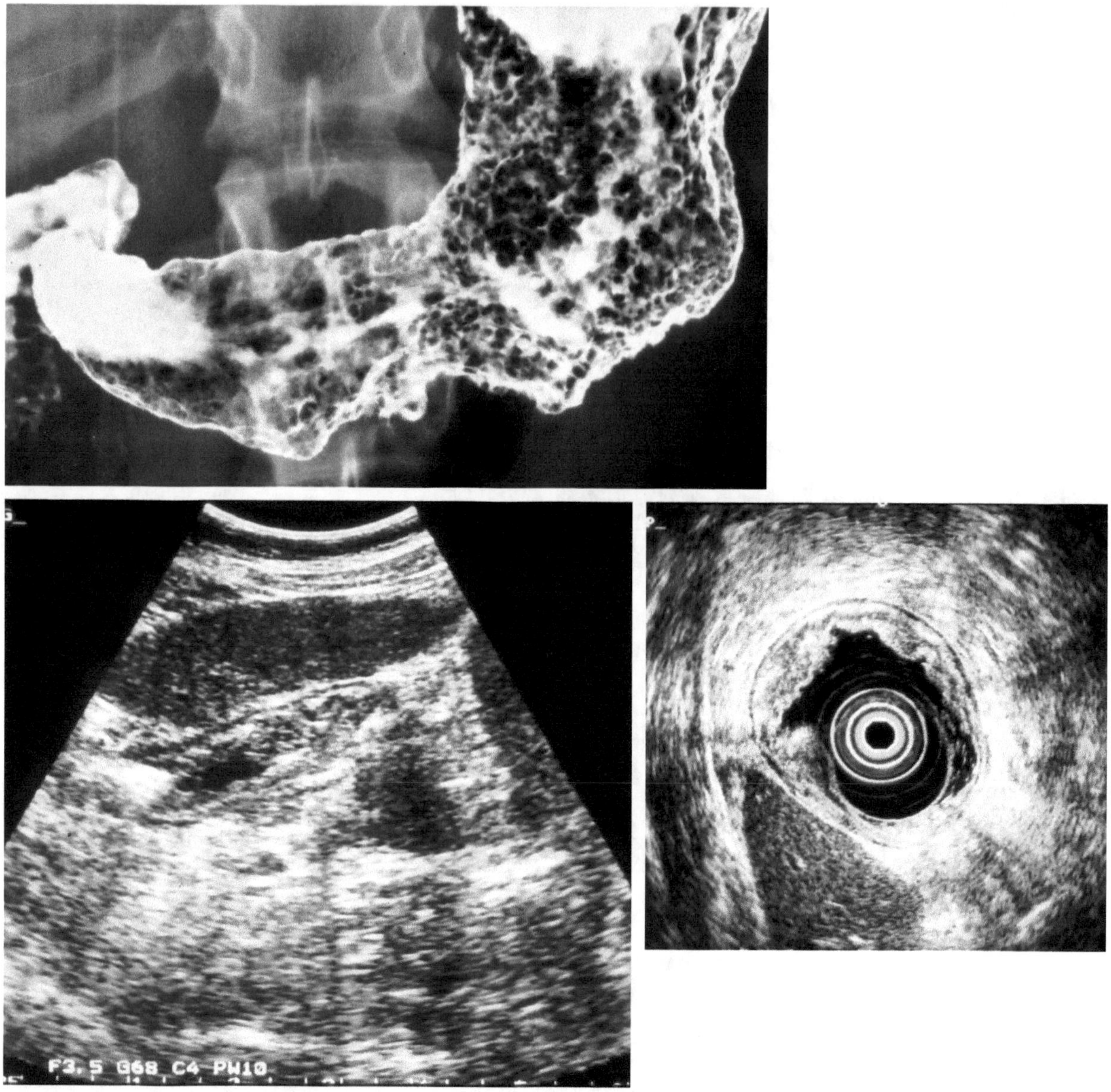

Fig. 2.16a–c. Crohn's Disease of the stomach. Double Contrast barium study (**a**) shows distortion of the normal gastric mucosal pattern with marked nodularity and multiple aphthous lesions. Note the irregular scalloping affecting the greater curve, due to active Crohn's Disease. Ultrasound (**b**) and Endoscopic-ultrasound (**c**) show marked transmural thickening of the gastric wall. The muscularis propria is intact

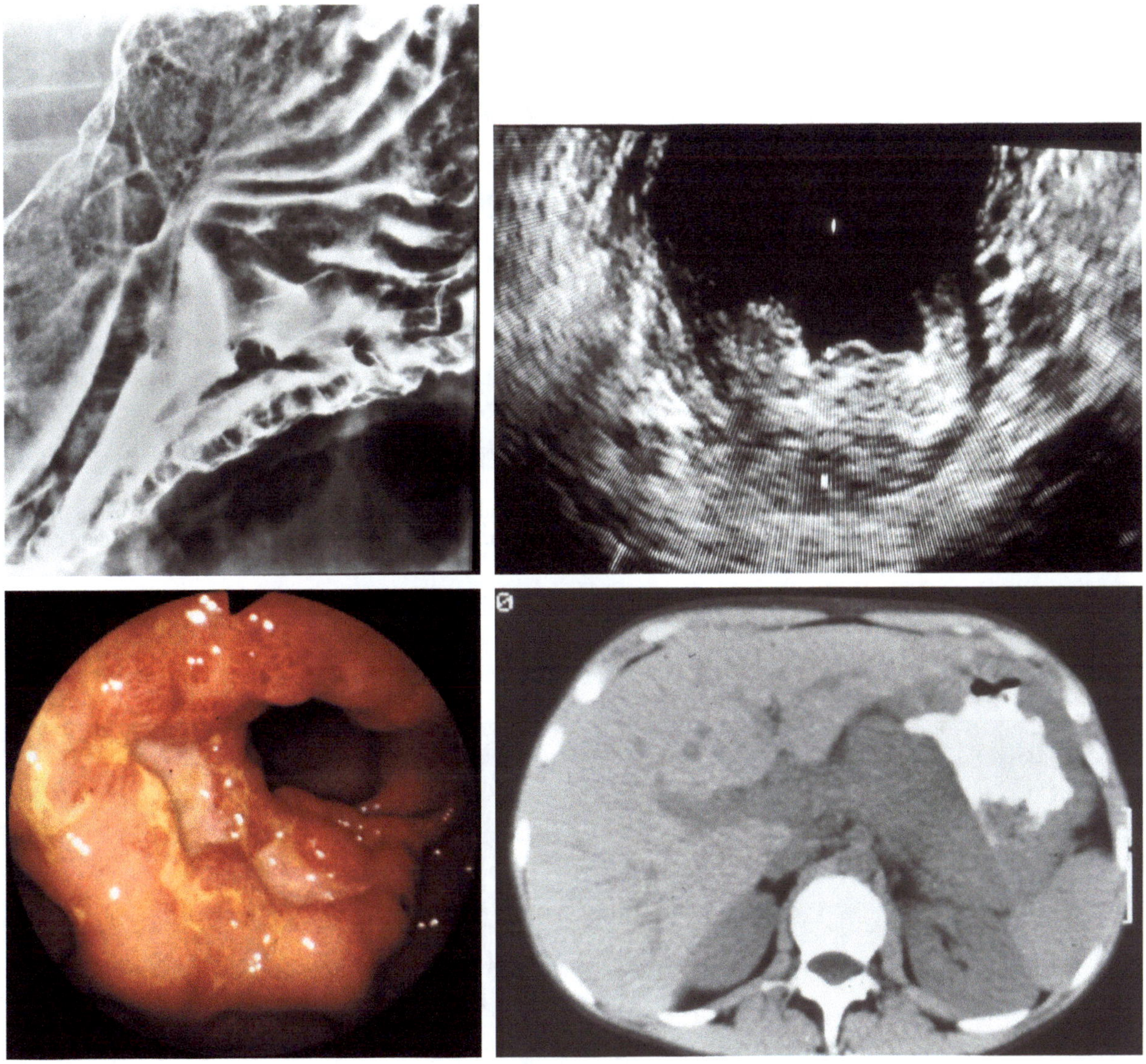

a b c d

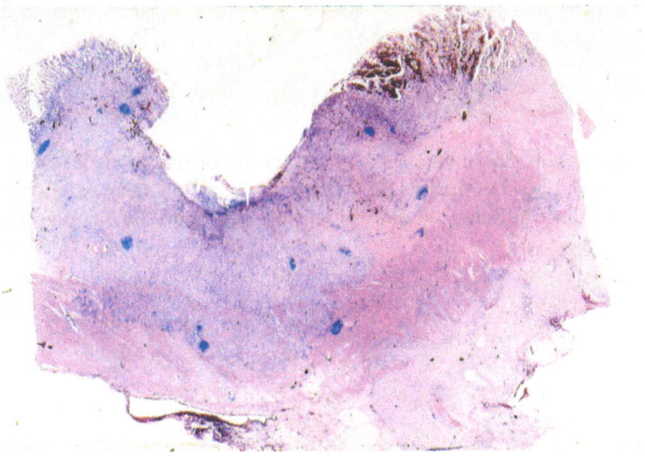

e

Fig. 2.17a–e. Non Hodgkin Lymphoma (NHL) of the stomach. Double Contrast barium study (**a**) demonstrating thickened radiating gastric folds on the posterior wall of the body of the stomach, with a central ulcerated elevation of mucosa. Endoscopic-ultrasound (**b**) performed two weeks after (**a**) confirms ulcerated nodular elevation of the gastric wall. Endoscopy (**c**) shows nodular gastric mucosal elevations with central ulcerations. At CT (**d**) marked asymmetric gastric wall thickening is present. Histopathologic resection specimen (**e**) confirms NHL

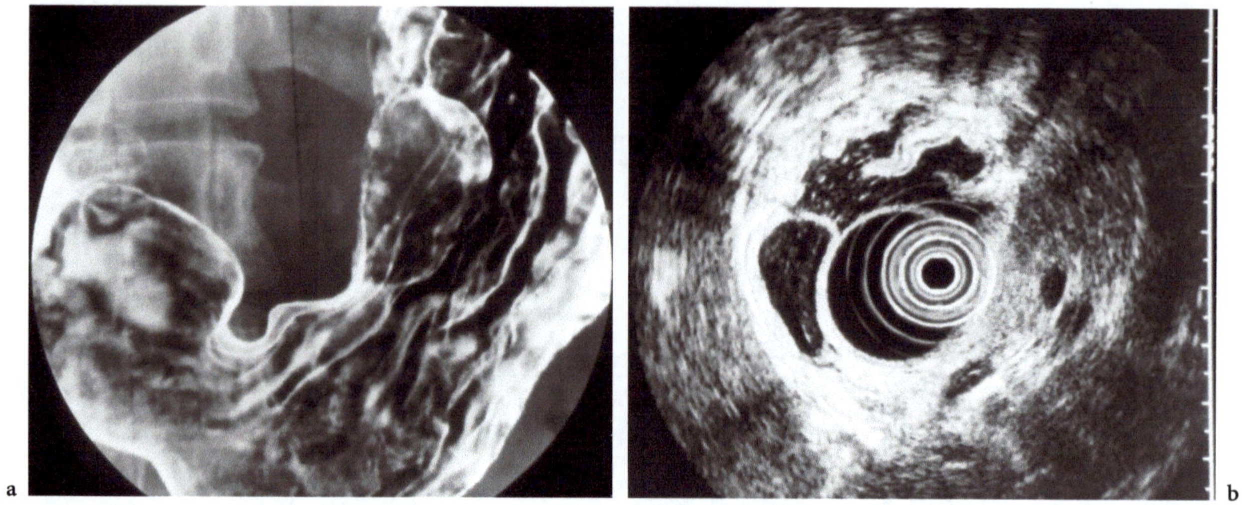

Fig. 2.18a,b. Benign Cyst of the stomach. Double Contrast barium study (**a**) demonstrates a half-round protrusion into the gastric lumen which arises from the lesser curve aspect of the stomach. Endoscopic-ultrasound (**b**) confirms its fluid nature, compatible with a benign cyst, such as a gastric retention cyst

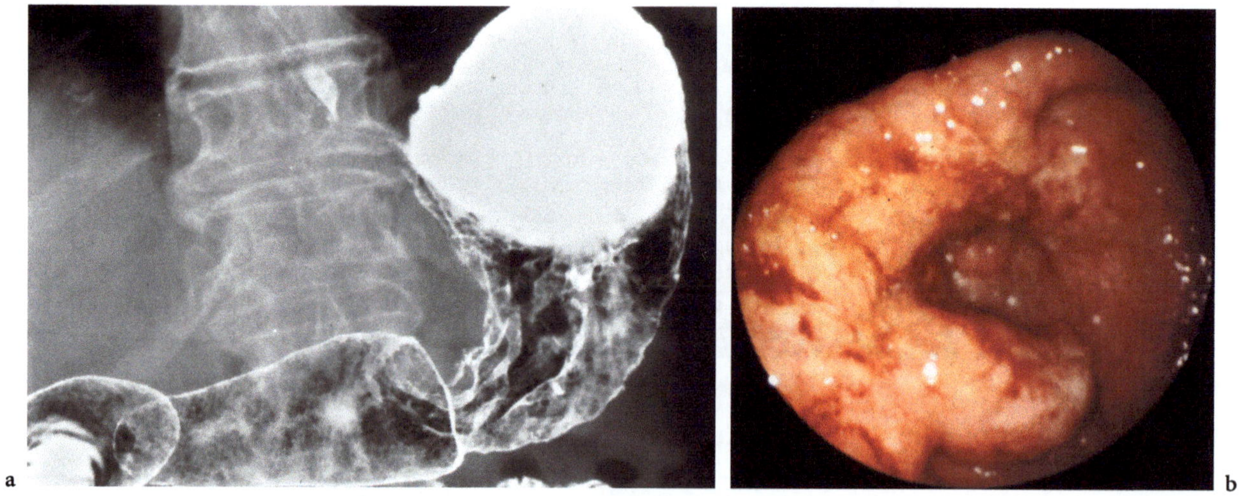

Fig. 2.19a,b. Borrmann 4 Adenocarcinoma of the stomach. Double Contrast barium study (**a**) demonstrates an irregular constriction affecting the body of the stomach, due to an extensive malignant process. Endoscopy (**b**) confirms the ulcerated irregular cauliflower lesion which is oozing blood. Biopsy revealed an adenocarcinoma of the stomach

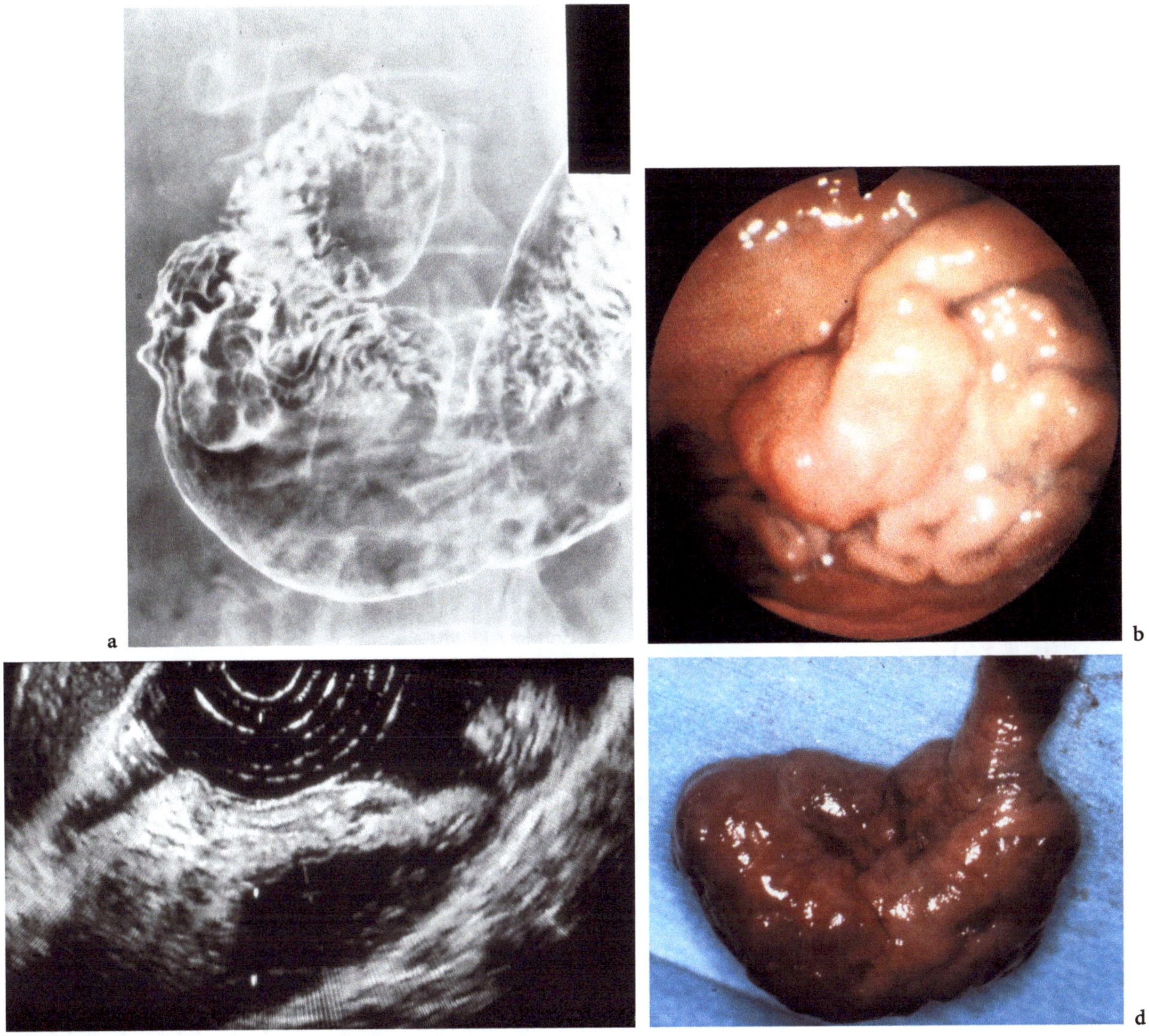

Fig. 2.20a–d. Gastric Polyp. Double Contrast barium study (a) demonstrates a large pedunculated polyp in the antrum of the stomach. Endoscopy (b) and Endoscopic-ultrasound (c) confirm the pedunculated polyp which was confirmed as a non ulcerated fibroid polyp on histopathology (d)

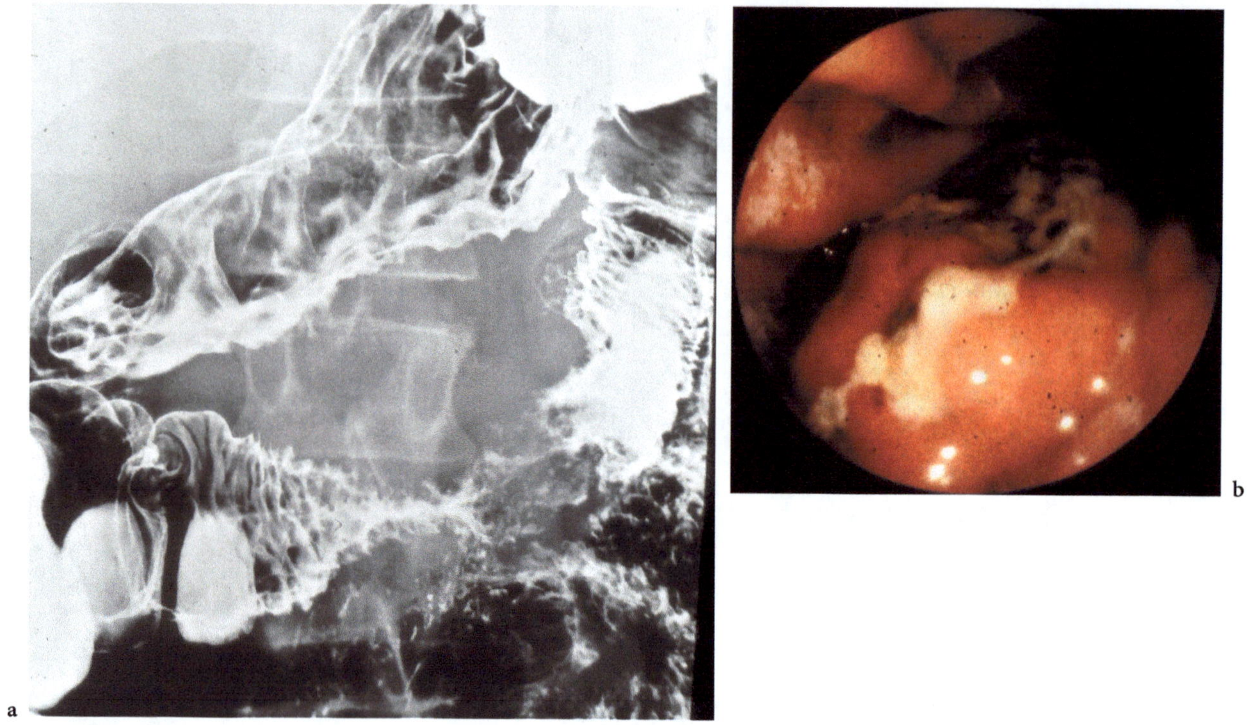

Fig. 2.21a,b. Metastatic Invasion of the stomach. Double Contrast barium studies of the stomach and colon (a). This image demonstrates irregularity of the greater curvature of the body and antrum of the stomach, together with a pinpoint tapered irregular stenosis of the transverse colon. Note the irregular transverse ridges, running perpendicular to the colonic axis. Gastroscopy (b) demonstrates an ulcerated nodular surface of the stomach. Diagnosis: Adeno-carcinoma of the colon with secondary metastatic ingrowth into the stomach

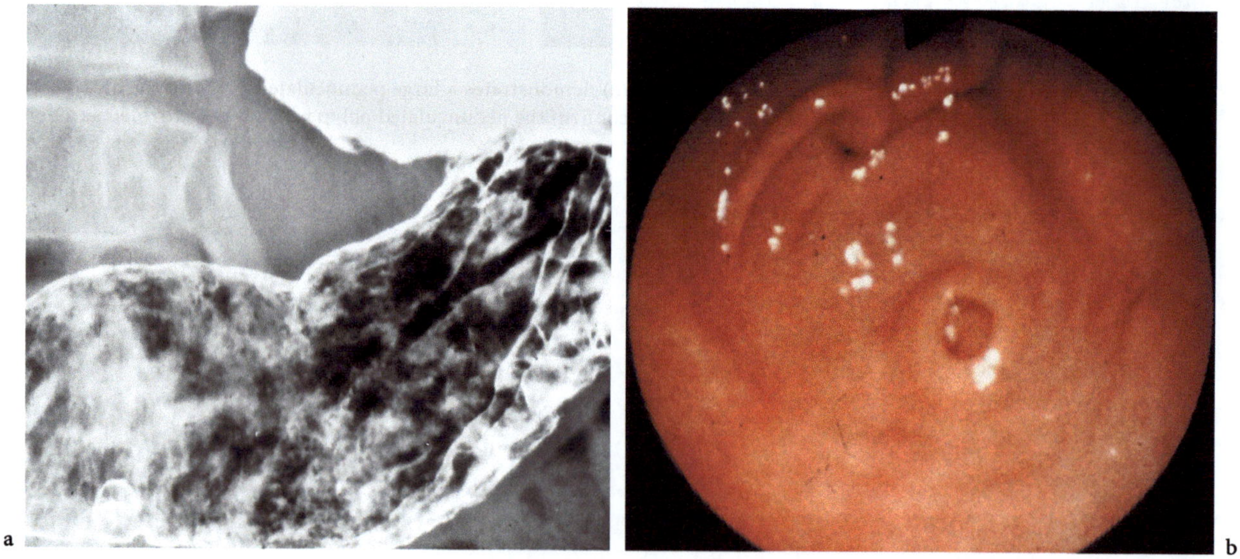

Fig. 2.22a,b. Ectopic Pancreas in the stomach. Double Contrast barium study (a) shows a small nodule in the antrum of the stomach (bottom left of image). Endoscopy (b) demonstrates the characteristic round umbilicated lesion situated a few centimeters proximal to the pylorus. Biopsy confirmed ectopic pancreas (pancreatic rest)

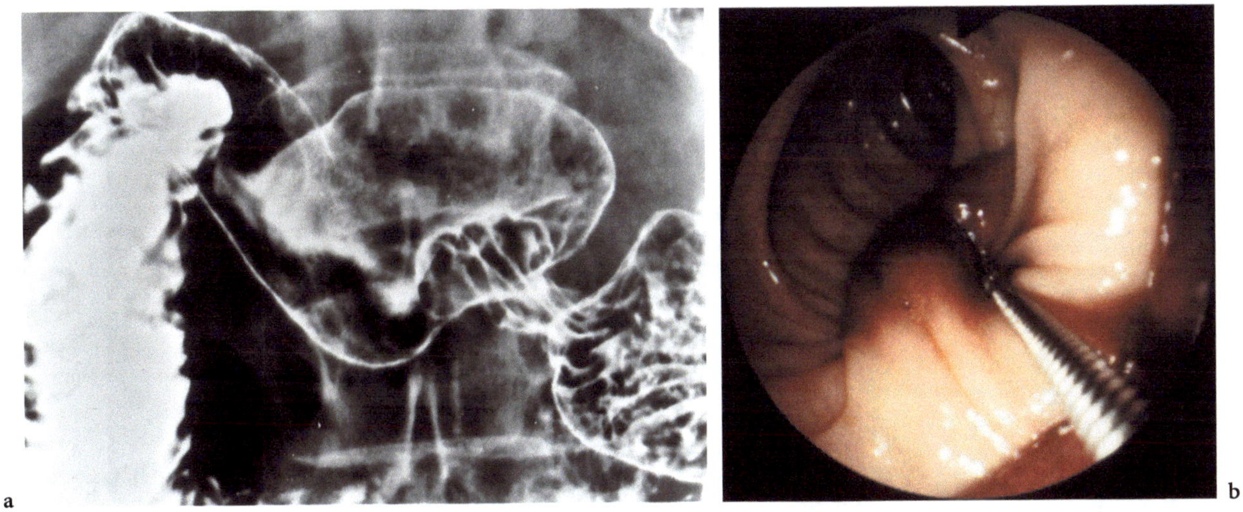

Fig. 2.23a,b. Antral Mucosal Prolapse. Double Contrast barium study (a) demonstrating prolapse of antral mucosa through the pylorus. Note the typical mushroom shaped deformity at the base of the duodenal bulb caused by this normal variant. Endoscopy (b) shows the prolapsed folds

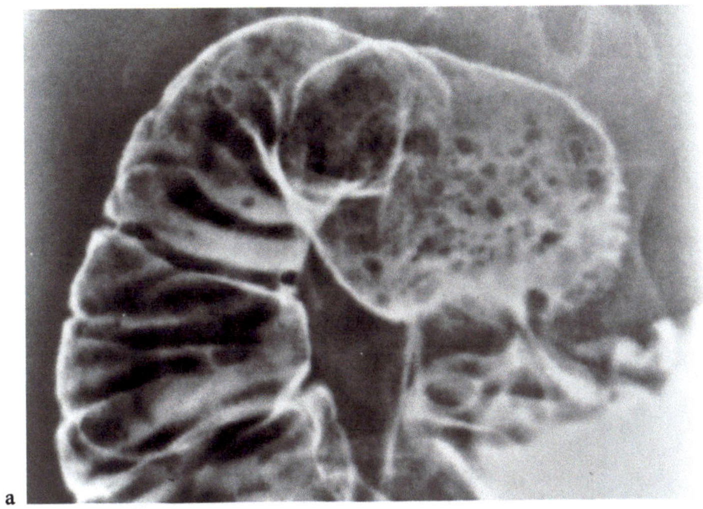

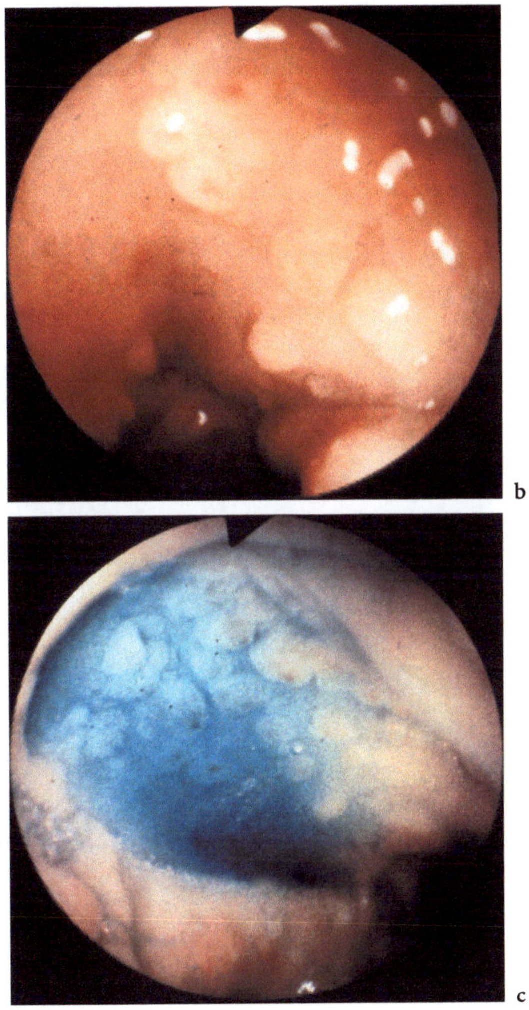

Fig. 2.24a–c. Duodenal gastric heterotopia. Double Contrast barium study (a) shows multiple hexagonal mucosal islands in the duodenum, classically situated at the base of the duodenal bulb. These are confirmed at endoscopy (b) and particularly well seen after staining with methylene-blue (c). Diagnosis: Gastric heterotopia

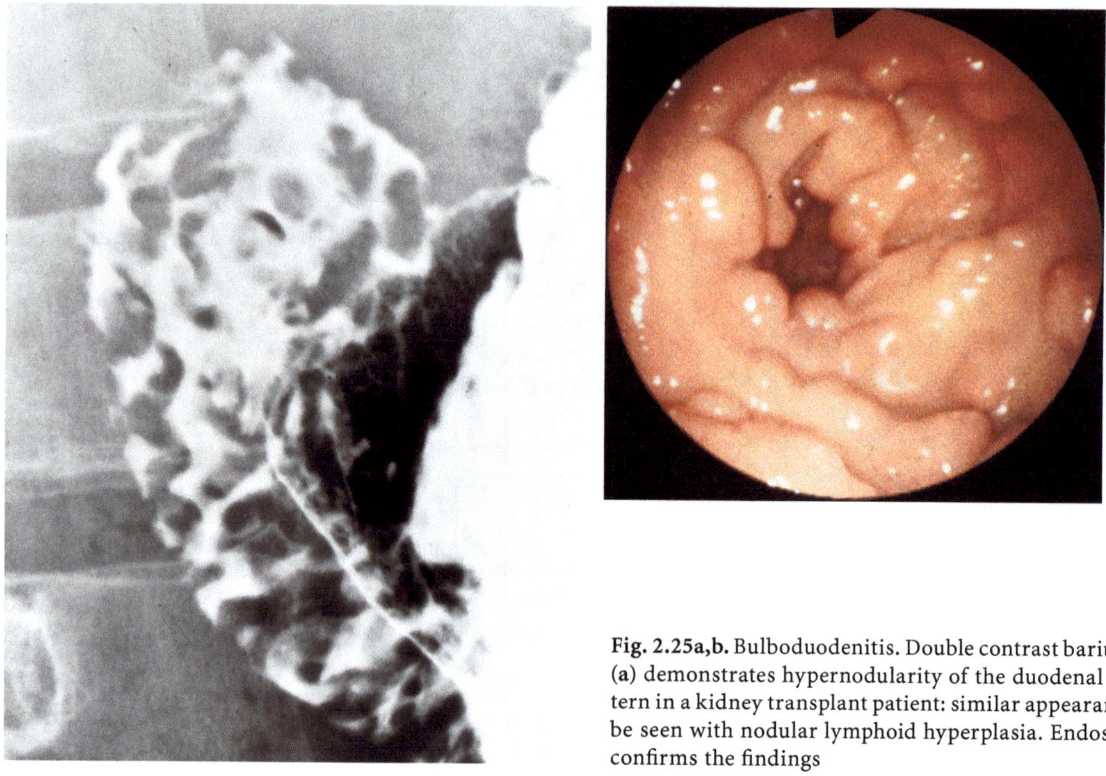

a b

Fig. 2.25a,b. Bulboduodenitis. Double contrast barium study (**a**) demonstrates hypernodularity of the duodenal fold pattern in a kidney transplant patient: similar appearances may be seen with nodular lymphoid hyperplasia. Endoscopy (**b**) confirms the findings

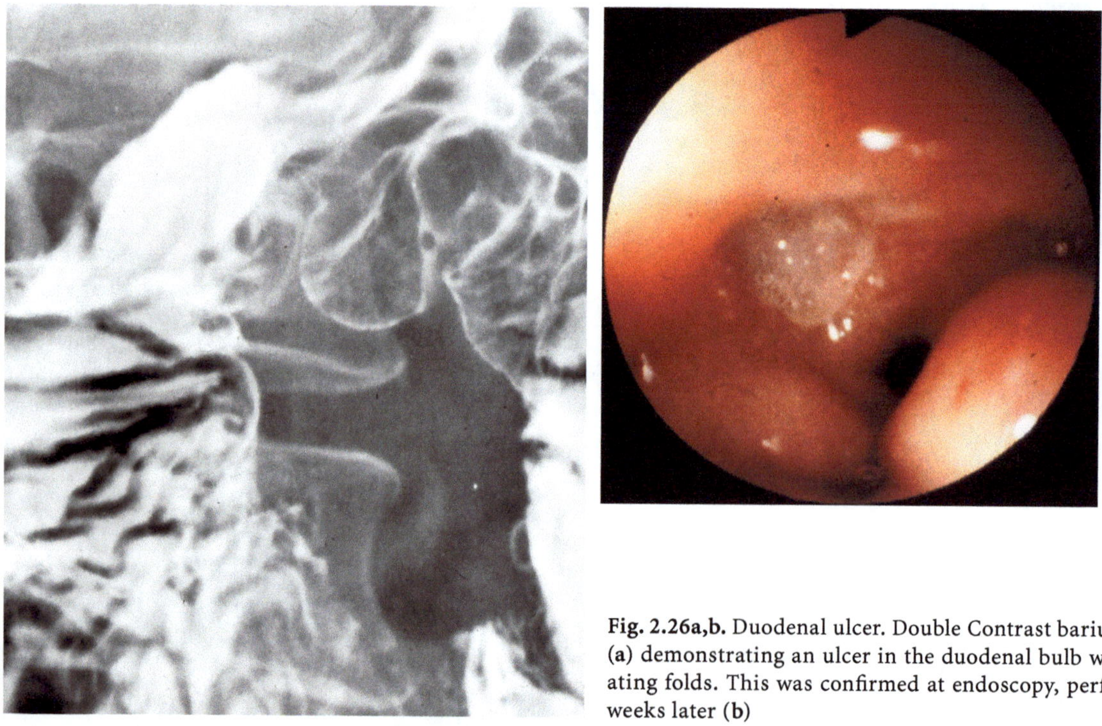

a b

Fig. 2.26a,b. Duodenal ulcer. Double Contrast barium study (**a**) demonstrating an ulcer in the duodenal bulb with radiating folds. This was confirmed at endoscopy, performed 3 weeks later (**b**)

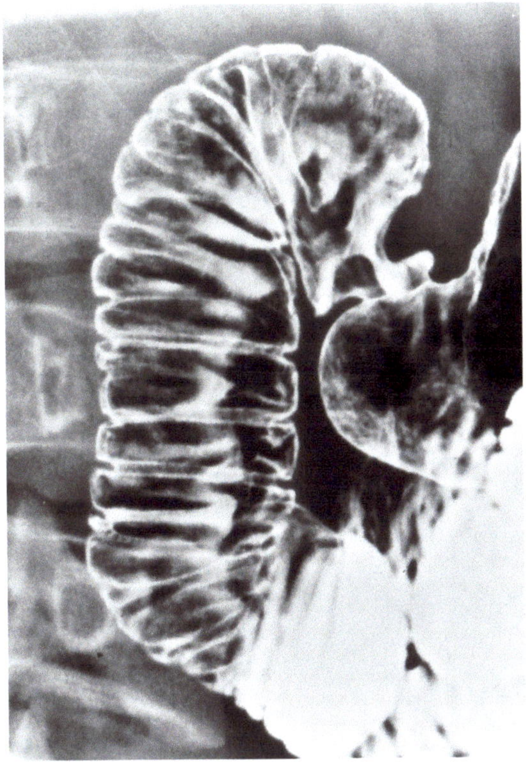

Fig. 2.27. Duodenal ulcer with scarring. Marked deformity of the base of the duodenal bulb after healing of a duodenal ulcer. Note the resulting pseudodiverticulum immediately adjacent to the pylorus

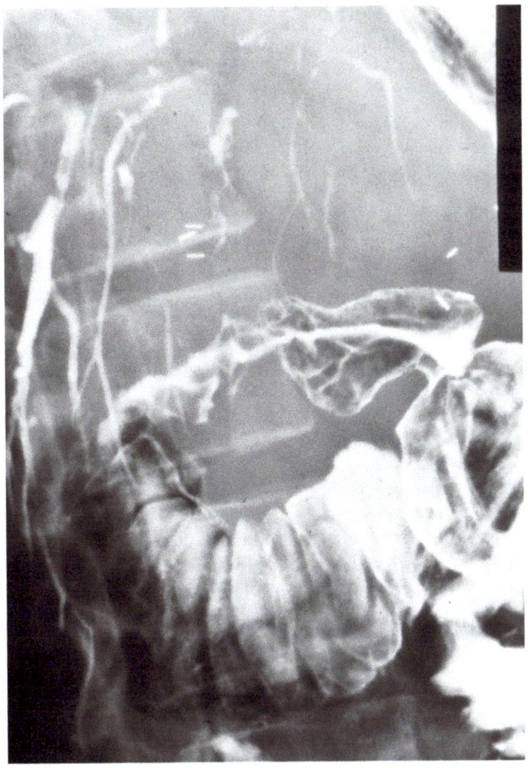

Fig. 2.29. Crohn' s stenosis and Duodenal fistula. Double Contrast barium study shows an irregular narrowing of the postbulbar duodenum due to lonstanding Crohn's duodenitis. There is also a duodenal-biliary fistula occurring as a complication of the Crohn's disease. Cholecystectomy clips are noted

a

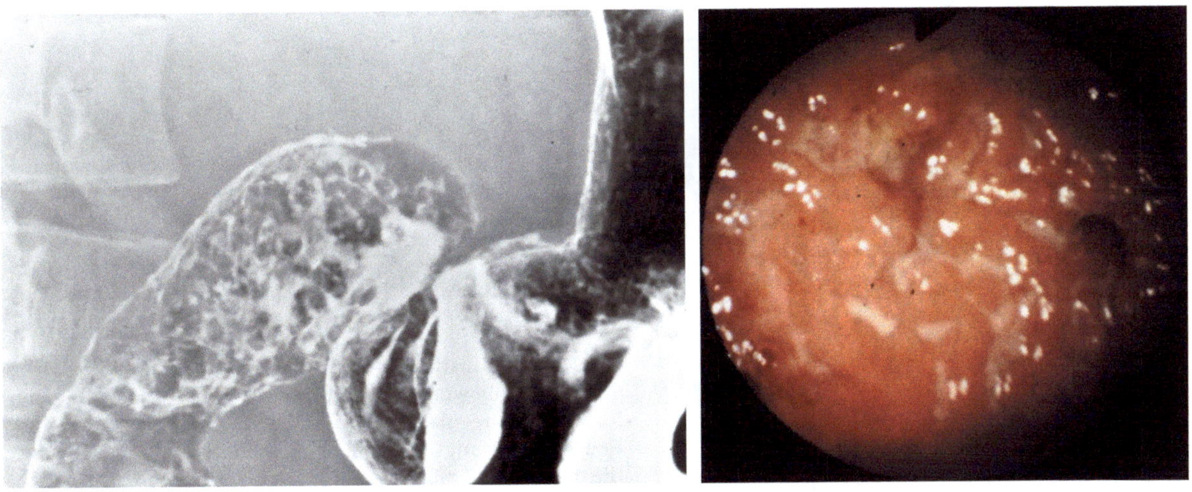

b

Fig. 2.28a,b. Crohn's duodenitis. Double Contrast barium study (**a**) shows multiple serpiginous lesions with aphthous ulcers in the duodenal bulb, due to active Crohn's duodenitis. This was confirmed at endoscopy (**b**)

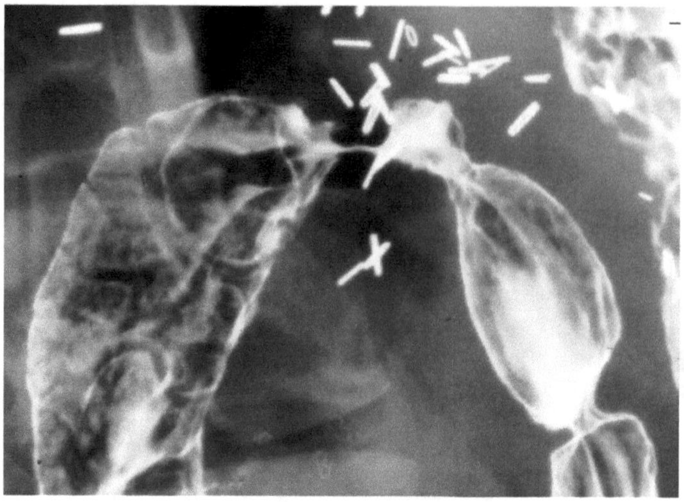

Fig. 2.30. Ischaemic duodenal stenosis. Double Contrast barium study which demonstrates a pinpoint stenosis in the post-bulbar region of the duodenum. This has resulted from ischaemic change four months after right nephrectomy for benign disease. Note the surgical clips

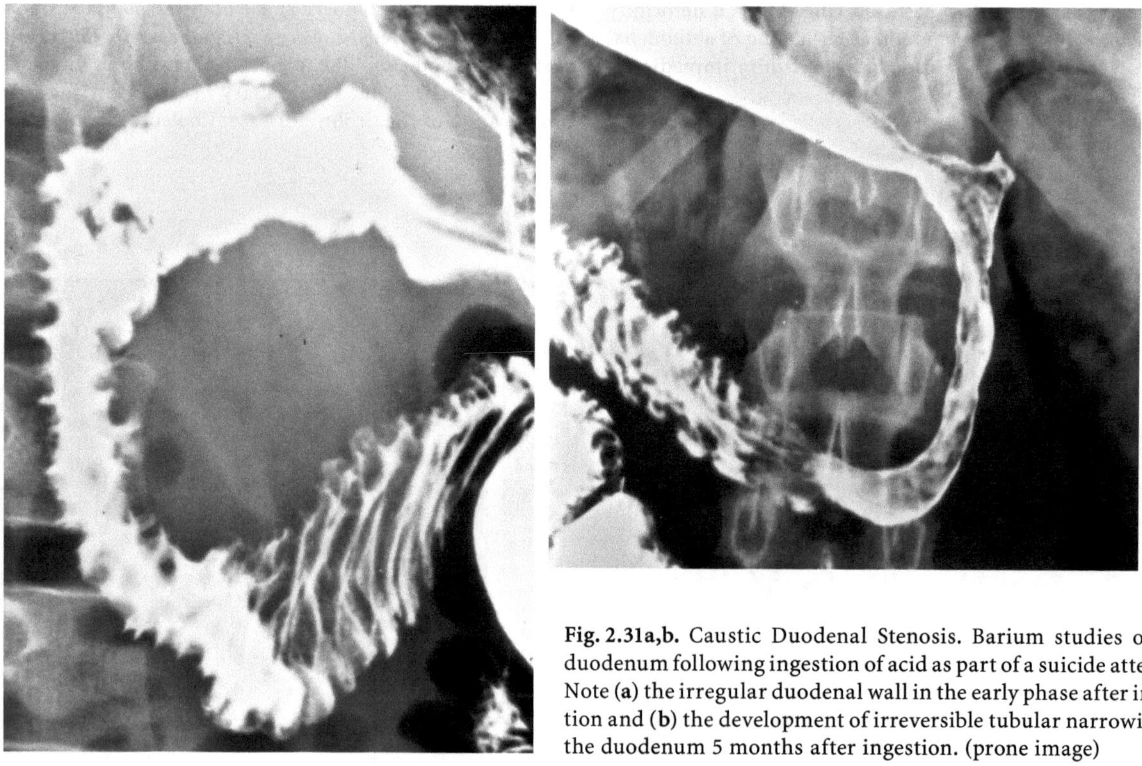

b

a

Fig. 2.31a,b. Caustic Duodenal Stenosis. Barium studies of the duodenum following ingestion of acid as part of a suicide attempt. Note (a) the irregular duodenal wall in the early phase after ingestion and (b) the development of irreversible tubular narrowing of the duodenum 5 months after ingestion. (prone image)

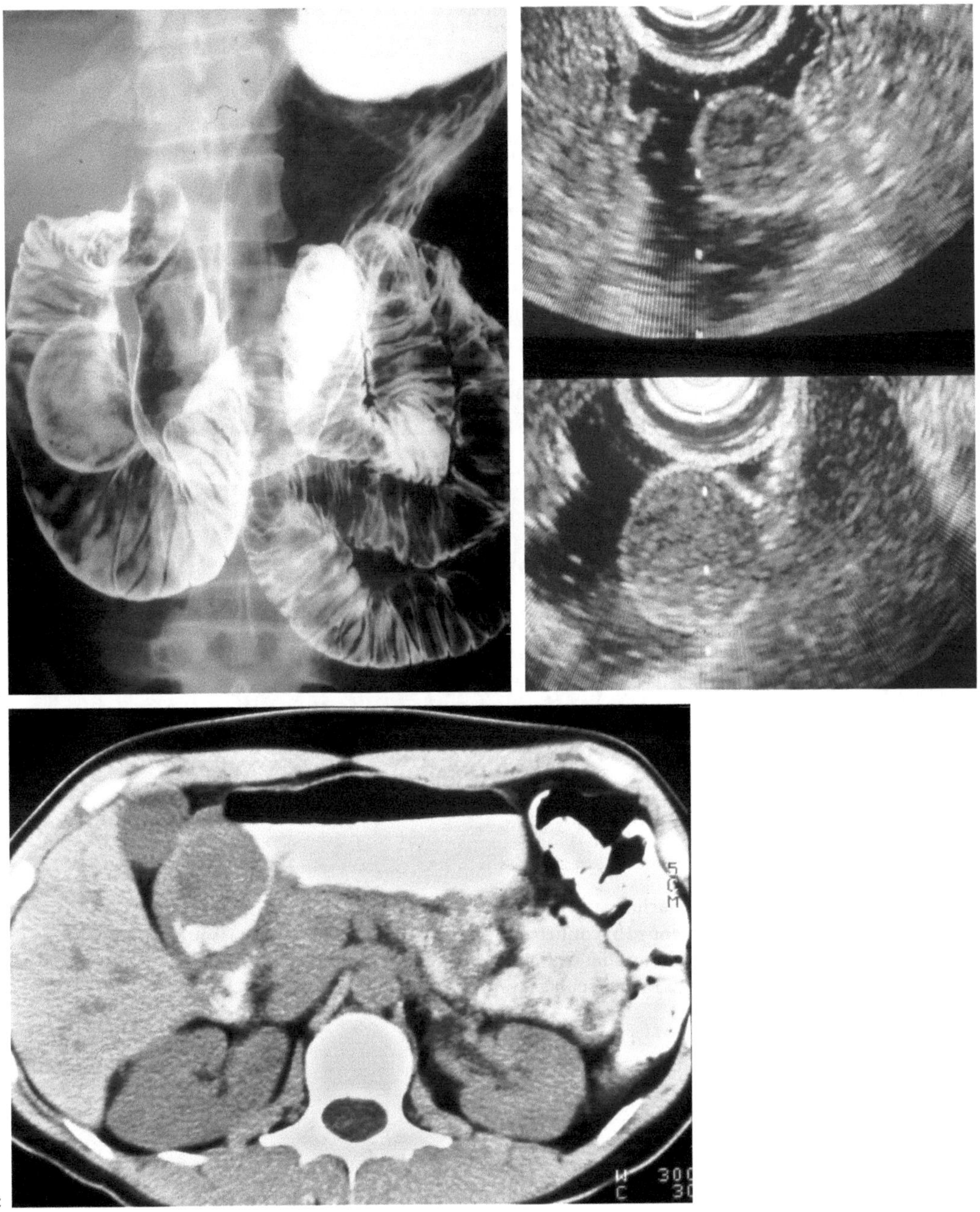

a b c

Fig. 2.32a–c. Leiomyoma of the duodenum. Double Contrast barium study (**a**) shows a round well delineated non-ulcerated lesion in the second part of the duodenum, bordering the major papilla. Endoscopic-ultrasound (**b**) demonstrates the submucosal lesion, typical of a benign leiomyoma. A CT examination (**c**) of another patient demonstrates the typical smooth impression of a duodenal leiomyoma

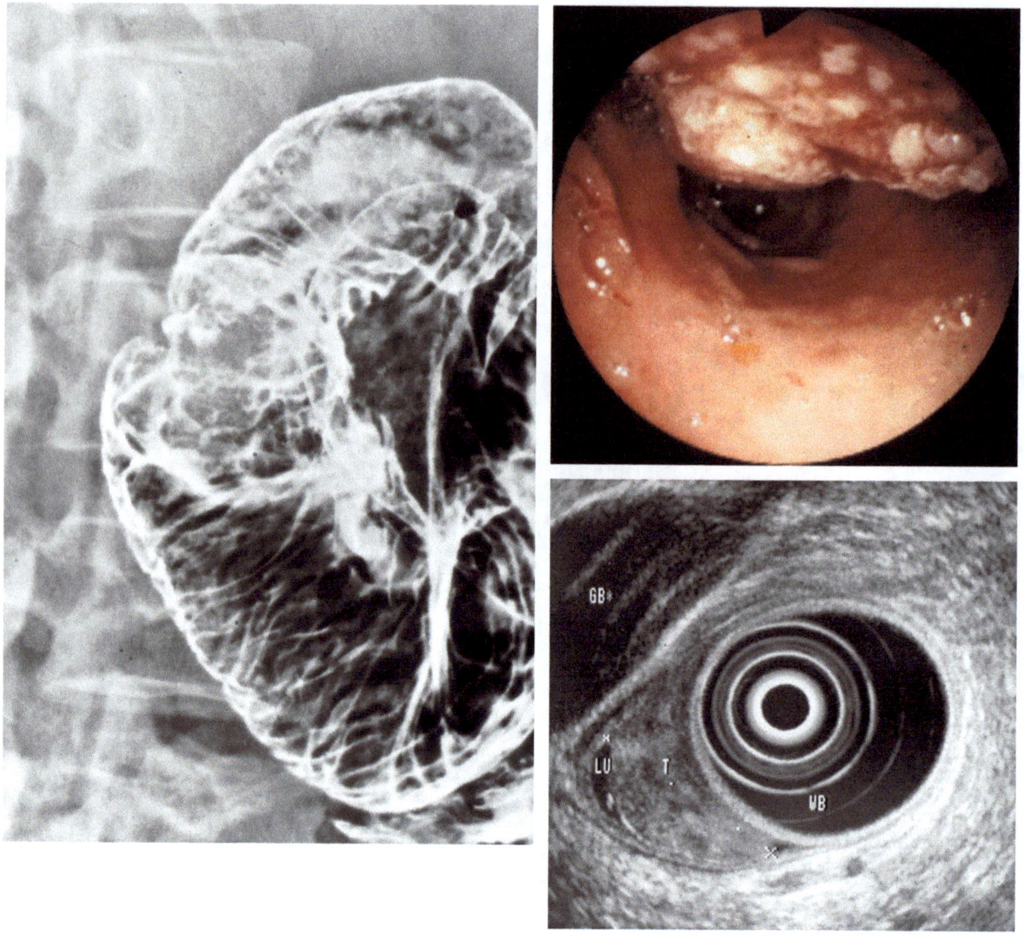

Fig. 2.33a–c. Duodenal Cancer. Double Contrast barium study (**a**) demonstrates a large bulky villous type mass extending into the duodenal lumen. Endoscopy (**b**) confirms the ulcerated bulky tumour mass protruding into the duodenal lumen which proved to be an adenocarcinoma at biopsy. Endoscopic-ultrasound (**c**) shows that the solid mass penetrating through the muscular layers of the duodenal wall

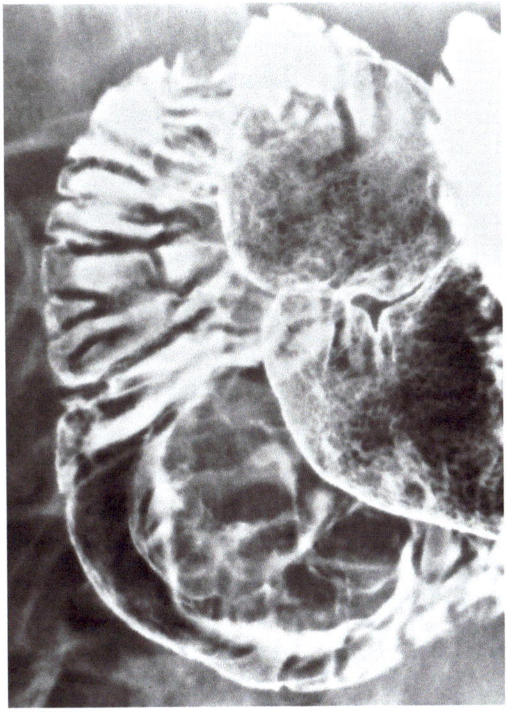
a

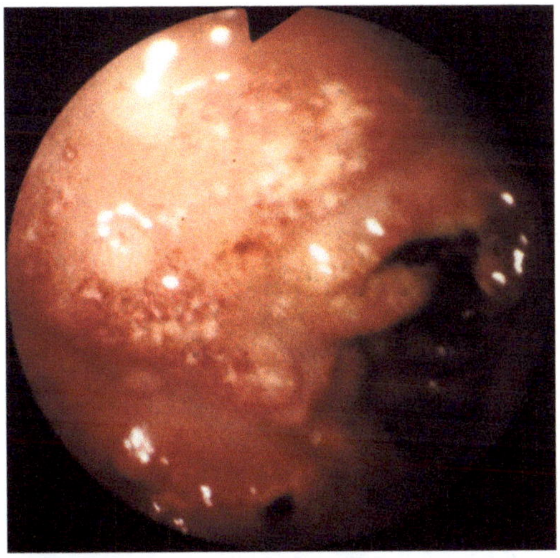
b

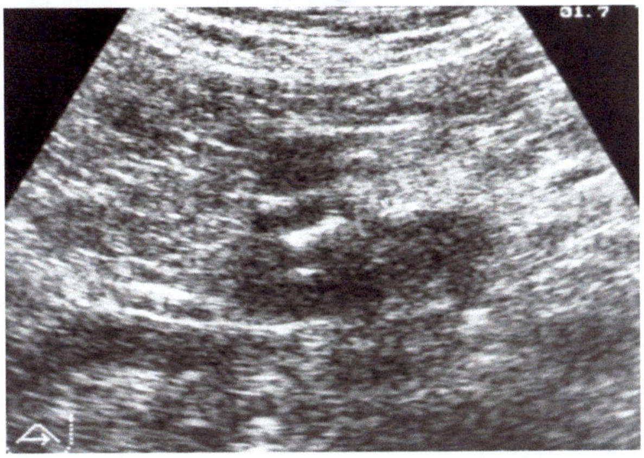
c

Fig. 2.34a–c. Carcinoid tumour of the duodenum. Double Contrast barium study (**a**) demonstrating a bulky rounded mass, protruding into the lumen of the duodenum. This caused marked narrowing of the lumen on endoscopy (**b**) and on ultrasound (**c**). The biopsy proven diagnosis was a carcinoid tumor

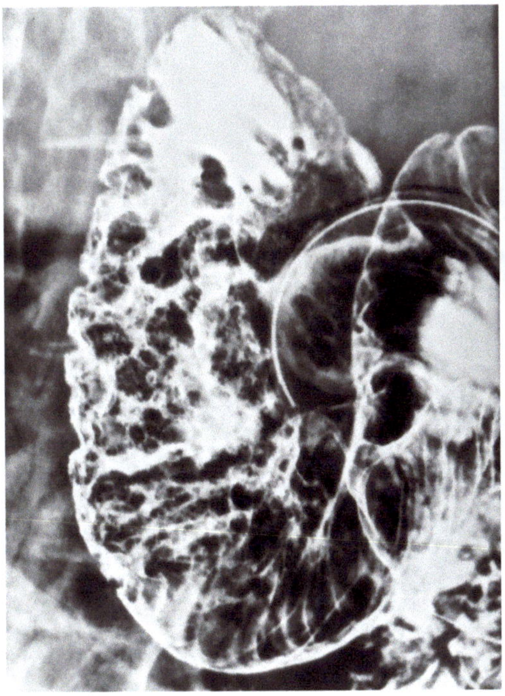
a

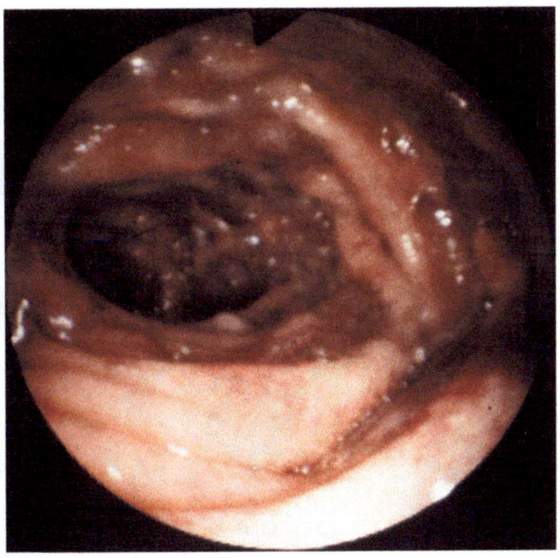
b

Fig. 2.35a,b. Kaposi's sarcoma of the duodenum. Double Contrast barium study (**a**) demonstrating an extensive and diffuse nodularity of the duodenum, due to Kaposi's sarcoma. This was confirmed at endoscopy (**b**)

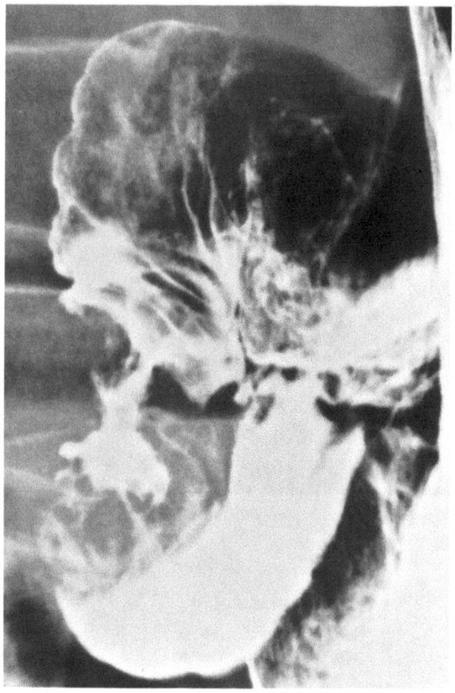

Fig. 2.36. Metastatic ingrowth into the duodenum. A Double Contrast barium study demonstrates irregular circumferential narrowing of the duodenum with marked ulceration, due to involvement by a large pancreatic head cancer

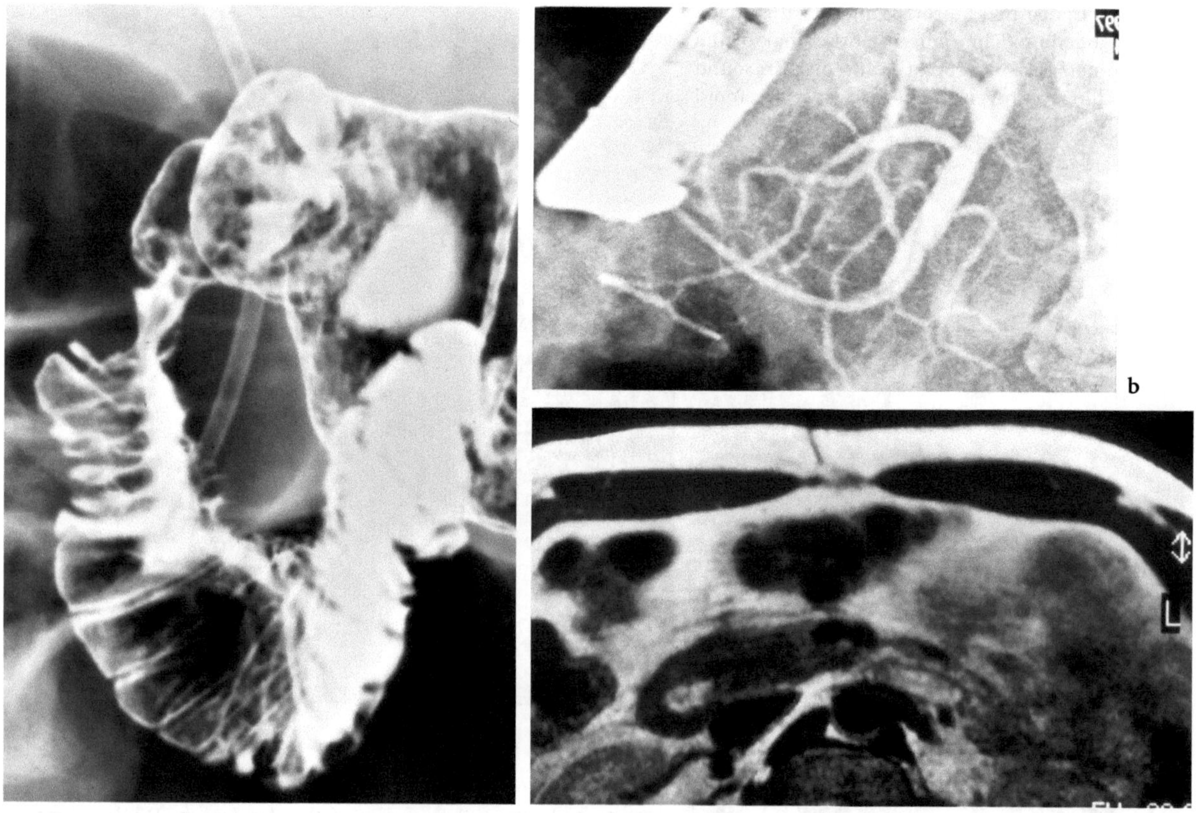

a b c

Fig. 2.37a–c. Annular Pancreas. Double Contrast barium study (**a**)demonstrates semicircumferential narrowing of the duodenum due to an annular pancreas. Note the biliary stent. ERCP (**b**) shows the pancreatic ductal system encircling the duodenum. MRI (**c**) shows the pancreatic head, folded around the duodenal lumen

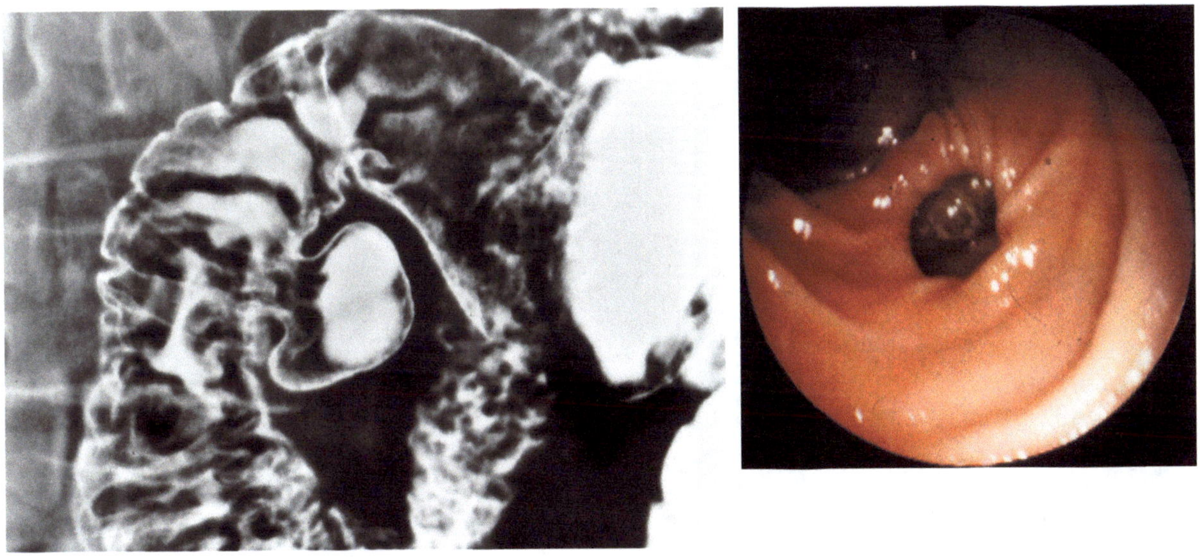

a b

Fig. 2.38a,b. Duodenum Diverticulum. Double Contrast barium study (a) and endoscopy (b) clearly show the diverticulum. Note the common peri-ampullary location

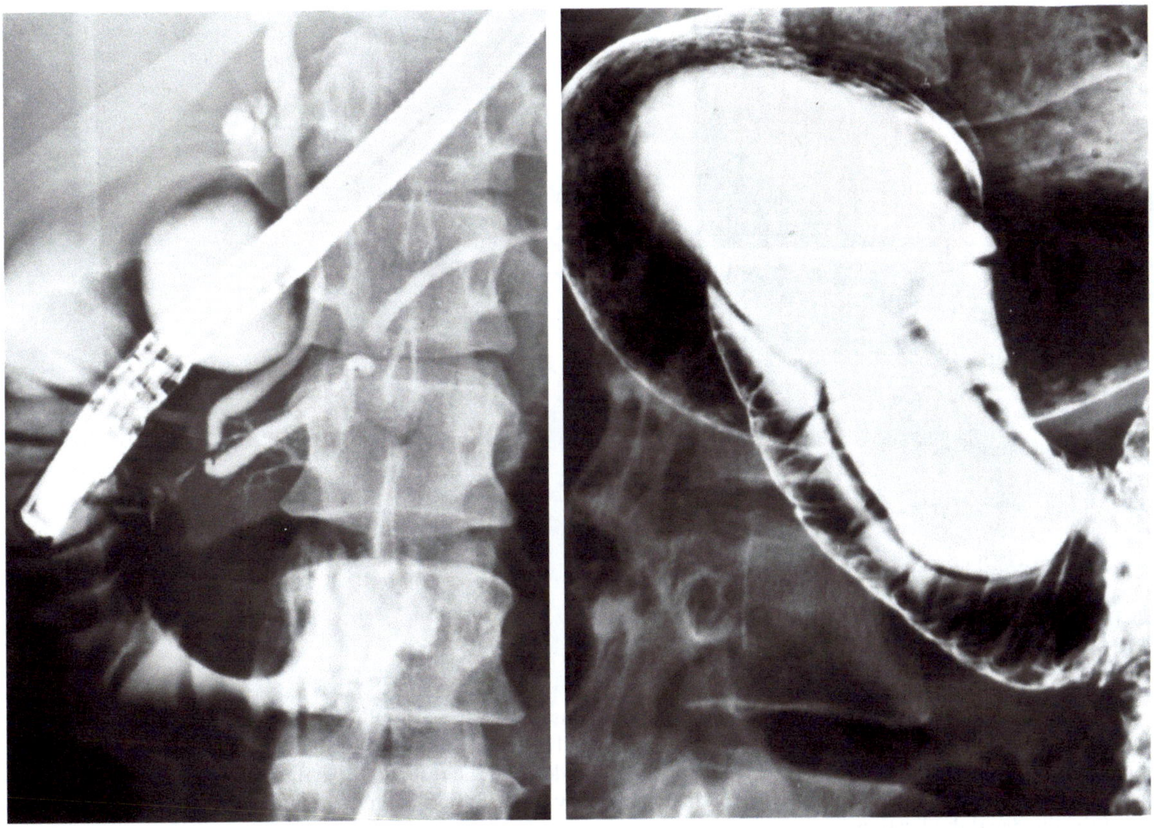

a b

Fig. 2.39a,b. Intraluminal Duodenal Diverticulum. ERCP (a) demonstrates a smooth well-delineated air collection extending caudally from the region of the major papilla, shown against a background of contrast in the rest of the lumen. The patient presented with intermittent bouts of acute pancreatitis. Subsequent Double Contrast barium study (b) demonstrates the inner and outer border of the diverticulum, which exhibits the typical “windsock” sign

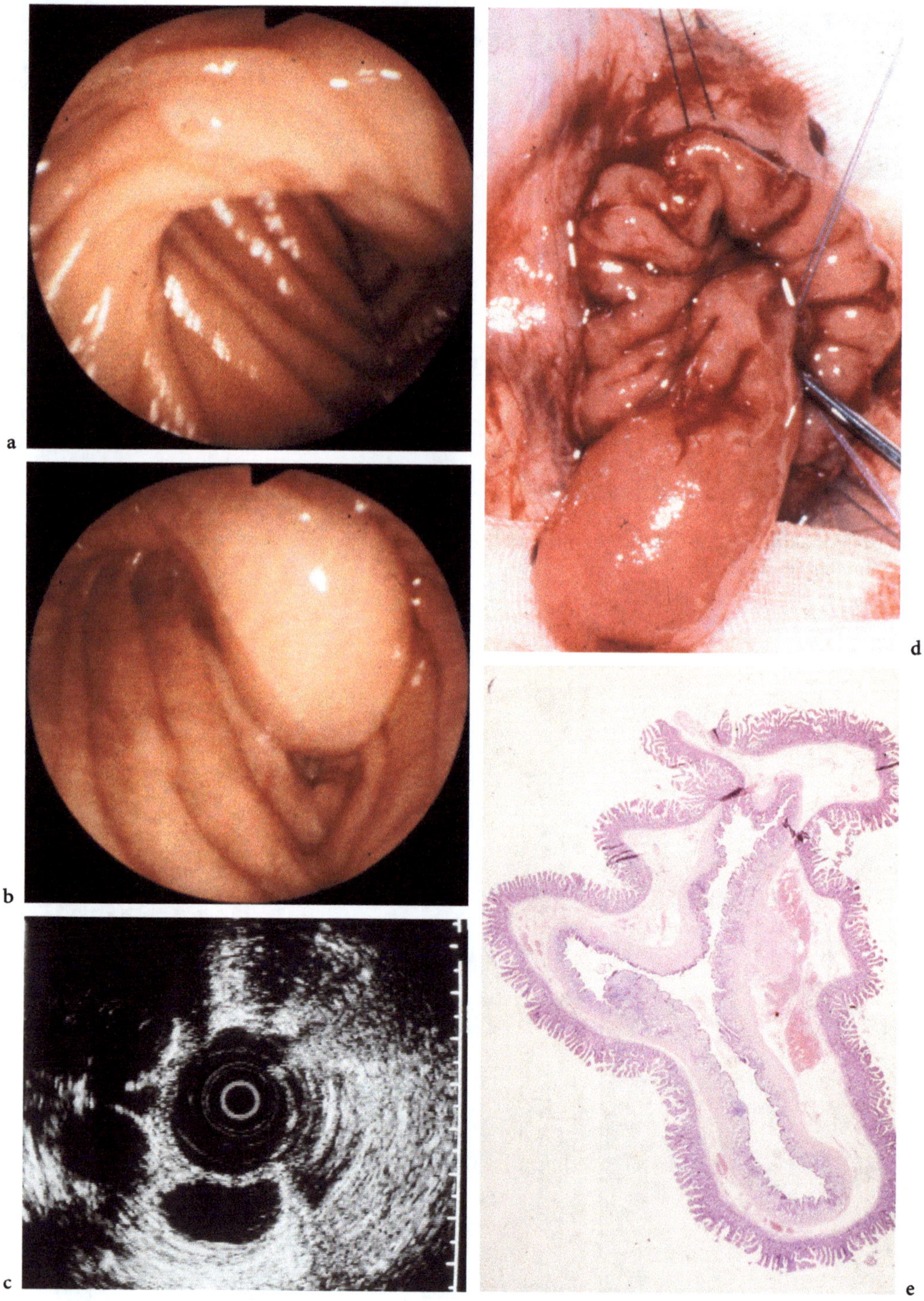

Fig. 2.40a–e. Duodenal Duplication Cyst. Endoscopy (**a,b**) demonstrates a smooth submucosal mass extending caudally from the major papilla, covered with normal mucosa. Note the normal papilla (**a**). Endoscopic- ultrasound (**c**) confirms the cystic nature of the lesion. The resection specimen (**d**) shows the intraluminal component of the cyst and histopathology (**e**) the inner- and outer epithelial lining of the duodenal duplication cyst

Endoscopy of the Upper Gastrointestinal Tract

3

Frans-Thomas Fork

CONTENTS

F.-T. Fork, MD
Department of Diagnostic Radiology, Malmö University Hospital, SE-20502 Malmö, Sweden

3.1 Introduction

The understanding of gastrointestinal diseases has changed dramatically during the past four decades. Many of these changes may be attributed to successful technical and pharmacological developments, typified by fibre-optic techniques and the detection and eradication of *Helicobacter pylori*. Endoscopic investigation of the gastrointestinal tract and endoscopic treatments continue to play increasing roles. During the same period radiology has contributed to the understanding of motility disorders, tumour biology, and the spread of tumour.

Endoscopy of the gastrointestinal tract not only facilitates education and training in gastroenterology through the visualisation of lesions in a full range of colours, but has also made the detection of early malignant lesions possible. This has opened the possibilities of treatment by endoscopy which is often curative and at low cost to society.

3.1.1 Indications

All patients with upper gastrointestinal tract (GIT) symptoms are eligible for gastroscopy. Gastroscopy is also indicated in patients with symptoms of iron deficiency anaemia and/or clinical suspicion of enteropathy, and may be indicated in some asymptomatic patients; i.e. healthy members of families with hereditary polyposis syndromes, most typically familial adenomatous polyposis (FAP). Finally, gastroscopy is indicated in follow-up programmes of ulcer treatment, cancer surveillance, dilation procedures, etc.

There are no exclusion criteria for gastroscopy in patients with a clinically sound indication. Gastroscopy in psychotic patients with vague indications may be postponed as might gastroscopy in severely ill patients, in whom any endoscopic finding would only result in a questionable change of management. There are no age limitations, and pregnancy is not a contraindication.

3.2 Examination Technique

Endoscopy of the upper GIT is possible to perform in almost all patients, the very few exceptions being patients with fractures to the facial skeleton and those with severe destruction of the cervical spine secondary to rheumatoid arthritis. In others, an advanced Zenker's diverticulum and a tight Plummer-Vinson membrane at the oesophageal inlet may create technical obstacles to proceeding, whilst obstructing lesions further down in the oesophagus and stomach may lead to an incomplete examination. Naturally, these endoscopic diagnoses may be important clinical findings.

The stomach should be empty before examination. This is usually achieved by an 8-hour fast. In patients with signs of gastric outlet obstruction and/or large acute gastric bleeding, a large-bore nasogastric tube is preferably put down before the examination to rinse and empty the stomach.

3.2.1 Pre-Treatment

Gastroscopy is invasive in nature and is found unpleasant by most patients. Insertion of a tube into the throat causes nausea and provokes vomiting, which many patients will find unbearable. Most centres will therefore offer sedation, usually in the form of an intravenous injection of a sedative such as Hypnovel or Diazemuls. It is important to retain intravenous access both during and after the procedure in order to be able to administer antidotes if necessary. Most centres will offer an alternative strategy of topical anaesthetic sprayed to the back of the throat. This has the advantage of the patient being left in full command of their faculties after the examination; i.e. car driving, going to work, etc.

Neonates and children up to the age 15 are always examined under general anaesthesia, usually by administering an infusion mixture of propofol and fentanyl. This combination is also used in adults with great anxiety. However, in the majority of patients simple sedation is sufficient, i.e. Hypnovel at a mean dose of 2.5 mg, range 2–10 mg or Diazemuls at a mean dose of 5 mg. In Europe butylscopolamine is often given to induce aperistalsis. In painful procedures like dilatation of strictures or removal of large foreign bodies, analgesia is achieved by an intravenous injection of pethidine, 25–50 mg or ketobemidone, 2.5–5.0 mg.

Premedication slows respiration and induces a transient fall in oxygen saturation. Young and healthy individuals are able to tolerate this, whereas the elderly with pulmonary and/or cardiac diseases are at risk. Hence, supplementary oxygen is routinely given during the examination and oxygen saturation is monitored by a pulse-oximetry device, until the patient recovers.

Endoscopic intubation and treatment also induce a transient bacteraemia which does not harm the healthy patient but may be dangerous to individuals who are immunodeficient or have heart valve prosthesis. Each endoscopic unit has its own recommendations of antibiotic pre-treatment, usually combinations of Gram-negative and broad-spectrum antibiotics. The current international trend is to save this pre-treatment for patients in whom endoscopic treatment will be applied, i.e. dilatations, injection treatment, diathermy, etc.

3.3 Anatomy

It is worth remembering that endoscopy of the GIT offers a means of inspecting the mucous membranes and therefore diagnosing mucosal lesions, but unlike radiology cannot be used to gain knowledge of deeper wall layers or structures beyond the gut wall. This is why it is often difficult to relate findings to surrounding landmarks.

A normal gastroscopy comprises deep intubation down to the inferior duodenal flexure. In certain cases this may be extended to the horizontal part of the duodenum; i.e. biopsies for possible cases of enteropathy, although it is increasingly recognised that this diagnosis may be excluded by a biopsy from the descending duodenum. The third part of the duodenum may also need to be inspected in cases of upper GIT bleeding arising from a more distal location, but the area beyond this point becomes the territory of dedicated small bowel enteroscops with or without balloons.

3.3.1 Hypopharynx and Cervical Oesophagus

Structures belonging to the pharynx and hypopharynx are well demonstrated, i.e. the tonsils, the base of the tongue, the epiglottis, the vocal cords, and valleculae. Contrary to radiology the piriform sinuses are not possible to inspect in detail due to the physiologic reason that the hypo-pharynx closes with passage of the instrument. Openings of pharyngeal diverticula are overlooked when small, as are shallow membranes at the oesophageal inlet. Cricopharyngeus, the lower component of the inferior stricture muscle marks the demarcation with the cervical oesophagus and is usually closed. Negotiation of this is normally simple but problems may occur with cricopharyngeal dysfunction.

3.3.2 Thoracic Oesophagus

The aortic arch creates a shallow indentation in the upper third of the oesophagus in the elderly. Sometimes a slight indentation in the mid-oesophagus is also encountered, caused by the adjacent left main bronchus. At its distal end the oesophagus tapers slightly to the left just before it enters the stomach. Another identifiable landmark in subjects with a hiatal hernia is the diaphragmatic inlet, which varies in width with respiration.

When distended with air the distal oesophagus demonstrates the margin between the pale squamous epithelium of the oesophagus and the reddish cylindrical epithelium of the cardia (Fig. 3.1a). This margin or transition zone is referred to as the "Z-line" because of the interdigitations of the mucosa. In healthy individuals the "Z-line" is normally found close to the diaphragmatic inlet, usually at 40 cm from the incisor teeth. The identification of the Z-line is important in the diagnosis of hiatal hernia, oesophagitis, and pre-malignant intestinal metaplasia, i.e. Barrett's oesophagus. The Z-line is difficult to depict at radiological examination; even on high-quality double-contrast oesophagograms (Fig. 3.1b), because of the subtle change of mucosal surface structure between the squamous and columnar epithelial lining.

The normal surface of the squamous epithelium is even, though slightly elevated islands of glycogen deposits may be seen (Fig. 3.2). These appear whitish and tend to increase in size and number with advancing age (glycogenic acanthosis). On contrast studies these deposits may be difficult to distinguish from candidiasis, which shows up as irregular pale yellowish plaques on endoscopy.

Normal submucosal vessels are faintly seen in the oesophageal body but are more prominent in the elderly with mucosal atrophy. Distinct, parallel threadlike vessels are regularly seen above the Z-line, most obvious in young patients (Fig. 3.3). Their relation to early oesophagitis is disputed.

3.3.3 Stomach

Easily recognised endoscopic landmarks in the stomach are the cardia, the greater curvature marked by its tortuous longitudinal folds (Fig. 3.4), the incisura angularis, and the pylorus (Fig. 3.5). Less obvious landmarks are the even surfaces of the lesser curvature and gastric antrum. These landmarks may all change in disease. In large men the stomach is sometimes found in a horizontal position or even found upside-down, whereas it is J-shaped in tall and slim individuals.

The structure of the gastric mucosa shows a faint, regular mosaic pattern, which is enlarged and prominent in conditions of gastropathy and correlates to the areae gastricae well known to radiologists (Fig. 3.6). This may be particularly marked in the condition of portal gastropathy, which is associated with portal hypertension, also evidenced by tortuous fundic veins in more severe cases. Submucosal vessels are not seen in healthy individuals, but become apparent in cases of gastric atrophy.

3.3.4 Duodenum

The antral fold converges towards the pylorus, which is a narrow muscular channel a few millimetres long that constitutes the lower gastric sphincter. It is located between the lesser and greater curvature but is often found in a more eccentric position towards the lesser curve aspect of the antrum. In its relaxed state the pylorus measures 10 to 15 mm in diameter, and is easily traversed by an ordinary gastroscope.

The duodenal bulb or first part of the duodenum is wide, and its mucosa yellowish and even. The superior duodenal flexure demarcates the commencement of the second part of the duodenum, and this is normally well recognised. From this point onwards the mucosal pattern is characterised by folds of Kerckring (Fig. 3.7). Most of the folds measure around 1 mm in height and run in a semicircular way with small longitudinal folds in between. A distended gallbladder may cause an indentation of the proximal duodenum.

In the mid-point of the second part of the duodenum, a normal-sized papilla of Vater may be identified with a forward-viewing gastroscope (Fig. 3.8), but is better appreciated by the use of a side-viewing instrument. Transition to the third or horizontal duodenum is marked by the inferior duodenal flexure, which is also easily defined.

The horizontal part of the duodenum is in most instances possible to reach with a standard gastroscope. Aortic pulsation is easily recognised in its mid-portion. It should, however, be born in mind that routine gastroscopy does not include the duodenum beyond the papilla of Vater and indeed in some instances may only include the duodenal cap. This is particularly important as during the performance of enteroclysis this part of the gut is not opacified, in order to minimise reflux of barium into the stomach. As a consequence significant malignant duodenal lesions may be easily missed by both groups.

3.4 Physiology

Because of its invasive character and thickness of the tube, gastroscopy is not suitable for monitoring motor function of the oesophagus, stomach, and duodenum, or for pressure recordings. However parietal cell function can be evaluated endoscopically by means of the Congo red test, a dye-spraying method (see below).

3.4.1 Chromo-Endoscopy

The natural mucosa offers a spectrum of colours, which facilitates detection of abnormalities to a higher degree compared to the grey scale offered by double-contrast barium investigations. A subtle change may be even more obvious by coating the mucous membrane with a dye, and this may aid the detection of epithelial metaplasia including premalignant areas of dysplasia (Fig. 3.9).

Thus chromo-endoscopy plays a useful role in advanced endoscopy. Improved detection is mediated through several ways. Firstly, a dye stains only the normal mucosa thereby leaving areas of dysplastic cell uncoloured. This is achieved when Lugol's solution, an iodine-based dye, is applied to the oesophagus. Normal mucosa with its typical glycogen content is stained dark brown, leaving non-glycogen-bearing dysplastic areas unstained.

A second technique is to enhance the normal delicate regular surface pattern of the mucous membrane. Indigo carmine is mainly used for this purpose, as it strikingly demarcates the normal from the abnormal which is coarse and irregular (Fig. 3.10). This dye is routinely used to ensure complete radical endoscopic treatment of flat, laterally spreading neoplastic lesions, and it readily displays any neoplastic part left behind.

A third dye, methylene blue, is absorbed by the cytoplasm of cells that have undergone intestinal metaplasia. The result may be difficult to interpret even for an experienced endoscopist, as the grade of absorption is unpredictable. A combination of Lugol's solution with methylene blue following water rinsing may be helpful for aiming the biopsy forceps at potential dysplastic areas.

A fourth dye is Congo red, which is used to test the secretory function of parietal cells of the stomach. After neutralising the stomach content with bicarbonate, the mucosal surface is evenly sprayed with the Congo red dye. The production of gastric acid is then stimulated by an i.v. injection of pentagastrin. In an acid environment, the red colour changes into blue. Congo red test without a colour shift unveils an environment of a pH over 3, i.e. achlorhydria. This is usually encountered in patients with B-12 vitamin deficiency, in those on acid reduction treatment, and after gastric antral resection. If change is still documented in the latter two patient groups, treatment is probably insufficient as there is still undesired gastric acid secretion.

In essence chromo-endoscopy is meant to help the endoscopist to detect areas of neoplasia but not to predict histology. It is thus mainly used to enhance the diagnostic yield of histology and cytology by improving the accuracy of obtained tissue specimens and brush smears.

3.5 Oesophageal Pathology

3.5.1 Hypopharynx and Cervical Oesophagus

One of the commonest problems encountered in this area is a Zenker's diverticulum (posterior pharyngeal pouch) usually found in the middle aged and elderly group. It is sometimes full of retained debris. Unfortunately the opening of the diverticulum is wide and tightly compresses the normal oesophageal inlet. This combined with its posterior position explains why the tip of the endoscope is more likely to enter the diverticulum. As the diverticulum is only lined by mucus membrane it is easily perforated, and the resulting mediastinitis presents a major clinical problem. Therefore, if a Zenker's diverticulum is suspected, a prior water-soluble contrast medium swallow is recommended. If endoscopy is still indicated, a slim paediatric gastroscope is used, preferably over a hydrophilic guidewire positioned under fluoroscopy.

Thin circular and semicircular membranes are frequently displayed on contrast studies but are incidental findings built up by mucosal and submucosal tissue components. These membranes are often single but may be multiple and readily dilated at endoscopy when symptomatic, i.e. when the lumen is 12 mm or less. They are usually not visualised at endoscopy as the pharynx is closed.

The Plummer-Vinson syndrome is an uncommon disease manifested by a combination of these proximal membranes with dysphagia, auto-immune disease and iron-deficiency anaemia. The syndrome is associated with an increased risk of carcinoma of the hypopharynx and upper GIT.

A final abnormality which may be encountered at the level of the pharyngo-oesophageal junction is cricopharyngeal achalasia, sometimes referred to as a cricopharyngeal bar. This results from cricopharyngeal hypertrophy and is a not infrequent cause of a failed endoscopy.

3.5.2 Thoracic Oesophagus

Ring formations are most often found in the distal oesophagus. Shallow rings located a few centimetres above the Z-line and covered by squamous epithelium are called A-rings and are usually asymptomatic. B-rings, or Schatzki rings, are more common and located at the Z-line, i.e. covered orally by squamous and aborally by columnar epithelium. They measure around 2 to 3 mm in thickness and are not associated with reflux oesophagitis. Patients typically complain of a long history of bolus obstruction.

When small, both A- and B-rings are probably easier to depict on contrast radiology. When symptomatic they are easy to treat by endoscopic balloon dilatation. It is however important to differentiate these rings from peptic strictures, as the latter need long-term acid reduction medication. Peptic strictures are usually recognised, as most of them are accompanied by other lesions secondary to reflux disease, i.e. erosions, ulcers, and irregular scar formations (Figs. 3.11, 3.12), together with secondary pseudo-diverticula formation. Gastro-oesophageal reflux disease, GORD, is most accurately evaluated by endoscopy.

3.5.3 Hiatus Hernia

Progressive weakness in the anatomic fixation of the distal oesophagus to the diaphragm may result in a hiatal hernia. The correct size of the hernia is easier to measure on contrast studies rather than to estimate endoscopically, due to the abundant landmarks on the radiograph (Fig. 3.13). The hernia itself is recognised by the width of the hiatal segment and the increasing number of red folds of gastric mucosa above the level of the diaphragm. Alternatively a hiatal hernia may be determined by cranial migration of the Z-line so that it is sited at less than 38 cm from the incisors.

The type of columnar epithelium in the hernia below the Z-line cannot be predicted by ordinary endoscopy. In order to distinguish normal fundic from transitional mucosa and the intestinal metaplasia in premalignant Barrett's oesophagus, dye spraying may be helpful (see above). In practice, however, tissue biopsies for microscopy are preferably obtained from each quadrant at 2-cm intervals.

In extreme conditions, most of the body of the stomach may be displaced into the thoracic cavity (an intra-thoracic stomach), forming complicated angulations often difficult to negotiate and a common cause of failed endoscopy.

3.5.4 Reflux Oesophagitis

The common condition of gastro-oesophageal reflux disease, GORD, is complex and clinically not fully understood (Stal et al. 1999). Whilst GORD is most accurately evaluated by endoscopy, the diagnosis is established by a pathologic 24-hour pH study. Minor episodes of gastro-oesophageal reflux are a normal finding in most individuals. Reflux is most often seen in patients with a hiatal hernia, but there is no absolute relationship between the presence of a hiatal hernia and GORD. Dysphagia and heartburn are typical symptoms, but nocturnal oral reflux may give rise to coughing, laryngospasm, and hoarseness.

Endoscopy is normal in up to 20% of patients with a typical medical history. Some endoscopists emphasise that erythema and increased vulnerability of the distal oesophagus are signs of early reflux disease, as is blurring of the Z-line, but others deny this. All agree that the presence of erosions, however tiny, shallow various-shaped ulcers demarcated by shiny red rims, and scar formations are lesions caused by reflux (Figs. 3.11, 3.12). See table below.

Irregularities of the oesophageal lumen secondary to ulcer deformities and scars are accurately depicted by high-quality contrast studies. Conversely erosions and shallow ulcers are easily overlooked; therefore patients with GORD should be evaluated by endoscopy. Complicating strictures are readily managed at endoscopy by the use of hydrostatic balloons.

The quality of lesions, their axial and circumferential spread, and the presence of complications form the basis of various classifications of GORD, lowest grade signifying just minute lesions and the highest grade circumferential lesions and deep ulcers. The current most popular classification is the Los Angeles classification (Table 3.1; Lundell et al. 1999).

This is mainly a classification of active disease and does not take complications of gastro-oesophageal reflux disease into account, i.e. scar formation and strictures. In dysphagic patients with no other symptom or sign of reflux oesophagitis, carcinoma of the oesophagus must be excluded.

3.5.5 Oesophageal Strictures

Longstanding superficial inflammation related to GORD may subsequently involve deeper wall layers,

Table 3.1. Los Angeles classification of oesophagitis (Lundell et al. 1999)

Grade	Los Angeles classification of oesophagitis One (or more) mucosal break(s)
A	No longer than 5 mm, not extending between the top of two mucosal folds
B	More than 5 mm long, not extending between the top of two mucosal folds
C	Continuous between the tops of two or more mucosal folds, but involving less than 75% of the circumference
D	Involving at least 75% of the oesophageal circumference

giving rise to fibrosis, scar formation, and narrowing. These strictures are usually found at the transitional zone in the distal oesophagus but may be encountered in the more proximal oesophagus in cases of columnar lining, as the stricture has migrated cephalad along with the transitional zone (Fig. 3.14).

Strictures secondary to contact damage by corrosive agents and medical compounds are often elongated and typically located at pressure points, i.e. aortic arch and left main bronchus.

The length and width of a stricture are preferably assessed on contrast studies, as some of these cannot be passed even by a small-diameter endoscope. A single-contrast oesophagogram shows the “true” physiologic size of a narrowed lumen, and should preferably be used for documentation.

A full anatomic description includes the distal part of the stricture, which may not be correctly delineated if the oesophagus distal to it is not fully distended with air. In such cases the length of the stricture is easily exaggerated.

3.5.6 Endoscopic Treatment of Strictures

Correct evaluation is important in order to choose the appropriate therapy. In most cases repeated dilatation procedures are performed. Short strictures are preferably dilated with hydrostatic balloons, whereas semisolid rods of various sizes are used in long and tough strictures. The advantage of balloons is twofold. Firstly they are applied through the working channel of the endoscope, allowing visual observation and function. Secondly they exert a radial and not an axial force, the former being less traumatic. The process is monitored fluoroscopically whilst the hydrostatic pressure of the balloon is increased, until the waist created by the stricture disappears. After deflating the balloon the success of treatment and the area and beyond are immediately inspected endoscopically.

The dilatation procedure aims to establish a lumen width of 20 mm. In most instances it is possible to do so in one setting, provided the initial width is around 8 mm or larger. If it is less than 8 mm it is advisable to perform stepwise dilatations over a couple of days in order to avoid a complete rupture of the wall. A late rupture, i.e. up to 36 hours post-procedure, is still a true risk even if all precautions have been taken. This life-threatening condition should be recognised and managed immediately, which means that the patient and caregivers must be aware of adverse symptoms.

3.5.7 Barrett’s Metaplasia

Gastric reflux induces inflammation of the normal squamous epithelium of the distal oesophagus. In patients with chronic reflux oesophagitis, metaplastic epithelium is seen. This metaplasia is thus an acquired condition as a tissue response to acid reflux. The secondary cephalad migration of the transition zone depends on the duration and severity of disease.

This sequence is a physiologic response to the initial inflammation and subsequent desquamation caused by reflux of gastric content. As re-epithelialisation occurs, the pale squamous epithelium is replaced by a specialised columnar epithelium which tolerates acidity much better (Fig. 3.15).

There are three recognised types of columnar metaplasia: (1) the fundic type of the normal gastric fundus; (2) the cardiac type with pyloric and cardiac glands and gastric foveolae, and (3) the intestinal-type Barrett’s mucosa. When present the latter is found bordering the transitional line from below. It carries an 8% risk of malignant degeneration. The cardiac type of metaplasia is located in between the Barrett’s and the fundic-type mucosa. Biopsy is necessary to establish which type is present and to rule out dysplastic degeneration. Radiology has nothing to offer in this respect.

In typical cases of Barrett’s when there is no concomitant oesophagitis, the normal pale squamous cell membrane of the oesophagus is sharply delineated from the pinkish metaplastic mucosa, where no vessels are seen. When oesophagitis is present the typical features of erosions, ulcers, exudation, and bleedings are seen.

As mentioned above strictures complicating GORD are found at the transition zone level as it migrates orally. Scar formation secondary to ulcer healing remains behind. It is evident from what has been previously stated that a complicating stricturing adenocarcinoma must be excluded.

Adenocarcinoma complicating long-standing Barrett’s metaplasia is usually found in the distal third of the oesophagus. Screening programmes have been initiated in order to find early and curable tumours. These include four quadrant biopsies every two centimetres starting just beneath the transition zone. Patients with dysplasia revealed at microscopy either enter a surveillance programme and are screened every 6 months, or are treated more aggressively if the dysplasia is severe. This may include formal surgical resection or submucous resection.

3.5.8 Other Oesophageal Ulcers

Ulcers may be superficial or deep and when deep can penetrate down to the muscularis propria. Aetiologies include infectious diseases such as candidiasis, herpes simplex, and cytomegalovirus as well as medications such as alendronate, tetracyclines, potassium chloride, etc. Deep ulcers are typically associated with post-sclerotherapy for varices and severe reflux oesophagitis.

Whilst ulcers are more readily diagnosed by endoscopy, radiology more accurately depicts complications such as fistula and stricture formations.

3.5.9 Varices

Cirrhotic liver disease causes high pressure in the portal vein and subsequent establishment of collaterals through which blood from the splanchnic veins reaches the systemic circulation. One of these collaterals diverts the venous blood through the coronary vein in the liver to mucosal venous capillaries and peri-oesophageal veins. From here the venous blood is shunted into the azygos and hemiazygos veins. Subsequently the oesophageal veins dilate and present as tortuous, fragile structures which easily bleed. In severe cases varices extend into the mid-oesophagus as well as down into the gastric fundus (Fig. 3.16). They are classified depending on size and extent (see Table 3.2) (Soehendra et al. 1998)

Bleeding from oesophageal varices is life-threatening and occurs in 30%–40% of those with varices. There is a 75% risk of re-bleeding within two years of the first episode.

At endoscopy oesophageal varices appear as axially running strings of blue-tinted sinuous structures, increasing in size aborally. Areas of diffuse redness and spots of haematin (Grade III) signify a 50% increased risk of bleeding.

Variceal bleeding is usually related to the severity of the disease and thus will be commoner with large tortuous vessels as well as signs of earlier bleeding and concomitant oesophagitis.

A total gastroscopy should always be performed, as there may be a further bleeding source from a synchronous caudal lesion. Bleeding episodes from ulcers in the pre-pyloric antrum and duodenal bulb or from gastritis is recorded in up to 50% of these patients.

Oesophageal varices have traditionally been managed by sclerotherapy. This therapy has proved efficient in controlling active haemorrhage but has no influence on the reduced life expectancy of these patients. The sclerosing agent is injected in repeated 1 to 2-ml aliquots in and around the varicose vein. Sclerotherapy controls the bleeding in up to 90%.

During the past seven years ligation of varices with rubber bands has gained increased popularity since the risk of treatment-induced bleeding is almost nullified. A transparent cylinder holding 5 to 10 tight rubber bands is mounted on the tip of a gastroscope. A varix is then sucked into the system and a band is released over it, resulting in a pseudopolypoid deformity of the vein that is instantly turned deep blue by stasis. Up to 10 rubber bands can be applied in severe cases at the first admission. Subsequently, fewer bands need to be applied with successful treatment, and one may resort to sclerotherapy for small residual veins.

In the event of unsuccessful treatment by the above techniques, or complete obliteration of view by blood, Sengstaken balloon compression may be applied.

3.5.10 Neoplastic Lesions

3.5.10.1 Benign Tumours

Benign tumours of the oesophagus are incidental and rare findings of which leiomyomas are the most common. These submucosal lesions are usually situated in the proximal part of the oesophagus. In contrast to gastric leiomyomas, oesophageal ones rarely ulcerate.

Papillomas are small pale lesions, single or multiple and difficult to distinguish from glycogen deposits. Adenomatous polyps are rare with the same features as adenomas elsewhere in the gastrointestinal tract.

3.5.10.2 Malignant Tumours

Malignant lesions of the oesophagus are diagnosed at endoscopy and confirmed by histological examination of the specimens obtained by endoscopic biopsy. In patients with a narrow and tight malignant stric-

Table 3.2. Classification of oesophageal and gastric varices (Soehendra et al. 1998)

Grade	Oesophagus	Gastric fundus
I	<5 mm across, straight, in distal oesophagus	<5 mm across
II	5–10 mm across. Mid-oesophageal extension	5–10 mm across. Single polypoid varices
III	>10 mm across, filling the oesophageal lumen. No normal mucosa. Red spots	>10 mm across. Conglomerate of thin walled polypoid varices

ture, brush cytology may improve the diagnostic yield. Tumour staging is achieved by CT examination, supplemented by endoscopic ultrasound (Fig. 3.17).

3.5.10.2.1 Squamous Cell Carcinoma

Sixty percent of all malignant tumours of the oesophagus are squamous cell in origin. There is an association with nicotine, intake of hot and noxious beverages, achalasia, corrosive oesophagitis, and Plummer-Vinson syndrome. The incidence varies world wide, from 5 to 100 per 100,000 inhabitants.

Dysphagia occurs late in the disease, when the tumour has reached a length of 3 to 4 cm and has narrowed the lumen to less than half (Fig. 3.18a). At this stage most tumours have infiltrated beyond the muscularis propria and are likely to demonstrate lymph node involvement.

A barium swallow readily describes the tumour as to location, size, and morphology but as mentioned above both CT and endoscopic ultrasound are needed for staging purposes. Three main morphologic types are identified: (1) the most common polypoid-exophytic form, (2) the depressed-ulcerative form, and (3) the least common, that of a stricture from diffuse infiltration.

All three types are friable, necrotic, and bleed easily. Hence intubation with an endoscope should be performed gently in order to avoid damage and perforation.

When small in size the first two types occupy only a sector of the mucous membrane, whereas large tumours tend to be circumferential. Endoscopically a clear demarcation is seen between the unaffected, normal mucosa and the discoloured, easily bleeding tumour.

In cases of infiltrated carcinoma there is eccentric narrowing of the lumen without obvious mucosal destruction. The malignant part of such a stricture may easily be overlooked early in the disease process, as the covering mucosa on the oral side looks normal. All strictures should therefore be subject to brush cytology as well as thoroughly biopsied.

3.5.10.2.2 Adenocarcinoma

The incidence of adenocarcinoma has increased during the last decades and it numbers almost 20% of all oesophageal carcinomas. The majority of adenocarcinomas arise at the oesophago-gastric junction. Second types of adenocarcinoma are associated with Barrett's oesophagus, and arise from the level of the displaced transition zone.

The common type of adenocarcinoma is infiltrative in character and causes narrowing of the lumen, sometimes without an obvious tumour mass. The underlying tumour is then difficult to detect, and multiple biopsies should be obtained in order to rule out the diagnosis. At this stage the disease may be difficult to differentiate against simple achalasia. Balloon dilatation, which is a standard treatment of achalasia, should always be postponed until a benign diagnosis is safely proven.

The surface of the tumour is vulnerable, erythematous, and bleeds easily although in early disease it may be manifest by just a slight change in colour. When ulcerated a tiny adenocarcinoma may already be histologically advanced.

Adenocarcinomas arising from Barrett's metaplasia may start as polypoid masses and then grow into infiltrative and stricturing lesions. Sometimes tiny satellite tumours are seen adjacent to the main tumour. Biopsies from the oesophagus inferior to the tumour may establish its metaplastic origin.

Tumours arising from structures close to the oesophagus may cause dysphagia through an extrinsic compression of its lumen, i.e. lung and mediastinal tumours. Also, submucosal metastases may give rise to compression. In these cases the covering oesophageal mucosa is normal. The correct diagnosis is established by CT and/or endoscopic ultrasound guided biopsies.

3.5.10.2.3 Early Oesophageal Cancers

The poor prognosis of oesophageal cancers when they become clinically symptomatic has called for endoscopic programmes to identify them at an early histological stage and whilst still curable. Some endoscopists have implemented surveillance programmes for patients at increased risk, such as heavy smokers and drinkers, those few survivors from earlier treated head and neck tumours, and patients with Barrett's oesophagus. However the cost-benefit of these programmes is questionable as the yield of early detected malignancies is still low. In practice there are no useful selecting criteria for selection, which leaves us with the challenge to identify the early lesions in patients on routine lists.

Early carcinoma may have no endoscopic features and is detected by chance on biopsies from patients with metaplastic epithelia of the distal oesophagus. The following macroscopic features should be looked for: (1) a localised vulnerable erosion with or without erythema, (2) a discrete area of irregular nodules and papillary structures, and (3) a small irregular and shallow ulcer. Typically these lesions all bleed easily when lightly touched, for instance after brushing the epithelial surface. When in doubt dye spraying with Lugol's solution may be helpful by improving detection (see above).

3.6 Endoscopic Treatment of Oesophageal Pathology

3.6.1 Endoscopic Dilatation of Malignancies

Advanced tumours cannot be cured, and treatment aims at relieving dysphagia. This is achieved by repeated dilatation procedures, more or less painful and with a risk of perforation. Good conscious sedation and analgesia of the patient as well as an experienced endoscopist are prerequisites for success of treatment.

After pre-medication the dilatation is initiated by gently advancing a hydrophilic floppy guide wire through the tumour area under fluoroscopic control, until its tip reaches the stomach. Semisolid rods or balloons are then passed over the wire to traverse the tumour area.

If balloons are used they are filled with diluted iodine contrast solution, and the dilating procedure is controlled fluoroscopically by noting the stricture effect on the balloon (Fig. 3.18b). For rods there are radio-opaque markers at the tapering tip to guide the operator as to whether or not the tumour has been passed. The dilating force is applied by hand which gives a reliable indication as to the tightness of the tumour. The treatment aims to achieve a lumen diameter of 20 mm. In cases with pain and/or in firm and extensive tumours, this width cannot be reached in one setting.

Often the dilatation is followed by other treatments such as coagulation of tumour tissue or deploying a tumour-bridging prosthesis, i.e. a stent (Fig. 3.18c). Laser, argon plasma, and heat cause coagulation. Injection of alcohol in small aliquots starting at the distal part of the tumour is a cheap alternative, but may be very painful. Brachytherapy with intraluminal irradiation is said to be efficient. All these procedures may keep the lumen open until death, but have usually to be repeated, and they all come with an increased risk of bleeding, necrosis, and perforation. Spontaneous tumour fistulation into the bronchial tree as well as perforations secondary to treatment are not uncommon complications, which may be managed by the use of covered stents to seal the openings.

3.6.2 Endoscopic Stent Treatment

Before implanting a prosthesis the length of the tumour must be charted. The size of the cuff ends are then added to this length. If the oral cuff of the stent ends in the upper oesophagus close to the hypo-pharynx, then there is a great risk that the patient will not tolerate the prosthesis. There is also a risk of a stent inserted proximal to the level of the carina to exert a compression force to the trachea via displacement of the tumour, causing a high respiratory embarrassment. In order to avoid this calamity, pre-ballooning of the tumour area to at least 20 mm is advisable. If no coughing is provoked then the implantation is probably safe. If respiratory stridor presents after deployment of a stent, this should be immediately retracted, but this is often extremely difficult or impossible. If a respiratory complication is created, the endoscopist must then be prepared also to stent the trachea.

Both plastic and self-expanding metal stents exert a radial force that initially may cause chest pain. Over time there is a risk of tumour overgrowth either at the ends of the stent or through its mesh, thus blocking the lumen. These problems are solved by coagulating the in- and overgrowing tissue or by inserting new stents through the old one.

3.6.3 Oesophageal Foreign Bodies

Organic lesions of the oesophagus may cause impaction of food and foreign bodies. Such lesions are ring formations, strictures, and intraluminal tumours. Defective muscular function, as in achalasia, may also cause impaction.

A water-soluble contrast study will readily demonstrate the level of obstruction. The obstructing material is then removed endoscopically by means of a Dormia basket, a polyp snare, or grasping forceps. Under no circumstance should the foreign body be pushed down into the stomach, as this manoeuvre may cause perforation to the lesion beyond the impaction.

Sharp and pointed bodies should be covered by an endoscopic overtube before removal in order to avoid damage to the mucous membrane (Fig. 3.19) Even a large solid foreign body may be mobilised endoscopically. In such cases it is advisable to have ready a laryngoscope and a pair of slightly curved pliers with which to grasp and retrieve the foreign body. The airway must be protected during this procedure. Large bodies in the hypopharynx and proximal oesophagus might best be removed through a rigid large-calibre oesophagoscope under general anaesthesia, and this is really the realm of the ENT surgeon.

The cause for an impaction should always be sought. At endoscopy tissue biopsies should be obtained from the level of impaction in order to disclose any early malignancy. It may be necessary to perform contrast radiology to exclude subtle rings and motility dysfunction.

3.7 Gastric Pathology

3.7.1 Ulcer Tears

Mucosal tears at the level of oesophago-gastric junction are known as Mallory-Weiss tears. Increased intra-abdominal pressure from episodes of forceful belching and vomiting are said to be causative factors. These tears tend to bleed in the acute phase and heal rapidly and are often found in alcoholics. The tears are elongated, around 5 mm long but sometimes rather extended, and located distally to the Z-line. They do not penetrate past the submucosa. At initial endoscopy an adherent blood clot may be shown covering a whitish and necrotic mucosal defect. Similar tears may be found in the body of the stomach at the level of the diaphragmatic opening in patients with a diaphragmatic hernia (Fig. 3.20). These ulcers, known as Cameron ulcers, have the same characteristics as Mallory-Weiss tears, including rapid healing. Hemostatic treatment is only advised if active bleeding is observed.

3.7.2 Gastritis

The normal mucosa of the stomach is pink in colour with no visible vessels. The mucosa shows gastric folds extending in parallel from the fundic region along the greater curvature of the body. No folds are seen in the distended, normal gastric antrum. The folds are soft and flatten by distension.

3.7.2.1 Hypertrophic Gastritis

Thickened gastric folds cause difficulties in differential diagnostics, as they may be normal, related to inflammation, or secondary to a diffusely infiltrating malignancy, i.e. linitis plastica or gastric lymphoma. The accuracy of forceps biopsies is low, as causative diseases are located in deep wall layers. In order to define which wall layer is enlarged, endoscopic ultrasound may be helpful. Thickening of mucosal and submucosal layers are more suggestive for an adenocarcinoma, whereas thickening of layer two indicates a benign disease (Mendis et al. 1994).

Endoscopic signs of gastritis include widespread hyperaemia of the mucous membrane and patchy distributed whitish metaplasia in between red areas of the gastric antrum. Small raised erosions are also seen (Fig. 3.21). The areae gastricae are irregular and prominent. The mucous membrane is swollen in more acute conditions and atrophied in long-standing situations, allowing the vascular pattern to become more apparent. Petechiae, submucosal bleedings, and necrotic erosions are seen with no proven correlation with the severity of disease.

Acute gastritis may be subdivided on the basis of the endoscopic appearance into mild and advanced gastritis. The former exhibits a generalised oedema, moderately swollen folds, limited mucosal bleedings, and small erosions. The stomach wall is less pliable with reduced distension. The same, but more extensive and pronounced signs are found in the advanced form of gastritis, sometimes referred to as erythematous gastritis. Exudate may cover the mucosa and bile is found in dependent parts of the stomach. Bile reflux into the antrum is allegedly blamed for the hyperaemic, red antrum folds seen converging towards the pylorus resulting in the so-called chemical gastropathy. Food retention is seen in advanced cases. Many of these changes are related to *Helicobacter pylori* infection (see below).

3.7.2.2 Atrophic Gastritis

Due to atrophy of the mucous membrane, normal gastric folds are flattened and vessels in the stomach wall become apparent. The surface is slightly irregular and adenomatous polyps may be seen. Grey-white plaques in the gastric antrum are associated with intestinal metaplasia, which is considered to be a precancerous condition. The same might be true for patients with pernicious anaemia who have atrophic gastritis and achlorhydria.

3.7.2.3 Gastritis Secondary to Medication

The gastric mucosa is sensitive to certain medical compounds such as aspirin and other nonsteroid-anti-inflammatory (NSAID) drugs. In addition to gastritis these drugs may cause chronic gastric and duodenal ulcers. The mechanism is mediated through depletion of prostaglandin, reducing the protection abilities of normal gastric mucous to the acid environment.

The endoscopic signs of NSAID-induced gastritis are the same as mentioned above. They are most often found in the distal gastric body and antrum. Erosions and petechiae are the early signs, often accompanied by red varicose folds converging toward the pylorus (Fig. 3.22). Medication induced ulcers may become large and typically are not accompanied by concomitant oedema or obvious erythema. Bleeding stigmata are frequently found.

The clinical benefit of prophylactic treatment with acid-reducing medication to patients on long-term NSAID treatment is still unclear.

3.7.2.4 Ménétrier's Disease

Although strictly speaking this is more of a gastropathy rather than gastritis, it is included here because in some instances there may be a prominent inflammatory response. This disease is characterised by grossly thickened and tortuous folds mainly located in the fundus and body of the stomach. Histology demonstrates hyperplasia of the goblet cells and widening of the glandular structures. This causes the fold thickening. The surface is covered by a surplus of mucus. Diagnostically, infiltrative carcinoma and lymphoma must be excluded. Endoscopic ultrasound is recommended followed by obligatory deep biopsies.

Glandular hyperplasia is also seen in cases with an overproduction of gastrin, i.e. in Zollinger-Ellison syndrome. The gastric folds are thickened but less so than in Ménétrier's disease but again the proximal body is the area most commonly affected. Gastric ulcers are a relatively infrequent finding.

3.7.3 Peptic Ulcer and Helicobacter Pylori

It is important to detect *H. pylori* infection because of its association with nonjunctional gastric adenocarcinoma, gastritis and duodenal ulceration, B-cell lymphoma, and reflux oesophagitis. There are a number of mechanisms for its detection. The urea breath test is the most accurate noninvasive test with an accuracy of 96% (Cohne et al. 1999). The rapid urease test or CLO test is performed at the time of endoscopy and has a 97% accuracy and an 80% sensitivity. This can indicate infection within minutes. Combining the CLO test with microscopy of tissue specimens, the detection rate comes close to 100%, emphasizing the importance of several biopsies from the gastric antrum (Gur et al. 1998).

If the infection is present it is thus logical to attempt eradication therapy, as it has been shown that not only do the large inflammatory folds (Fig. 3.23) come back to normal, together with acid secretion and fasting serum gastrin levels (Yasunaga et al. 1994), but there is also better healing of peptic ulcers. This is so even if there is no concomitant acid suppression (Treiber and Lambert 1998). Furthermore it has been shown that complications such as haemorrhage, perforation, and late pyloric stenosis are largely eliminated if the infection is eradicated (Macri et al. 1998).

Eradication therapy is mainly carried out as a one-week triple therapy, i.e. a proton pump inhibitor (PPI) combined with amoxicillin and clarithromycin or metronidazole. Bismuth or Ranitidine bismuth citrate triple therapies are also prescribed, as these two regimens have not caused any antimicrobial resistance. A high eradication rate and reduced risk of resistance are achieved by adding a PPI to the antibiotics (Lind et al.1999).

Long-term studies after eradication showed that 6% of patients still had a positive urea breath test and that 110 patients out of 170 were still symptomatic. Of those 31 were complaining of heartburn and 12 stated that this symptom was new (Fraser et al. 1998). The risk of recurrent ulcer disease after eradication is low, and then often found in younger patients within the first six months and after low-efficacy therapy. It has been postulated that the recurrence is a result more based on recrudescence than reinfection (Gispert et al. 1998).

According to recent epidemiologic studies, the prevalence of *Helicobacter pylori* infection is decreasing in the developed world and not all gastroduodenal ulcers are related to this infection (Blaser 1999; Tytgat 2000). In a multicentre study comprising 2,300 patients, it was shown that 27% of endoscopically confirmed duodenal ulcers were unrelated to *H. pylori* or NSAIDs (Ciociola et al. 1999). At the same time an increase in gastro-oesophageal reflux disease was recorded, as was Barrett's oesophagus and oesophageal adenocarcinoma.

3.7.4 Benign Ulcer Disease

The pathogenesis of benign gastric ulcers is not fully understood but is related to a weakness in the mucous barrier towards acid and pepsinogen. Some etiologic factors are recognised, i.e. *Helicobacter pylori* infection that is also associated with gastritis and duodenal ulcer disease, NSAID medications, Zollinger-Ellison syndrome, and stress.

In the majority of cases benign ulcers are single, measuring less than 10 mm across. Multiple benign ulcers are usually located in the gastric antrum and are often secondary to NSAID treatment. Giant ulcers, i.e. those larger than 30 mm are often induced by medications.

Benign ulcers are most commonly found in the distal part of the stomach, along the lesser curvature of the body and in the gastric antrum (Fig. 3.24). A second benign ulcer may be found on the opposite wall, a so-called kissing ulcer, and sometimes there may be an associated duodenal ulcer. In elderly patients, ulcers are frequently located in more proximal parts of the stomach (Fig. 3.25). This probably is a consequence of both the normal age-related cephalad migration of the fundopyloric mucosa transition zone as well as the development of chronic atrophic gastritis.

Examination of the stomach aims at verifying or excluding a clinical suspicion of a mucosal disease, to exclude signs of malignancy and to estimate risk of bleeding and perforation. There is no role for radiography, because serious complications of gastric diseases such as bleeding and malignancy cannot be ruled out with certainty by this method. By contrast, gastroscopy is not only highly sensitive in these aspects but in addition offers an efficient and simple means for tissue sampling and treatment.

At endoscopy a benign ulcer is recognised by its light yellow-grey granular base of desquamated epithelium and fibroid tissue. In the acute phase, the ulcer base is sharply demarcated by a shiny, slightly oedematous and erythematous zone with no signs of regenerating epithelium. Dark spots of haematin and coagulated blood indicate risk of ulcer bleeding, and this is substantial in cases where a visible vessel is seen (Fig. 3.26).

In the healing phase a growing zone of granular regenerating epithelium is seen covering the ulcer edges. The initial surrounding erythema and oedema of the acute phase vanishes, and normal mucosa folds can be followed up to the edge of the ulcer without evidence of any deformity (Fig. 3.27). The ulcer base is progressively covered by red, regenerating epithelium, rich in capillaries and raised to the surrounding surface (Fig. 3.28). Finally it contracts, leaving a scar behind which pales over time.

Current ulcer treatment is highly efficient. Even large ulcers with signs of bleeding heal within a couple of weeks. Deep ulcers heal with extensive scar formation that may end in pronounced local deformity with convergence of mucosal folds. One such deformity, known since the dawn of gastrointestinal radiology, is the so-called Lilja deformity or purse bag stomach, in which shortening of the lesser curve aspect of the gastric antrum brings the pylorus close to the gastric angle. The end result is a bag-like deformity of the stomach complicated with gastric outlet obstruction and retention.

A minute deformity may pass unnoticed or ignored as just a triviality. Such a small deformity may however be the only evidence of an early malignant lesion. That is why the stomach should be examined both with good air distension as well as slightly collapsed, as any deformity will become more obvious.

3.7.5 Malignant Ulcer

An ulcer that is large, irregular in shape, with an uneven irregular margin and found outside the ordinary locations of benign ulcers runs an increased risk of being malignant. The endoscopic sensitivity in differentiating malignant from benign ulcers measures around 80%, and only single ulcers elude correct classification when not properly biopsied. The diagnostic sensitivity for ulcerated early gastric cancer (EGC) is examiner-dependent, and it may be easily overlooked. In routine hands the detection rate of EGC is still rather low as the diagnosis is based on identification of subtle irregularities at the ulcer rim. A typical benign ulcer has a "punched out", sharp margin all around, whereas the mucosal rim around a malignant one shows granular irregularities and patchy discolorations. Unlike an acute benign ulcer there is no obvious oedema or erythema encircling a malignant one. Some of the surrounding folds running up to the edge of a malignant ulcer are split close to the ulcer and reveal a "mouse eaten" appearance, while others exhibit a club-like deformity, sometimes fused and ending at a short distance from the ulcer crater (Fig. 3.29).

3.7.6 Histopathology

Benign-looking ulcers of the pylorus or in the prepyloric antrum do not have to be examined histologically. In these cases testing for *Helicobacter pylori* infection is enough. Tissue biopsies from all other ulcers should be obtained in order to rule out any dysplasia. Several biopsies from the ulcer rim are recommended; especially from areas of discolouration or surface irregularities. In order to increase the chance to obtain positive biopsies from a latent carcinoma, some authorities postpone biopsies from the ulcer until after the treatment has commenced. The theory is that the benign part of an ulcer heals whilst the malignant part remains unaffected (Fig. 3.29).

Cytology is also helpful, obtained by brushing not only the ulcer crater but also the rim. In some departments a cytologist is in attendance to dry and fix the specimens, thus ensuring quality and adequacy of the specimens.

3.7.7 Neoplastic Lesion of the Stomach

3.7.7.1 Benign Polyps

Gastric polyps are mainly small and an incidental finding, although large ones may prolapse and cause retention-like symptoms. They are divided into non-neoplastic (Fig. 3.31) and neoplastic (Fig. 3.32). Of the former 85% are glandular cysts and hyperplastic polyps, the rest inflammatory fibroid polyps and hamartomas.

3.7.7.2 Hyperplastic Polyps

Hyperplastic polyps are the most common polyps of epithelial origin and as a rule are multiple and found throughout the stomach. They have an association with chronic fundic gastritis, and although this presents an increased risk for malignancy, hyperplastic polyps themselves do not have a malignant propensity. At endoscopy these polyps present from small nodules to 15-mm proliferative lesions, with or without a stalk (Fig. 3.30). Biopsy is only necessary in large polyps to establish their true nature.

3.7.7.3 Neoplastic Polyps

Neoplastic polyps are epithelial in 90% of cases, the rest being endocrine, mainly carcinoid lesions. About 7% of all gastric polyps are frankly malignant according to a large series of 4,852 patients with gastric polyps (Stolte et al. 1994).

3.7.7.4 Gastric Adenoma

Five to ten percent of all polyps are adenomatous and thus have malignant potential, and, if the polyp is larger than 2 cm there is a 40% risk of malignant degeneration. Most of them are single and located in distal parts of the stomach (Fig. 3.31). There is an association with chronic atrophic fundic gastritis, and these are the same polyps found in FAP.

Histologically three subtypes are identified, i.e. tubular, tubulovillous (Fig. 3.32), and villous type. As in the colon, the latter two types show increased risk of malignant deterioration. The villous type is often located in the gastric antrum and may cause gastric outlet obstruction.

At endoscopy these polyps are elevated lobular structures which may be semi-pedunculated, usually of a darker colour than the surrounding mucosa. Erosions and ulcers are signs of malignancy.

3.7.7.5 Adenocarcinoma

Gastric adenocarcinoma constitutes 75% of all gastric malignancies and afflicts mainly patients age 50 and older. The aetiology is not fully known but genetic and dietary factors play a role, as does infection. Patients with adenomatous polyps, pernicious anaemia, chronic antral gastritis with intestinal metaplasia, and Billroth II resections have an increased risk of developing gastric cancer (Figs. 3.34, 3.35). The five-year survival rate for gastric cancer exceeds 90% when the disease is diagnosed at an early stage but less than 10% when it is advanced. In countries with a high prevalence of gastric cancer and an ongoing program for screen detection, up to one out of three detected cancers are early ones. However in low prevalence areas this percentage is much lower.

Depending on their macroscopic features carcinomas are classified into four subgroups. The type 1 adenocarcinoma is polypoid in shape, and 60% are located in the gastric body. These tumours represent around 20% of all gastric cancers. They are well demarcated from the surrounding mucosa, and have an irregular, friable, and easy bleeding surface. Their successful removal gives a five-year survival rate of around 30%.

The type II adenocarcinoma is a rather well demarcated malignant ulcer. It is seen in up to 40% of gastric cancers and has a five-year survival rate of around 60% after curative treatment. When small, this type II cancer is easily misinterpreted as a benign ulcer (Fig. 3.35). Multiple biopsies from all quadrants are usually needed to confirm malignancy. Type II cancers are further subdivided into types IIa, IIb, and IIc (see below).

Type III carcinoma is a diffusely infiltrating lesion dominated by a large ulcer of several centimetres in diameter. This may partly be surrounded by normal mucosa that explains the difficulties of obtaining representative forceps biopsies. Again, multiple specimens from all around the ulcer edge are recommended. These tumours are seen in up to 15% and have a poor five-year survival rate of less than 15%.

The type IV adenocarcinoma is a diffusely infiltrating one and is highly malignant, with almost no patient surviving five years. Most of these are local tumours in the fundus and body. The diffusely infiltrating type throughout the stomach, so-called linitis plastica, is seen in less than 30% of the type IV-cancers (Fig. 336). It usually involves most parts of the stomach wall but not the mucosa. Distension of the stomach by air inflation is increasingly diminished, and the tumour is disguised by benign appearing mucosa. It may therefore be overlooked at endoscopy. Biopsies should be aimed at scattered focal ulcers, if any are present, and toward areas of irregular mucosa in order to increase the microscopic yield. When suspected a high quality double-contrast barium meal is the method of choice to verify its existence (Fig. 3.37a).

Circumscribed and elevated tumours are obvious and offer no diagnostic problem. Ulcerated lesions as well as diffusely infiltrating ones may cause great diagnostic problems. As emphasised earlier it is important to examine the stomach both fully distended with air as well as slightly collapsed to enhance fold architecture and surface pattern. Displaced, thickened, and tortuous folds may point to an alleged lesion, as might an area of coarse nodularity and surface irregularity. These features are difficult to detect at conventional radiography.

3.7.7.6 Early Gastric Cancer, EGC

The Japanese Society of Gastroenterology has defined the main endoscopic types of early gastric cancers – that is to say a cancer whose invasion is limited to the mucosa and submucosa. In these cases the dysplastic area is strictly limited to the mucous membrane and its total thickness should be less than twice that of the surrounding mucosa. As noted above Type I is a polypoid cancer and type III an ulcerated one. Type II is subdivided into three. It may be slightly elevated (type IIa), true flat (type IIb), or depressed (type IIc) (Fig. 3.37). Combinations of these are common.

The early lesions do not cause symptoms and are thus incidental findings. Radiography is impracticable and endoscopic detection difficult as the prevalence is low in Western society. In our material from southern Sweden we find less than 1 case per 250 gastroscopies, i.e. 10–20 cases annually, in spite of the fact that we have had a special interest in these lesions for a long time.

At endoscopy EGCs are recognised as slightly discoloured areas, from dark red to yellowish pink, with a deranged surface pattern and sometimes a central depression. Vital dye spraying with methylene blue or indigo carmine (see above) helps to identify the lesions (Fig. 3.38), as does examination during various grades of distension.

3.7.7.7 Gastric Lymphoma

Lymphomas constitute approximately 24% of all gastric malignancies. Most of them are non-Hodgkin's lymphoma and part of disseminated disease. Primary gastric lymphoma belongs to the localised form. Constitutional symptoms, such as fever, night sweats, and weight loss tend to be less obvious in gastric lymphoma than in Hodgkin's lymphoma. The prognosis and response to treatment are significantly influenced by histopathology, stage of disease, and tumour markers. Patients with favourable disease may survive more than 7 years.

At endoscopy it may be difficult to distinguish a gastric lymphoma, which is an infiltrating lesion with ulceration, from an adenocarcinoma and even a prominent benign ulcer. The infiltrating part creates a coarse surface pattern with broad based, flat, hillock-like elevations (Fig. 3.39). Greyish discoloured areas of increased nodularity may be seen without any obvious ulcer. The infiltration may progress and simulate linitis plastica. A diagnostic feature of a lymphomatous ulcer is the dendrite-like extensions connecting these ulcers to their surroundings (Fig. 3.40). The ulcers may show bleeding stigmata, are usually multiple if not very large, and later form a raised, volcano-like crater (Fig. 3.41a,b). A primary gastric lymphoma is usually easy to disclose with double-contrast examination of the stomach, which also gives useful information of the extent of disease (Fork et al. 1984).

Histopathology is crucial in establishing the correct diagnosis. Multiple forceps biopsies may be supplemented by brush cytology to cover an extended suspicious area. As gastric lymphoma infiltrates superficially, there is a high reward from tissue biopsy and brush cytology (Fork et al. 1985).

3.7.7.8 Other Gastric Tumours

There are a variety of tumours which originate from supporting tissue components of the gastric wall, and which are mainly submucosal in distribution covered by normal mucosa. The most common are gastro-intestinal stromal tumours (GISTs) formerly known as leiomyomas and leiomyosarcomas. They comprise about 5% of gastric neoplasms (Fig. 3.42a,b).

Small GISTs are a quite a frequent finding in the proximal stomach, measuring 15 mm or less but occasionally several centimetres. They may present because of dysphagia or bleeding from a centrally located ulcer. There are no good criteria for differentiating benign from malignant, and many authorities regard them all as potentially malignant. However tumours under 25 mm are unlikely to metastasise. Leiomyosarcomas in particular may have a large extra-gastric portion best appreciated at CT, which also assesses involvement of adjacent tissue compartments and organs.

Gastric carcinoids are small lesions and represent less than 2% of all gastric polyps. They are usually multiple and flat, sometimes with an ulcer. At endoscopy they cannot be differentiated from other polyps.

Kaposi sarcoma is basically a hemangiosarcoma with proliferating endothelium of capillaries. At endoscopy these tumours are recognised as intensely red elevated lesions, varying in size and numbers. They may be polypoid with or without a depressed ulcer, or spread diffusely. Biopsies are often negative when the lesion is mainly located in the submucosa.

Metastases to the gastric wall originate from primary cancers in the lung, breast, pancreas, testes, and ovaries, but also from malignant melanoma. The last named is classically demonstrated as brown or black submucosal nodules, often with a central necrotic ulceration (Fig. 3.43). Metastases from breast carcinoma may infiltrate diffusely, most typically in the antral area.

Lipomas are rare tumours in the stomach, identified by their yellow colour and soft shape that change with the patient's position.

Hamartomas are incidental findings without any morbidity. They cannot be distinguished with any degree of certainty from other polyps. Other polypoid lesions with a firm consistency and without specific endoscopic criteria are adenomyoma, fibroma, neuro-fibroma, eosinophilic granuloma, and those caused by parasites, for instance *Anisakis marina*, a worm found in raw fish.

Although not a tumour, heterotopic pancreatic tissue is mentioned here as it may simulate a tumour mass. It is usually found as an incidental finding located n the gastric antrum on the greater curve aspect (Fig. 3.5). It is recognisable as a slightly elevated, small horse-shoe like lesion with a central depression.

3.8 Endoscopic Treatment of Polyps and Tumours

3.8.1 Polypectomy

As a number of polypoid lesions are in fact carcinomas, it is essential to obtain tissue biopsies from all such lesions and to supplement these with biopsies from the surrounding mucosa before attempting any therapeutic procedure. Particularly large polyps must be removed surgically, while small ones may be excised using an endoscopic snare and diathermy. It is advisable to perform an endoscopic ultrasound examination before so that polyps with signs of infiltration into deeper wall layers may be identified. This is particularly important with larger lesions. All the excised material must be sent for histopathologic analysis in order to minimise the risk of leaving malignant tissue behind.

3.8.2 Endoscopic Mucosal Resection

A truly superficial neoplastic lesion, i.e. one limited to the mucosa may be successfully removed by the endoscopic route. The lesion is checked by chromoendoscopy and its borders marked out with small burns from a heater probe or hot biopsy forceps. The mucosectomy starts with injection of submucosal, 2-ml aliquots of saline around the lesion. When elevated sufficiently it is ensnared with an open polypectomy snare and removed, preferably in one piece. The specimen should then be mounted on a cork plate so that the histopathologist can scrutinise the cut surface for any sign of tumour infiltration. If this is present the patient should have a final surgical removal.

3.8.3 Endoscopic Treatment of Gastric Cancer

Surgery is the only means thus far to offer the patient a definitive cure. However, in patients with evidence of metastases to local or peripheral nodes, cure is not possible. Treatment then aims at keeping the gastric outlet patent. A total gastrectomy may be chosen, or in patients with antral disease a gastro-enterostomy might suffice. As an alternative to surgery treatment by a stent may be considered. The advantage of stenting a distal malignancy is that it is less invasive, saves the patient days in hospital and is less expensive. It should however be kept in mind that a stent does only allow liquid contents to pass.

3.8.4 Vascular Abnormalities of the Stomach

3.8.4.1 Haemangioma

Haemangiomas are circumscribed, intensely red and shiny flat spots measuring 1 to 10 mm. They are also called arteriovenous malformation, (AVM), angiodysplasia, telangiectasia, etc., and may be seen throughout the entire gastrointestinal tract (Fig. 3.44a,b). As small lesions may be difficult to differentiate from suction artefacts, it is wise to examine the mucous membrane in bleeding patients before endoscopic suction has been applied. An elevated lesion with a central depression usually contains a submucosal component.

Vascular abnormalities may be incidental findings but are also seen in various diseases such as von Willebrand's disease, collagenous diseases, and Osler-Weber-Rendu syndrome. They are also associated with aortic stenosis, post-irradiation situations, and chronic renal failure. The telangiectases associated with Osler-Weber-Rendu syndrome have a predilection for the gastric body and caecum.

Haemangiomas are potential bleeding sources. If there is active bleeding they may be treated with a form of coagulation, i.e. heater probe, bi-polar electrocautery, argon-plasma, YAG-laser, etc. Lesions larger than 5 mm have a risk of treatment-induced bleeding, which normally ceases with continuous coagulation.

3.8.4.2 Other Vascular Lesions

The watermelon stomach, or gastric antrum venous ectasia (GAVE), is characterised by areas of intense redness of the gastric antrum (Fig. 3.45a,b). These may be confluent or sometimes appear like varicose veins diverging from the pyloric region. The underlying abnormality consists of ectatic veins and partially thrombosed capillaries. The condition is related to portal hypertension in which the gastric vessels participate in portosystemic blood shunting. The antral mucosa is friable, bleeds easily, and may be successfully treated by argon plasma coagulation.

Gastric varices are rare and are usually located in the fundic region. They present as thickened tortuous folds, covered by normal looking mucosa. Isolated fundic varices may be secondary to thrombosis of the splenic vein as a result of pancreatic diseases. Unlike oesophageal varices, fundic ones may only be treated with injection of tissue glue in order to minimise the risk of bleeding when the thrombus cast is expelled.

A less common lesion is the so-called "visible vessel", which may be easily overlooked when not bleeding as it is not surrounded by an ulcer. These are often referred to as a Dieulafoy lesion and when bleeding are likely to demonstrate a pulsatile pattern. They are best dealt with by clipping, although injection of aethoxysclerol, adrenaline infiltration, heater probe coagulation, etc. are also successful.

Ischaemia of the stomach secondary to extensive arterial disease is a rare entity. The mucosa is eroded and the necrotic area is sharply demarcated from well-perfused mucosa. The naked surface may expose the muscle layer, which is discoloured by bleeding from different episodes.

3.8.5 The Management of Non-Variceal Bleeding

Upper gastrointestinal bleeding remains a common cause for acute admission to the hospital. It requires considerable medical resources and is associated with significant morbidity and mortality, especially in patients over the age of 75 (Rockall et al. 1995). The risk of re-bleeding is significantly increased in the elderly and in those with comorbidity, especially heart disease. The lowest mortality rate is shown in bleedings secondary to NSAID medication and from a gastric rather than a duodenal ulcer (Hasselgren et al. 1998).

A variety of classifications have been used in order to predict bleeding prevalence and recurrence. The Forrest classification is the most widespread and tested one, and is based on the endoscopic appearance of the ulcer base (Forrest et al. 1976).

Peptic ulcer bleeding stops spontaneously in 80% of patients. There is a greater risk of morbidity and mortality in those in whom it does not stop, or starts to bleed again. Active bleeding is sometimes subdivided into that which is pulsatile bleeding (Ia) (Fig. 3.46a,b) and that which is oozing (Ib). As might be expected there is a significant disparity in the visual interpretation of the lower-grade stigmata (Lau et al. 1997). Most endoscopists remove an adherent clot to examine the ulcer base, as an eroded vessel is detected in one out of three such cases. As there is an up to 45% risk of an ulcer with adherent clot and a visible vessel to re-bleed, this should be treated instantly.

3.8.6 Endoscopic Haemostasis

There are three types of endoscopic treatment available for haemostasis; namely injection, thermal, and mechanical methods (Fig. 3.47). The therapeutic end-points in those with active bleeding are cessation of bleeding and to reduce or eliminate the risk of re-bleeding. The role of endoscopic treatment as a prophylaxis in non-bleeders is less clear.

3.8.7 Injection Therapy

Injection therapy is widely available and cheap. Either saline or dilute epinephrine (0.1 mg/ml) may be used and is injected into the submucosa surrounding the bleeding source. Saline acts by compressing the local circulation whereas epinephrine acts by causing vasoconstriction and platelet aggregation as well as tamponade (Fig. 3.48). Relatively large doses of epinephrine can be used without any serious cardiovascular side effect, as long as the injected material is drained to the portal vein and metabolised in the liver (Sung et al. 1993). However, as epinephrine does not induce permanent thrombosis in one out of 8–10 cases, a second haemostatic method is recommended to obliterate the vessel.

Sclerosants used for variceal sclerotherapy such as aethoxysclerol and polidocanol have successfully been used to treat bleeding sources. These agents cause tissue necrosis and should therefore be used in small amounts only, preferable as the final sealing injection into the bleeding vessel itself, after preceding epinephrine tamponade. In practice this strategy is no longer recommended, as there are no convincing studies to support the clinical benefit of using sclerosants as a complement to epinephrine injection (Lau et al. 2000). Instead injection of human thrombin from pooled plasma is preferable. Thrombin initiates the clotting cascade without any risk of local tissue damage or any serious side effects. Indeed thrombin seems to promote ulcer healing, thus reducing the need for transfusion with attendant improvement in mortality rates (Kubba et al. 1996).

Table 3.3. Prevalence and risk of re-bleeding bleeding ulcers (Laine and Peterson 1994)

Endoscopic appearance	Forrest class	Prevalence % (range)	Further bleeding % (range)
Clean base	III	42 (19–52)	5 (0–10)
Flat spot	II c	20 (0–42)	10 (0–13)
Adherent clot	II b	17 (0–49)	22 (14–36)
Visible vessel, not bleeding	II a	17 (4–35)	43 (0–81)
Active bleeding	I	18 (4–27)	55 (17– 100)

An alternative agent which is efficient and tissue-friendly is fibrin sealant. However it is rather expensive and technically difficult to use. A dual-channel injector is needed through which 0.5 ml of fibrinogen and thrombin respectively are injected separately. The first channel is immediately rinsed by flushing through 1–1.5 ml of saline, which also squeezes the active compound into the submucosa. The glue is then injected while the needle is gradually withdrawn, and a tissue fibrin sealant is instantly formed. The injection is repeated four times close to and around the bleeding spot. A series in which this method was repeated until all endoscopic bleeding stigmata had disappeared showed a significant risk reduction for re-bleeding (Rutgeerts et al. 1997).

Absolute alcohol has also been used as a haemostatic agent as it is a very potent tissue-damaging compound. It should not be injected in larger aliquots than 0.2–0.4 ml, and then only to a total of 2 ml. Alcohol induces thrombosis that may lead to serious gastric necrosis and death.

3.8.8 Thermal Methods

Heat applied to living tissue creates coagulation of tissue proteins, contraction of arterial walls, and shrinkage of vessels. However, thermal energy may be dissipated by flowing blood with secondary loss of effect. This can be overcome by using contact thermal methods in which compression of the vessel walls brings blood flow to a standstill. They are then sealed together by heat. Vessels up to 2 mm in diameter can be successfully treated (Johnston and Jensen 1987). Both multipolar electrodes and heat probe devices have proven to be highly efficient (Hui et al. 1991).

Successful electrocoagulation requires a forceful tamponade with a large probe. The heat should have a low setting of not more than 25 watts, applied in 2-second pulses, and repeated 10–15 times over the ulcer bed.

Likewise tamponade is essential when using a heater probe, preferably 10 Fr size. The energy is delivered in a couple of 30 J pulses before the probe is retargeted.

Noncontact methods include YAG laser and argon plasma coagulation. The former is expensive, bulky, and not easy to use while the latter is the opposite. Because of blood flow, noncontact thermal methods are less effective in the treatment of actively bleeding ulcers. Instead these methods are used to finish off injection therapies by adding further coagulation.

3.8.9 Mechanical Methods

The initial technical problems of the deployment of metallic clips through a retroflexed and tangential endoscope have been overcome (Sabat et al. 1998). Metallic clips are used alone or after preceding injection therapy, and offer the best means of treatment for bleeding from large seized arteries. The clips are premounted on disposable devices and easy to deploy after some training.

3.8.10 Post-Haemostatic Management

Re-bleeding may occur as a result of an acid-peptic digestion of the thrombus that plugs the eroded artery. As acid suppression theoretically ought to prohibit episodes of recurrent bleedings, proton pump inhibitors in high doses are given intravenously to sustain a high intragastric pH (Schaffalitzky de Muckadell et al. 1997). Although solid cost-benefit data are still lacking, i.v. PPI treatment is widely recommended, especially in frail patients (Hasselgren et al. 1997).

Whilst some authors have demonstrated that there is a reduction in the risk of re-bleeding following successful treatment (Villanueva et al. 1994), this has not been verified by others (Messmann et al. 1996). Likewise, some authors have not been able to show that repeated treatment has any influence on mortality or need for surgery (Lin et al. 1996).

3.8.11 Management of Gastric Varices

Histoacryl, a cyanoacrylate, has been successfully employed for the endoscopic treatment of oesophageal varices and is the only recommended technique to treat fundic varices. When Histoacryl comes in contact with blood, e.g. when injected into the bleeding vessel, liquid Histoacryl instantly transforms into a solid substance and hence occludes the lumen. Histoacryl was randomly tested against a hypertonic saline-epinephrine injection treatment in 126 patients with bleeding ulcers. A mean of 1 ml Histoacryl was injected into the vessel, immediately followed with saline to ensure full delivery and clearing of the needle injector channel. Histoacryl treatment resulted in significantly less early re-bleeding episodes but no other advantages over the saline-epinephrine mixture (Lee et al. 2000). Instead a small risk of possible embolic complication was reported.

3.8.12 Percutaneous Endoscopic Gastrostomy (PEG)

The nonsurgical placement of a feeding gastric tube has been performed in radiology departments for a long time, and it is still indicated in patients with a tightly narrowed or completely obstructed oesophagus. However the endoscopic procedure has the advantage of offering an optimal intragastric view, and the majority of procedures are performed by this route.

3.8.12.1 Indication

The primary indication for creating a gastrostomy is to establish a means for long-term enteral feeding in patients with serious dysphagia but without impairment of the gastric outlet. Seriously ill patients with short survival expectancy do better with a nasogastric or nasojejunal tube (Park et al. 1992; Norton et al. 1996) and due to previous reported high 30-day mortality rates, strict procedure indications have now been agreed upon (Rabeneck 1997). These also include gastric decompression in patients with reversible disease, as well as feeding in patients with incurable disease but with a potential for extended survival and who require a regular change of nasogastric tube. A final consideration is home care of seriously ill patients.

3.8.12.2 PEG Sets

There are a number of different gastrostomy sets on the market. Internal fixation may be achieved by an inner retention disc, an inflatable balloon, or a mushroom-like end. The PEG tube is fixed to the external abdominal wall by a second, adjustable clipping device, sleeve, or bolster (Soehendra et al. 1998).

3.8.12.3 Patient Preparation

The patient should be fasting and the skin at the puncture site shaved and clean. Whether or not antibiotics should be given as prophylaxis is debated (Kozarec et al. 1986). Premedication with 2.5 mg of intravenous Hypnovel is usually sufficient. Occasionally i.v. opiates are given.

3.8.12.4 The PEG Procedure

The patient is intubated in the left lateral position and the stomach examined. The patient is then repositioned into a supine position, and the stomach is inflated to its maximum, apposing the anterior gastric and abdominal walls. The distended stomach displaces neighbouring organs, and a puncture site is chosen where transillumination of the abdominal wall is at its brightest. The puncture site is then anaesthetised, and a Wallace-type cannula is inserted into the stomach under endoscopic control.

The oral pull-on-string method is most widely used (Ponsky et al.1989). Here the sheath is left in position and the pull-through string inserted down it. This string is either snared or caught in a crocodile clip, and then the whole endoscope together with string is withdrawn whilst a second operator holds the other end of the string. The looped end of the string is then tied to the PEG tube and the PEG tube is pulled down the oesophagus by gentle traction on the string. Finally the tapered tube is pulled through the abdominal wall and fixed against the frontal abdominal wall with an external device.

Apposition between the gastric and abdominal walls must be close, but excessive traction causes blanching of the gastric mucosa and should be avoided (Aisenberg et al. 1991). The technique is safe with good long-term results (Grant 1993).

The Russell introducer method is probably faster but technically slightly more difficult (Russell et al. 1984; Hogan et al. 1986). This method is advantageous in patients with oesophageal obstruction too narrow for the inner bolster of the PEG to pass.

A gastroscope is inserted and the stomach inflated maximally. The puncture site is chosen in the same way as above. A flexible J-wire is inserted through the puncture needle into the stomach. A dilator within a peel-away sheath is introduced over the guidewire, and again introduced into the stomach. The dilator is exchanged with a gastrostomy tube with an inner balloon that is filled with water. The introducer sheath is peeled away and the tube placed in the sleeve of the outer retention disc and fixed to the skin with adjusted tension. The whole procedure is controlled endoscopically.

The inborn weakness with this technique is the push procedure of placing the PEG. If the set does not penetrate the stomach wall it displaces it with risk of leakage. The calibre of the set creates a rather large hole through which the stomach may deflate into the peritoneal cavity. The overall risk of complication has been shown to be greater with the Russell introducer method (Petersen and Kruse 1997).

3.8.12.5
Post-Procedural Care

The post-procedural PEG care includes nil by mouth during the first 6 hours and analgesia in case of wound pain. If there are no signs of complication, the patient may be discharged the same day with feeding through the tube. In order to maintain tube patency it is important to flush it with water after each feeding (Mathus-Vliegen 2000).

3.8.12.6
Complications

In a meta-analysis the success rate of radiologically placed gastrostomy is higher, 99.2%, compared to endoscopic placement, 95.7% and the procedure related mortality less, 0.3 compared with 0.5 ($p<0.001$). The 30-day mortality rates were equal, 15%. There was no difference in total complications, 13.3% and 15.4% respectively. However, less serious complications were recorded in the radiology group, 5.9% versus 9.4% (Mathus-Vliegen 2000).

Most complications include infection, and leakage of air and bowel content. It is therefore important to keep the wound clean and well dressed. Leakage is prevented by daily checking of the external bolster for loosening. Conversely, too tight fixation may cause pressure necrosis and dislocation of the internal bolster into the gastric wall.

Complications present early, particularly if the prerequisites for an optimal procedure are not present. The stomach should be kept well distended with air throughout the procedure in order to minimise the risk of interposition of either liver or large bowel. Transillumination must be bright and clear for the same reason. The needle puncture must be perpendicular to the abdominal and gastric walls to guarantee the shortest possible penetration for the PEG, thereby eliminating the risk of leakage. The patient and nursing team are instructed to contact the endoscopy unit as soon as possible if any tube- or wound-related complication should occur.

The PEG is easily removed by cutting the penetrating tube. Re-endoscopy is required to snare the internal bolster and extract it.

3.9
Pathology of the Duodenum

3.9.1
Deformities and Extrinsic Impressions

Neighbouring organs, when enlarged, may cause indentations of the duodenal bulb and loop. For example the ventrocranial part of the duodenal bulb may be displaced by a dilated gallbladder, as may its dorsocranial wall by a dilated common hepatic bile duct.

A pancreatic head carcinoma will bulge into and deform the medial wall of the duodenum, both above and below the level of the ampulla. This may be severe enough to prevent the passage of an endoscope.

A ring-like deformity of the mid-part of the descending duodenum is sometimes seen in cases of annular pancreas, i.e. incomplete rotation of the ventral component, leaving either a strand of pancreatic cells or just a fibrotic ring behind. This congenital defect is in most instances an incidental finding.

An inherent weakness of the duodenal wall is caused by the passage of the pancreatic and biliary ducts through its muscular component. As a consequence juxta papillary diverticula may develop and are commonly found in elderly patients. These are often multiple and of various sizes. If large, they may interfere with pancreatic and biliary drainage causing pancreatitis and biliary obstruction, particularly if they are full of inspissated food material. However most are incidental findings.

The horizontal part of the duodenum may be narrowed by extrinsic vascular causes; posterior narrowing from an aneurysm of the abdominal aorta and anterior narrowing from a tight superior mesentery artery.

Bulky malignant lesions adjacent to the duodenum may deform and compress the lumen, such as a cholangiocarcinoma arising from the gallbladder or extensive nodal disease at the liver hilum and in the hepatoduodenal ligament.

3.9.2 Duodenitis

This starts as mild inflammation of the mucosa, evidenced by patchy areas of erythema on the top of the folds. With increasing severity the superficial mucosa is desquamated to form complete erosions, and small petechial bleeding may then be seen (Fig. 3.49). This is often accompanied by more vigorous peristalsis than would be expected. Duodenitis is regarded as a precursor to duodenal ulcer disease, although this is not confirmed.

Some patients, especially those on long-term renal dialysis, may have a chronic low-grade duodenitis characterised by a pale mucosa studded with nodules of various sizes.

3.9.3 Peptic Ulcer Disease

Helicobacter pylori infection is identified as the main causative factor for duodenal ulcer disease, although the process is definitely aggravated by smoking and drugs such as NSAIDs.

Half of all ulcers are located on the ventral wall of the duodenal bulb, and twin ulcers are seen in almost 15% of patients. These may be on opposite walls, so called "kissing ulcers". Duodenal bulb ulcers measure normally less than 10 mm across and 2 mm depth, but the sizes range from 5 to 25 mm in diameter and 1 to 3 mm in depth.

When many small and shallow ulcers are seen spread on a background of surrounding erythema, the condition is referred to as "salami ulcers" due to its resemblance of the cut surface of the eponymous sausage.

Chronic ulcer disease is marked by scar formation caused by the healing of earlier ulcers that have penetrated into the submucosa. If there is continuous ulcer disease it will result in progressive fibrosis of the duodenal cap, creating a so-called "clover leaf deformity" from pseudodiverticulum formation (Fig. 3.50). Severe fibrosis may lead to pyloric stenosis and cause gastric retention. With this background any new ulcer may then be irregular in shape.

Gastrinoma-induced ulcers have the same features as others but may be observed in the more distal duodenum.

Modern ulcer treatment with eradication of *Helicobacter pylori* and PPIs rapidly induces ulcer healing. This may partly explain the reduced incidence of duodenal ulcers seen today.

3.9.4 Ulcer Complications

Duodenal ulcers are subject to the same complications as gastric ulcers with the added problem of scar-induced gastric outlet obstruction. The major acute complications are bleeding and perforation, with bleeding often of a profuse nature due to the proximity of large arteries. However the endoscopic treatment options are the same as described for bleeding from gastric ulcers (see above).

3.9.5 Crohn's Disease

Crohn's disease is said to involve the duodenum in 0.5%–4% of patients who have evidence of this disease elsewhere. The early appearance is of erythema followed by discrete aphthoid erosions and small ulcers surrounded by normal mucosa. Cobble stone deformity with deep and branching crevices may occasionally be seen, and strictures are evident in advanced cases.

3.9.6 Gluten Enteropathy

In mild disease the mucosa of the duodenum and the small bowel may be totally normal. In those with advanced disease the mucosa shows signs of atrophy, and the submucosal vasculature is increasingly well seen subsequent to the loss of villous architecture. At this stage so-called "scalloping" of the folds of Kerckring may be evident. The surface pattern is made more obvious by submerging the mucosa in water, i.e. by immersion endoscopy. Chromo-endoscopy with indigo carmine more clearly reveals scalloping of folds as well as the coarse mosaic pattern of the surface pattern in untreated cases.

3.9.7 Intestinal Lymphangiectasia

Not infrequently, small white spots may be seen on the top of the villous folds which may ooze a milky fluid if biopsied. These result from stasis in the fine lymphatic vessels of the villi and are a rather common but nonspecific finding and of no great significance (Patel and DeRidder 1990). This condition is reported in patients with severe disorders, primarily those causing immunodeficiencies such as malignancy and AIDS.

3.9.8 Vascular Abnormalities

Vascular abnormalities in the duodenum are much the same as in other parts of the GIT. Hemangiomas are quite commonly seen, and the telangiectases in patients with Osler-Weber-Rendu disease have the same features as elsewhere in the body. Varices are seen in patients with portal hypertension and in those with advanced tumour growth obstructing the normal venous drainage.

Duodenal ischemia is a rare condition characterized by loss of the normal fold architecture together with erythema and necrotic discoloration. A history of a recent serious fall in blood pressure usually supports the diagnosis.

3.9.9 Benign Tumours

Duodenal polyps are often multiple and are of inflammatory, metaplastic, or neoplastic origin. Inflammatory polyps represent residual mucosal rests after prior erosive inflammation of the duodenum and have the same colour as the normal surround. They measure up to 2 mm in size and are located in the proximal duodenum and duodenal bulb.

Gastric metaplasia appears as a slightly elevated irregularity of the base of the duodenal bulb and consists of gastric body mucosa harbouring both parietal and goblet cells.

Lymphoid hyperplasia may be seen throughout the duodenum, more often in childhood and young adults.

Hyperplasia of Brunner's glands is classically seen in the bulb and descending duodenum in the elderly.

Adenomatous polyps are most often located around the papilla of Vater. They may be single or multiple, usually small and never obstructing (Fig. 3.51). The relationship to polyposis syndromes, above all FAP and Gardner's syndromes, is well established. In these patients multiple polyps are found in the second and third parts of the duodenum, and as adenomatous lesions are precursors to periampullary carcinoma, they should be followed up if not removed.

Villous adenomas are also found in the duodenum and appear as sessile, carpet-like lesions with an irregular and whitish surface. They may show substantial lateral spread (Fig. 3.52) and, taking into consideration their high risk for malignancy, this indicates that they are not suitable for endoscopic removal.

3.9.10 Malignant Tumours

Primary carcinoma of the duodenum is rarely seen. It usually presents late as a multilobulated exophytic growth, which bleeds easily from a necrotic surface. It may be circumferential and as a rule is confined to the periampullary region (Fig. 3.53).

Secondary involvement by direct extension of tumour is most commonly encountered from a carcinoma of the head of the pancreas. This distorts the duodenum, and the mucosa may become breached both above and below the ampulla. The papilla itself may become swollen and oedematous, particularly with an ampullary carcinoma, but this sign is also seen with a gallstone obstructing the distal common bile duct.

Duodenal lymphoma is usually contiguous with gastric lymphoma and shows the same endoscopic features. These include scattered and confluent polypoid protrusions, sessile ulcerated lesions, and submucosal spread. (Fig. 3.54)

Finally GISTs may be encountered in the duodenum and display the same smooth submucosal appearance as shown in the stomach.

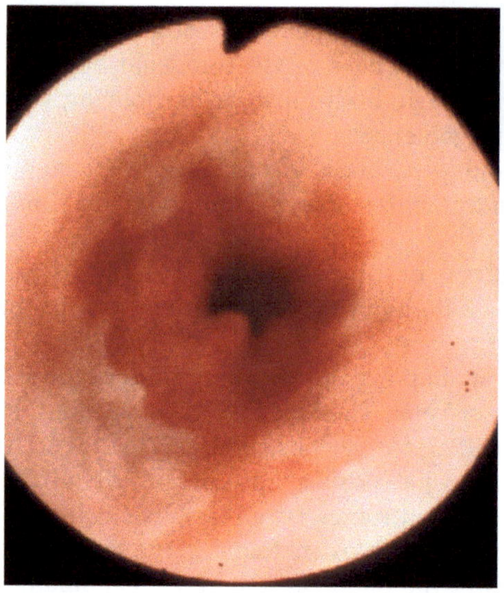

a

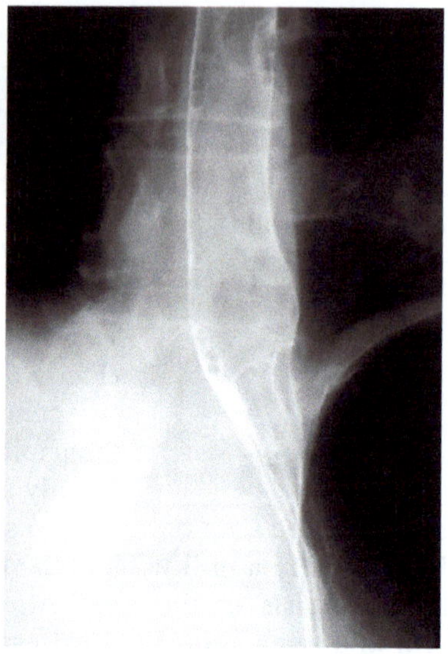

b

Fig. 3.1a,b. The normal oesophagogastric junction with a well demarcated Z-line as seen at endoscopy (**a**) and the equivalent radiographic view (**b**)

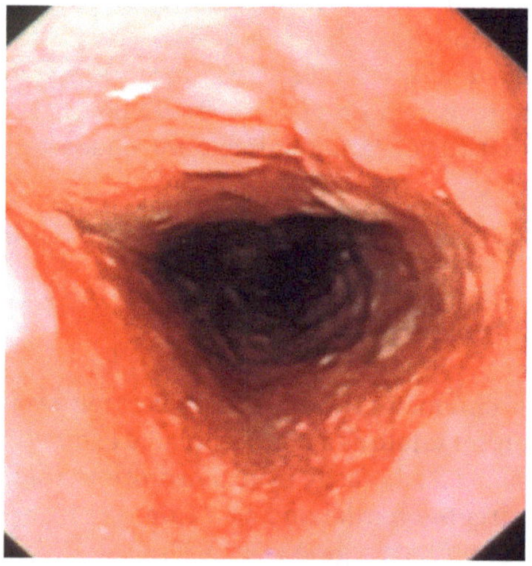

Fig. 3.2. Normal oesophagus with mucosal deposits of glycogen

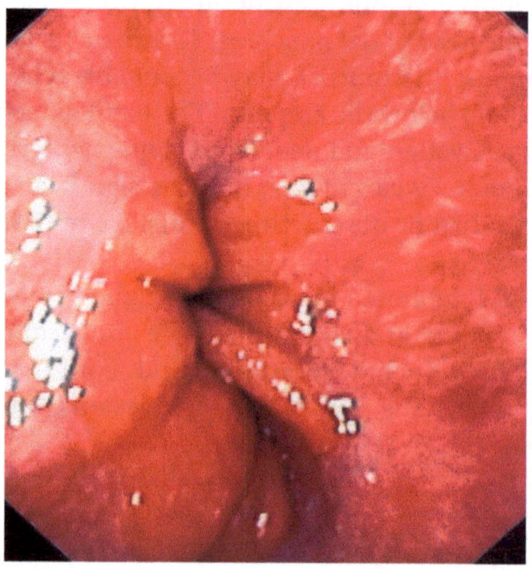

Fig. 3.3. Normal oesophagogastric junction in a young adult. Note the Z-line at the diaphragmatic inlet with a palisade-like vessel architecture above it

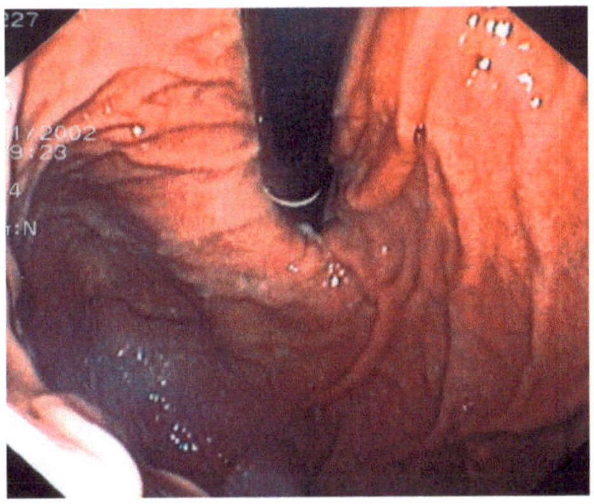

Fig. 3.4. Normal gastric fundus and body. The gastroscope is retroverted, demonstrating the instrument emerging through the gastric cardia

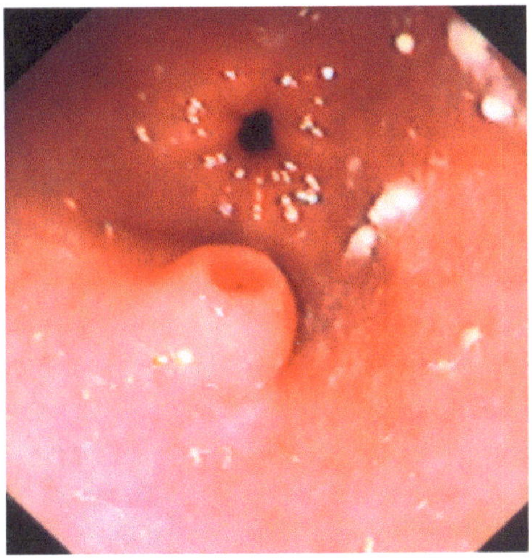

Fig. 3.5. The gastric antrum and pylorus. The small polypoid lesion with a central pit represents an aberrant pancreas or pancreatic rest

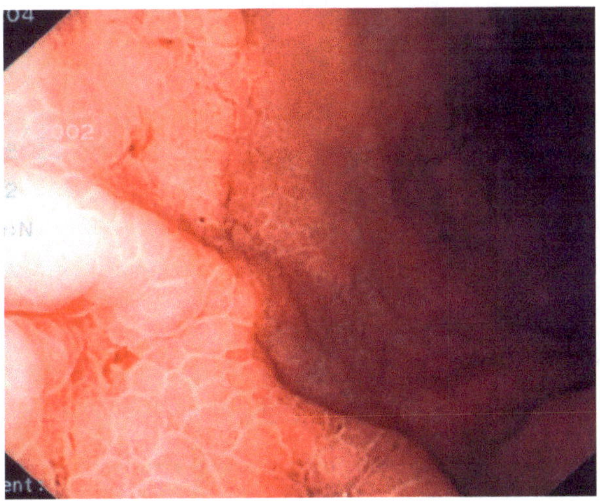

Fig. 3.6. Coarse area gastricae in a patient with chronic portal hypertension

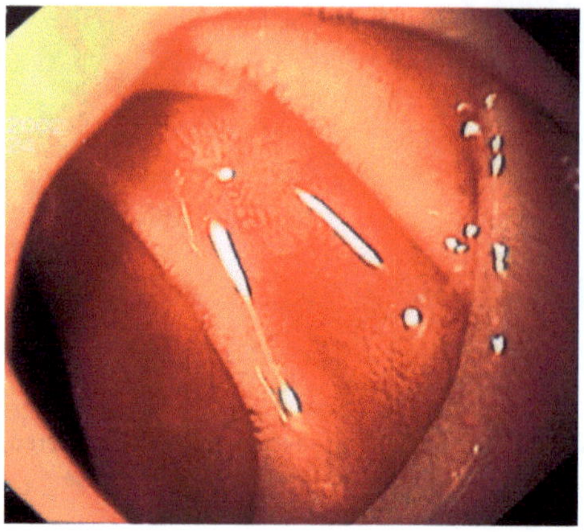

Fig. 3.7. Normal proximal small bowel mucosa demonstrating the folds of Kerckring

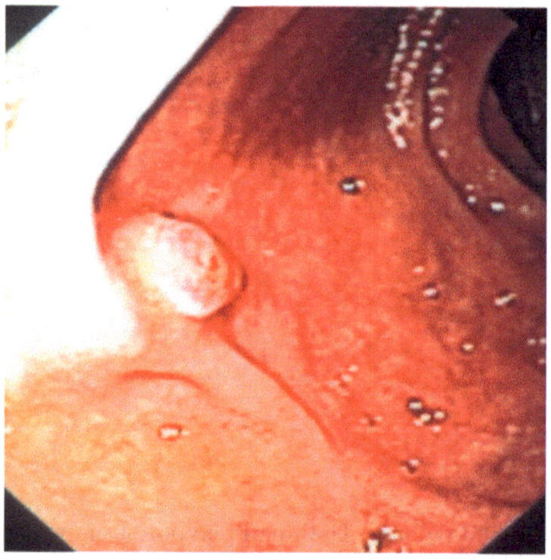

Fig. 3.8. Descending duodenum with the minor papilla

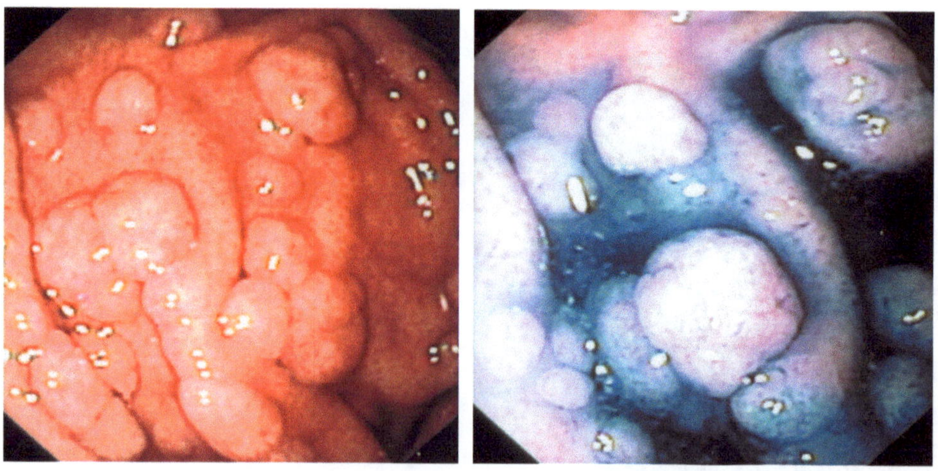

a b

Fig. 3.9a,b. Polypoid gastric mucosa which was confirmed as foveolar hyperplasia at microscopy. Note that the surrounding mucosa looks the same before (**a**) and after carmine dye staining (**b**)

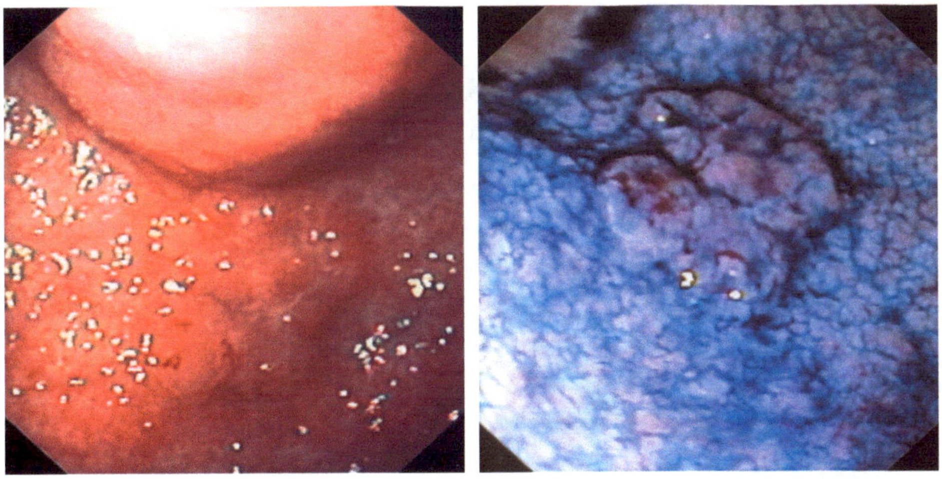

a b

Fig. 3.10a,b. A subtle small, ill defined structural change of the gastric mucosa (**a**), which becomes more evident following chromogastroscopy with indigo carmine (**b**). This proved to be a histologically advanced neoplasm

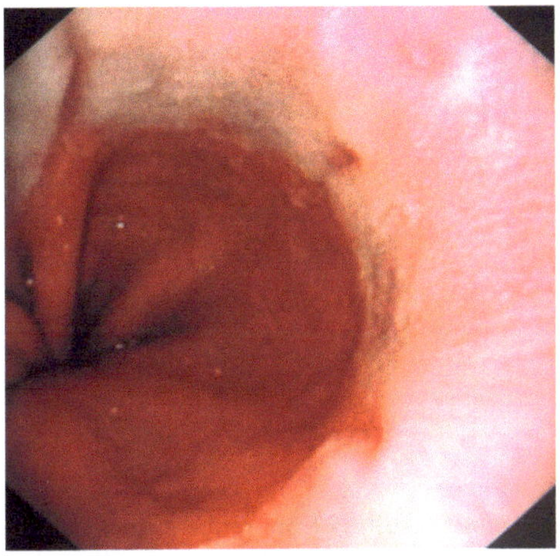

Fig. 3.11. Reflux oesophagitis with small and separate erosions, grade 1. Note the aboral location of the Z-line, which is likely to indicate short segment Barrett's oesophagus

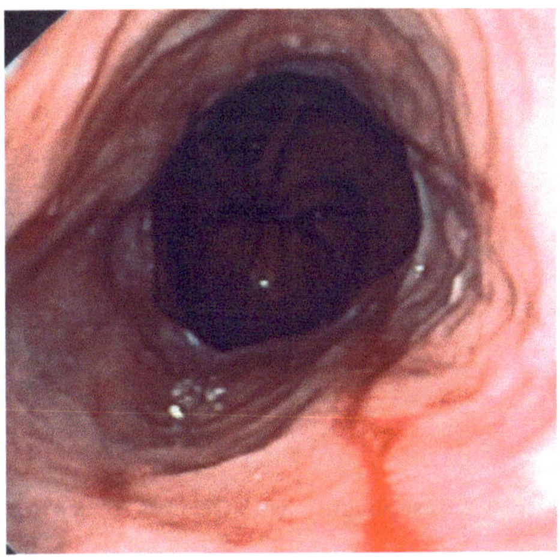

Fig. 3.12. Reflux oesophagitis with long erosions and scar formation indicating longstanding GORD

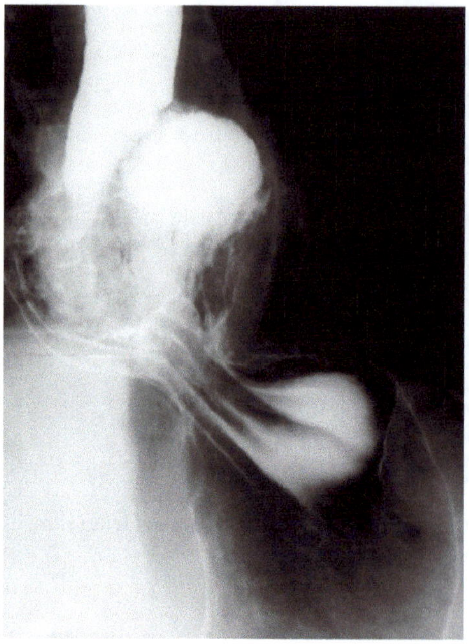

a

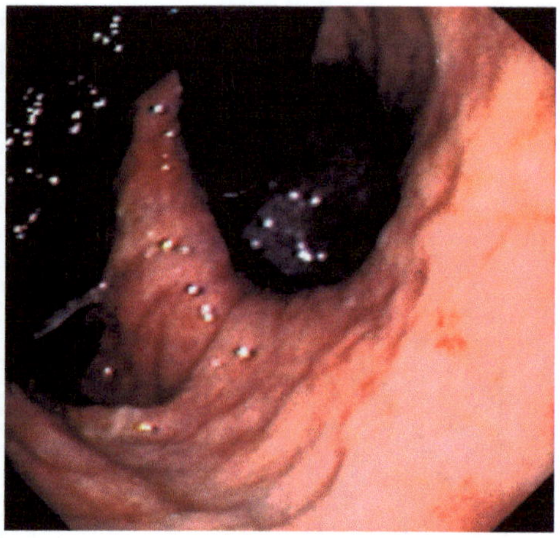

b

Fig. 3.13a,b. Large combined-type hiatus hernia with a significant rolling element as shown on a barium meal (**a**) Although its presence is appreciated at endoscopy by retroverting the endoscope (**b**), its actual size is better appreciated on the barium study

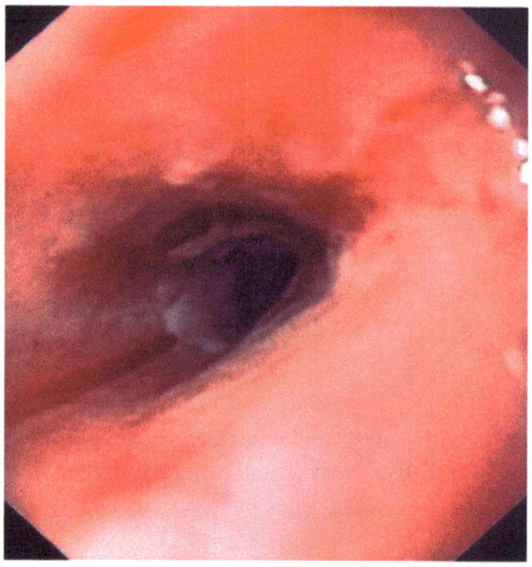

Fig. 3.14. A long segment stenosis resulting from reflux oesophagitis as viewed from above. The submucosal spot bleeding sites were secondary to the passage of an obstructing bolus

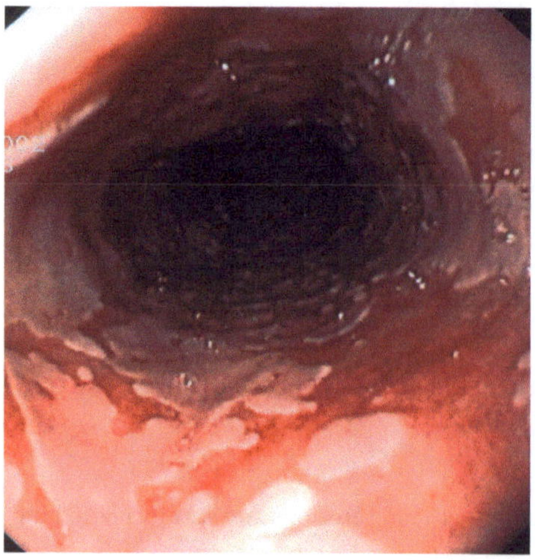

Fig. 3.15. Widespread Barrett's oesophagitis with islands of normal oesophageal mucosa

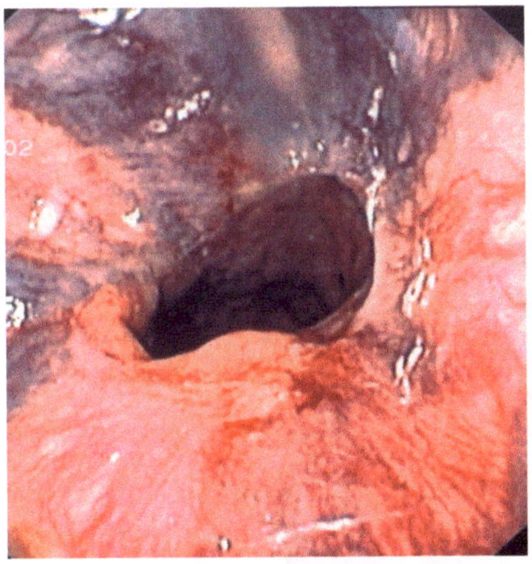
a

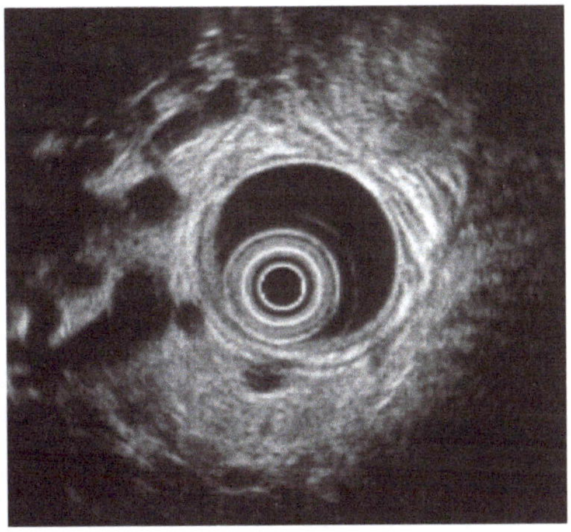
b

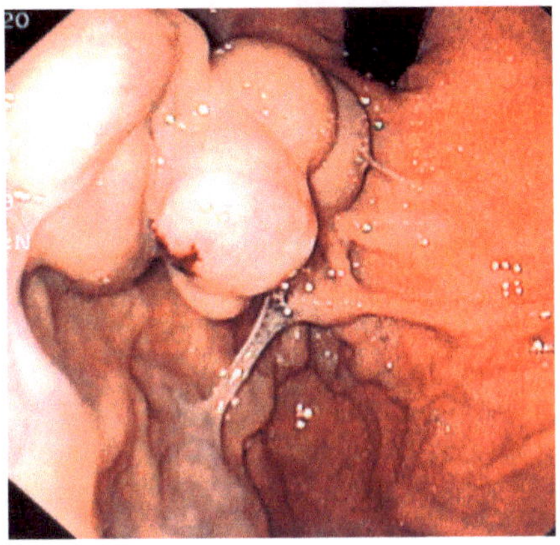
c

Fig. 3.16a–c Oesophageal varices. Note the purple dark oesophageal varices, almost confluent at the diaphragmatic inlet (**a**) Endoscopic ultrasound shows tortuous veins extending from deep peri-oesophageal structures (**b**) Fundic varices are also present in this patient (**c**). Note the small bleeding spot

Fig. 3.17a–c. Small polypoid lesion in the distal third of the oesophagus (**a**). Following chromo-endoscopy with methylene blue, numerous tiny satellite lesions were revealed (**b**). Endoscopic ultrasound showed thickened mucosal layers with slight irregularity of the superficial one-third of the submucosa (**c**). Histology revealed a carcinoma extending into the submucosa

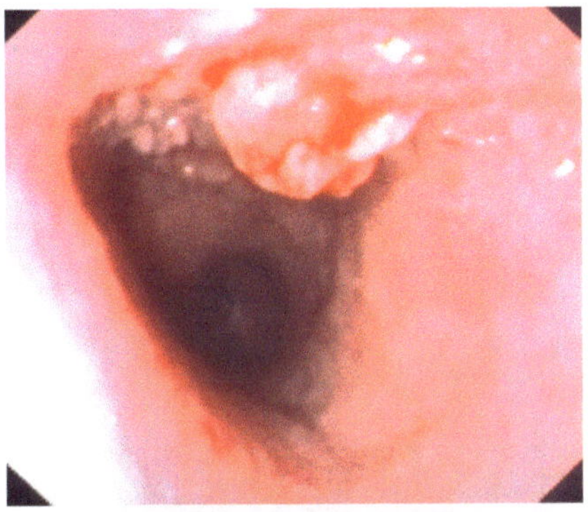
a

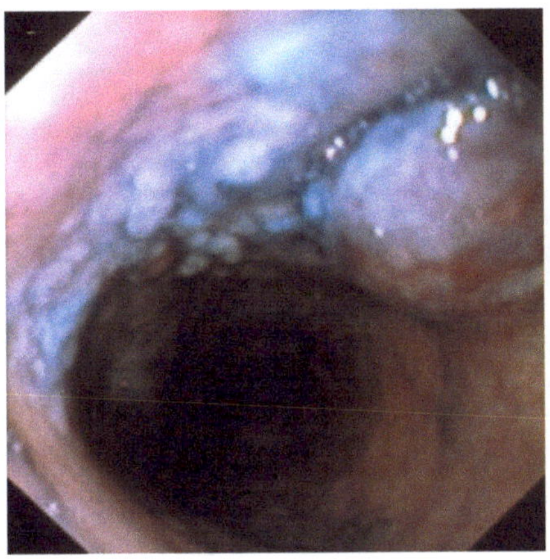
b

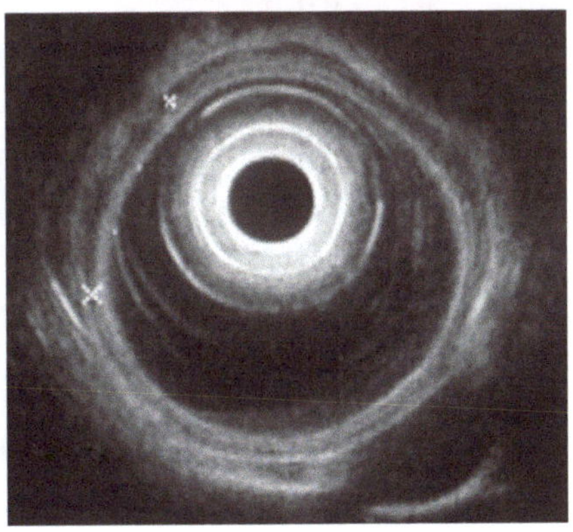
c

a b c

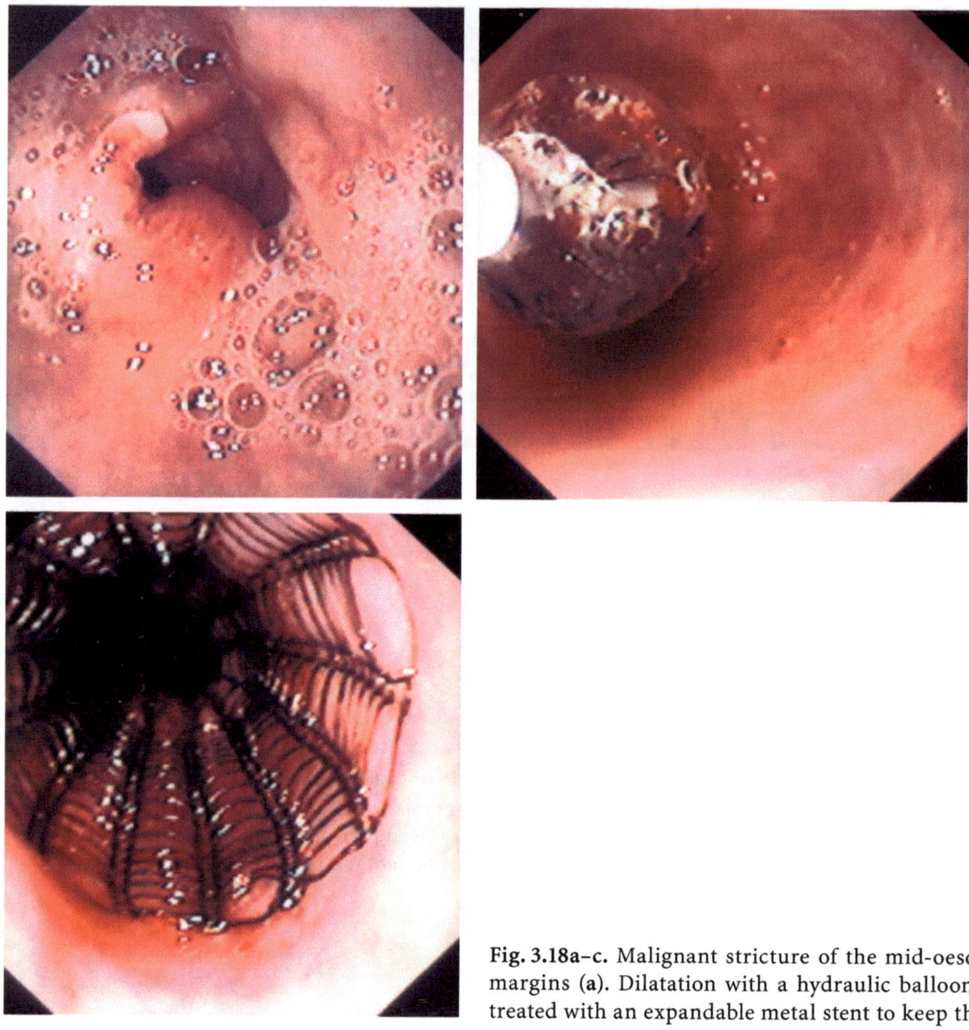

Fig. 3.18a–c. Malignant stricture of the mid-oesophagus with irregular margins (**a**). Dilatation with a hydraulic balloon (**b**), and permanently treated with an expandable metal stent to keep the lumen patent (**c**)

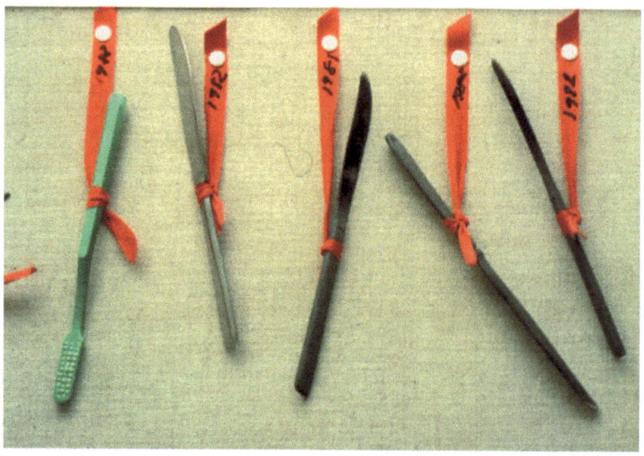

Fig. 3.19. Foreign bodies removed by endoscopy in our Endoscopy Unit. These include knives and a tooth brush

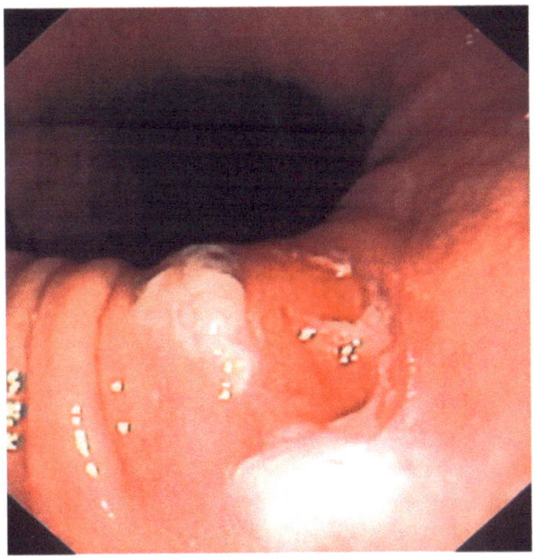

Fig. 3.20. A “Cameron ulcer”. A moderately large shallow ulcer within a hiatus hernia and just beyond the Z-line

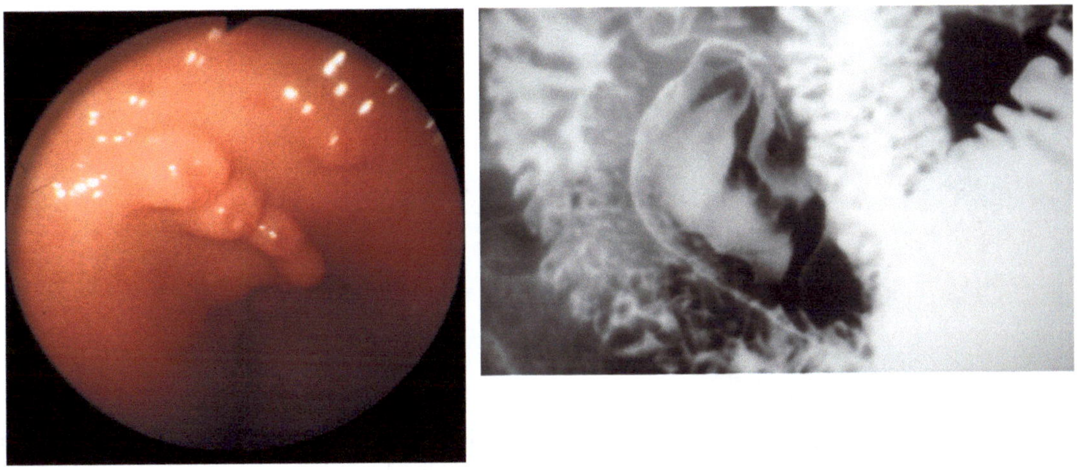

a

b

Fig. 3.21 a,b. Chronic antral gastritis with several rows of erosions converging towards the pylorus (**a**), also shown on the double-contrast barium meal (**b**)

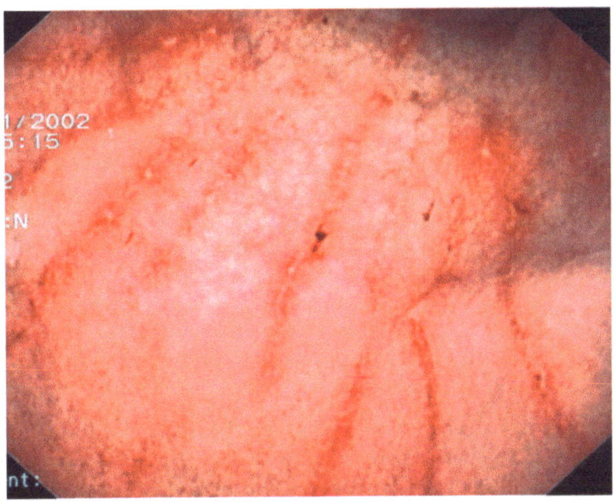

Fig. 3.22. Superficial and elongated erosions with spot bleedings. These are typical appearances seen secondary to NSAID medication

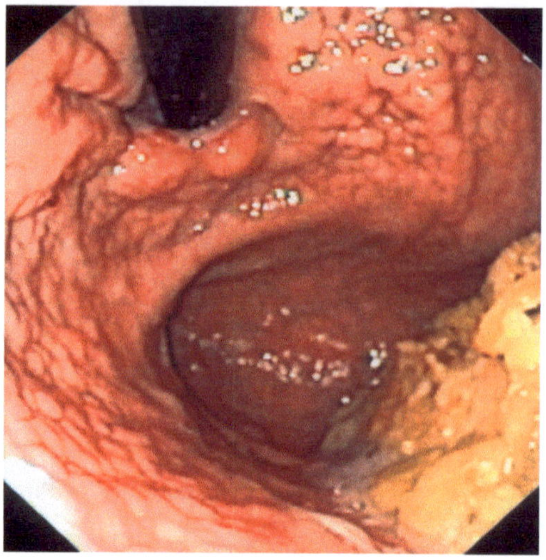

Fig. 3.23. Prominent and thickened gastric mucosa secondary to *Helicobacter pylori* infection. This view is of the fundus and proximal body. Note some gastric residue

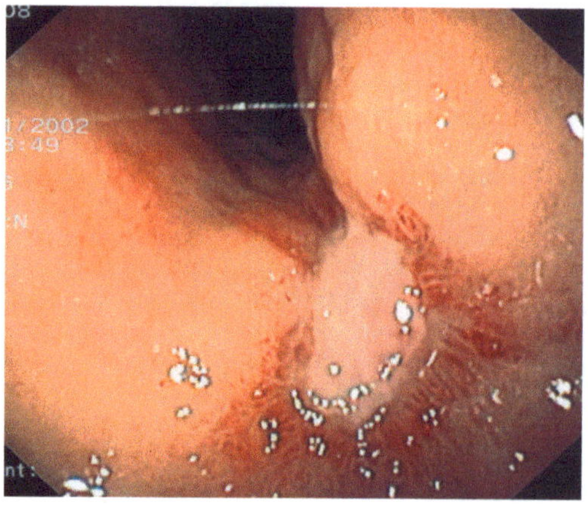

Fig. 3.24. Benign ulcer at the incisura angularis, demarcated by a hyperaemic, healing mucosa

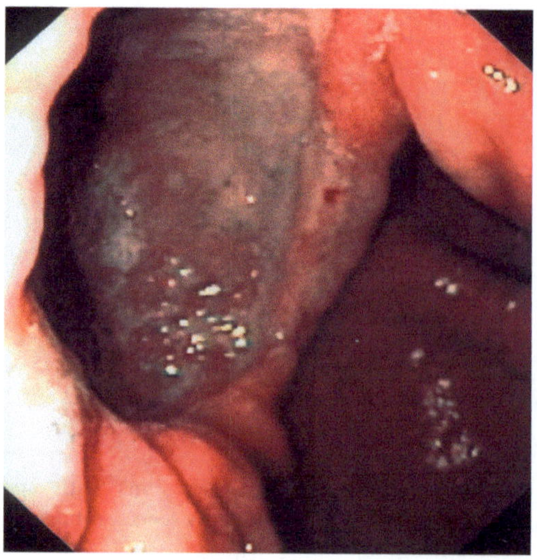

Fig. 3.25. An antral ulcer with a necrotic ulcer base and bleeding spots at the ulcer rim. The patient presented with iron-deficiency anaemia and was *Helicobacter pylori*-positive

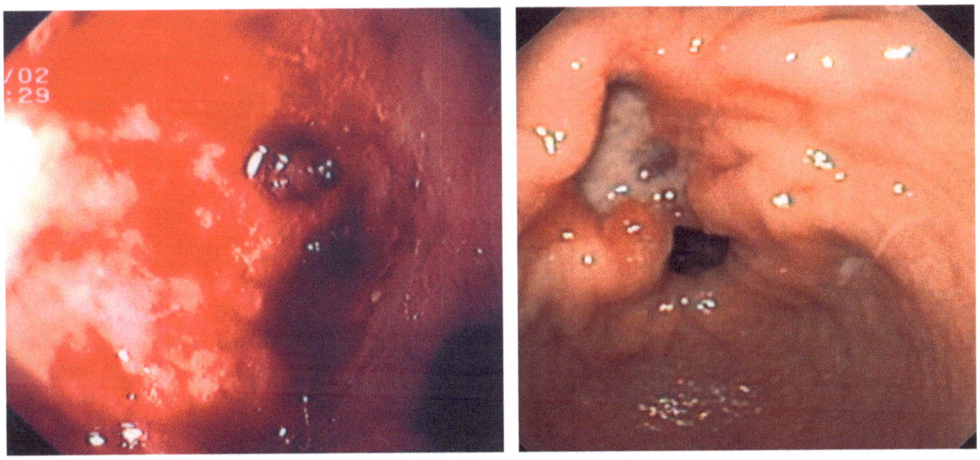

a b

Fig. 3.26a,b. Bleeding pre-pyloric ulcer with a shiny, visible vessel (**a**). The same ulcer in a final healing stage with convergence of folds and slight displacement of the pylorus (**b**)

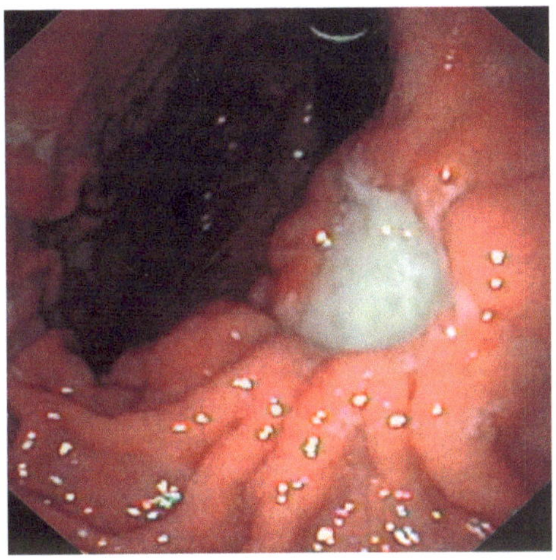

Fig. 3.27. A large 15-mm ulcer at the incisura angularis. Note that the folds are converging towards the ulcer with no mucosal discoloration or change of structure, indicating benign disease

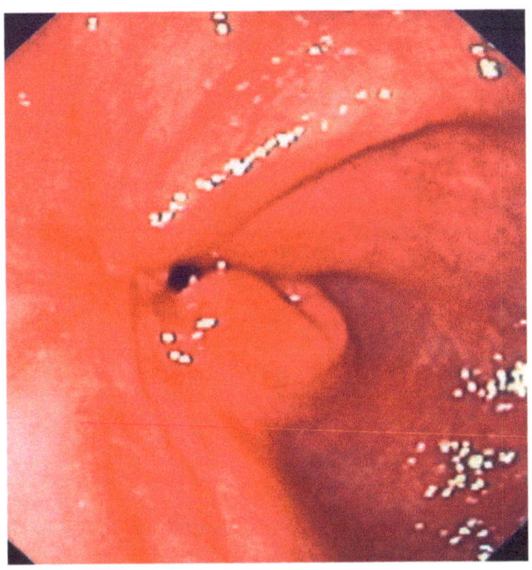

Fig. 3.28. Chronic antral ulcer with scar formation and narrowing of the pylorus, slightly displaced

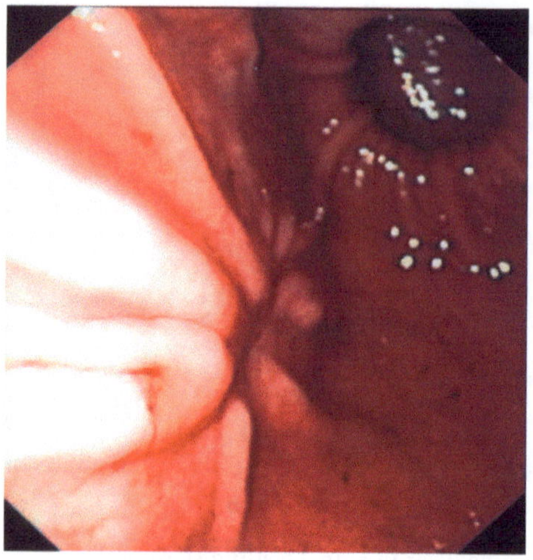

Fig. 3.29. A problem gastric ulcer. Initial biopsies were benign, and the benign part of the ulcer is healing with folds converging and clubbing close to the elongated ulcer scar. A new set of biopsies at this stage revealed an EGC. The explanation is that whilst the benign part of the ulcer heals, the malignant one increases in relative size, and is therefore easier to catch with the biopsy forceps

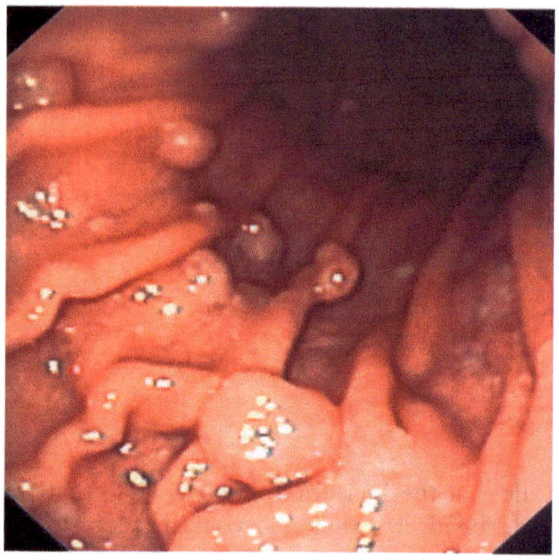

Fig. 3.30. Metaplastic gastric polyps, which as here usually present in large numbers

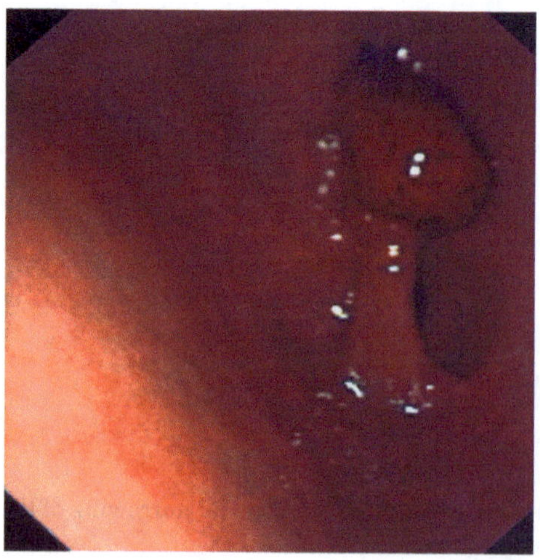

Fig. 3.31. An adenomatous polyp with a stalk, situated in the gastric antrum

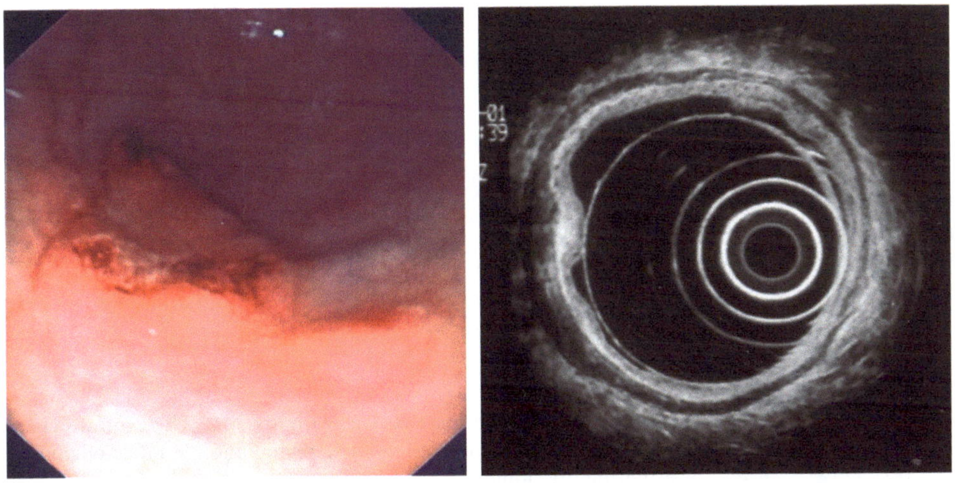

a b

Fig. 3.32a,b. A tubulovillous adenoma shown as a small elevated and irregular antral lesion with a superficial bleed (**a**). A 20-MHz endoscopic ultrasound showed thickening of the mucosal layers (**b**). Histology revealed a tubulovillous adenoma with severe dysplasia

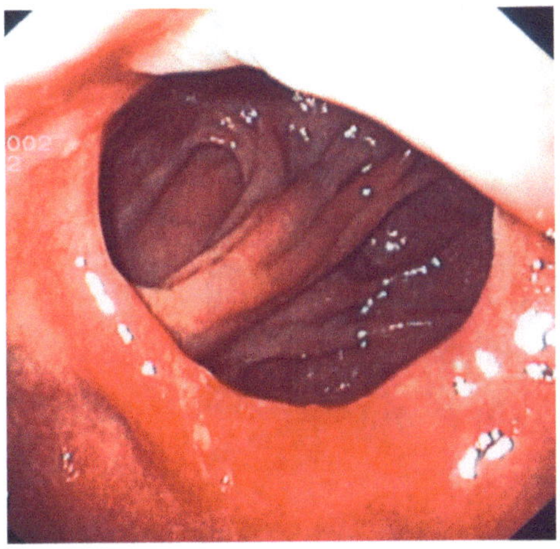

Fig. 3.33. A normal anastomosis following a Billroth II gastrectomy as seen from above. Note the typical fold architecture of the afferent and efferent jejunal loops

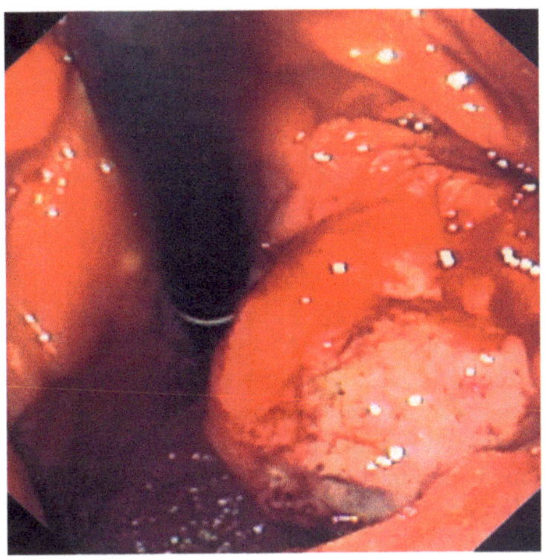

Fig. 3.34. A B-II stromal carcinoma demonstrated by retroverting the endoscope in the stoma

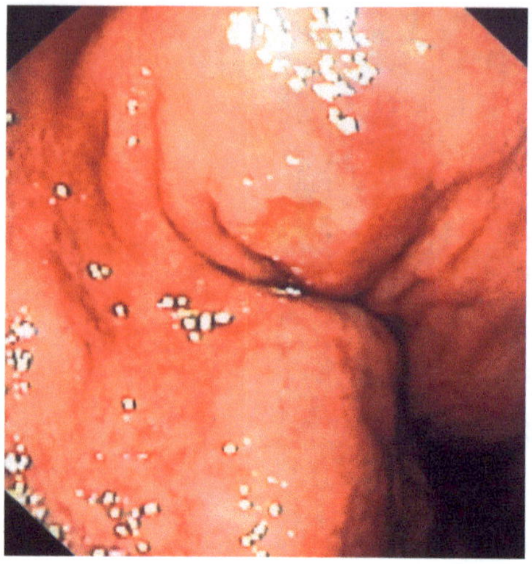

Fig. 3.35. A 65-year-old male patient with an EGC. The central depression, a sign that may indicate an early malignancy, is made obvious by desufflating the stomach

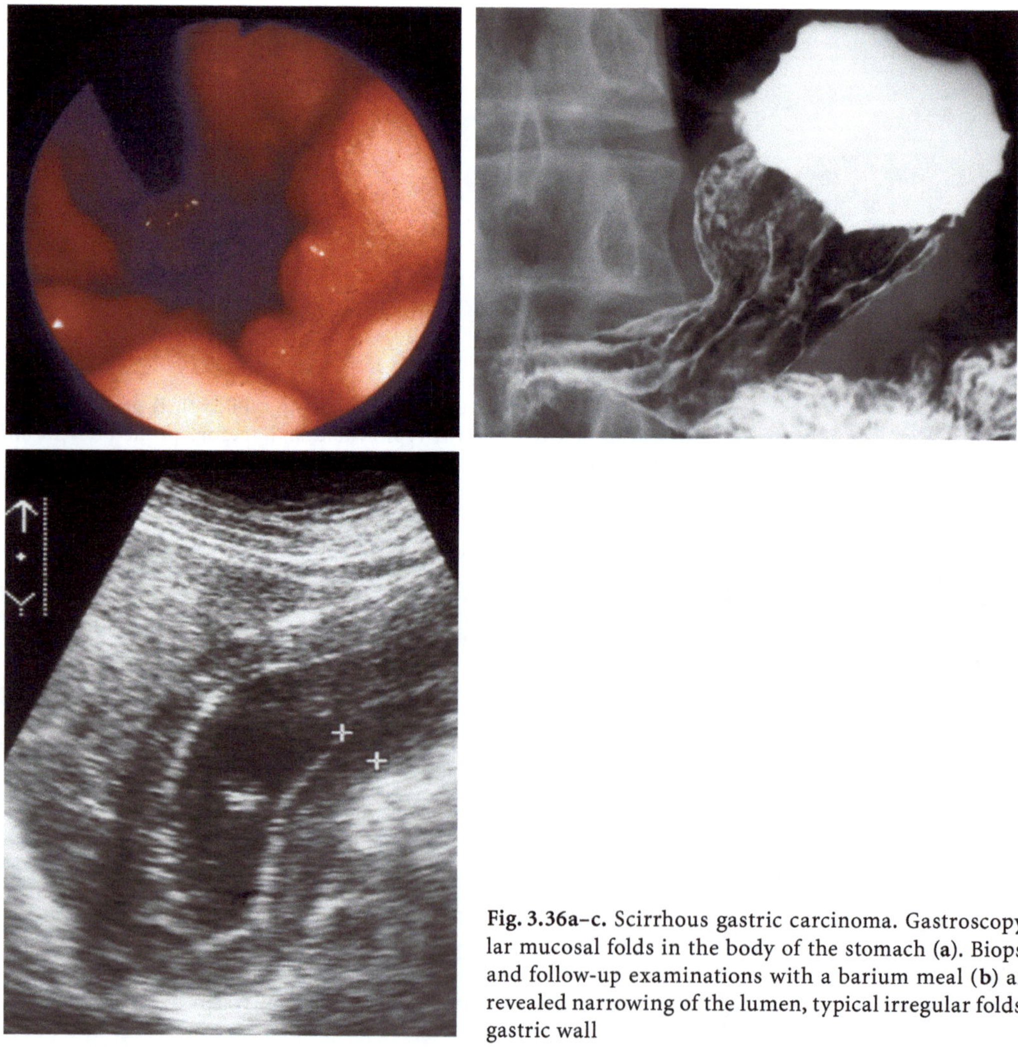

a b c

Fig. 3.36a–c. Scirrhous gastric carcinoma. Gastroscopy revealed irregular mucosal folds in the body of the stomach (**a**). Biopsies were negative and follow-up examinations with a barium meal (**b**) and ultrasound (**c**) revealed narrowing of the lumen, typical irregular folds, and a thickened gastric wall

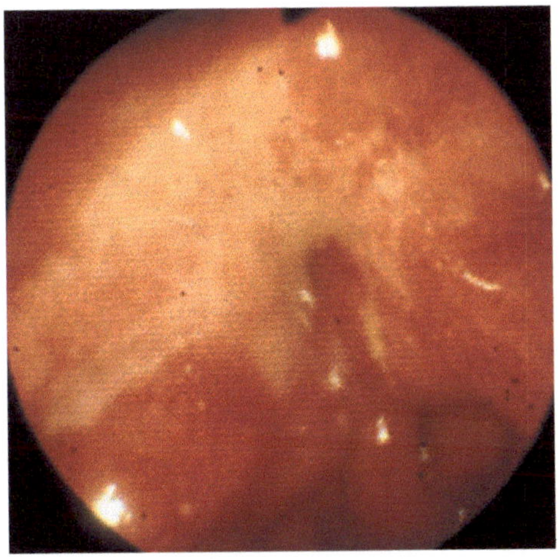

Fig. 3.37. A discoloured and small superficial antral carcinoma with a slightly depressed, irregular surface. Histology however revealed infiltration through the submucosa

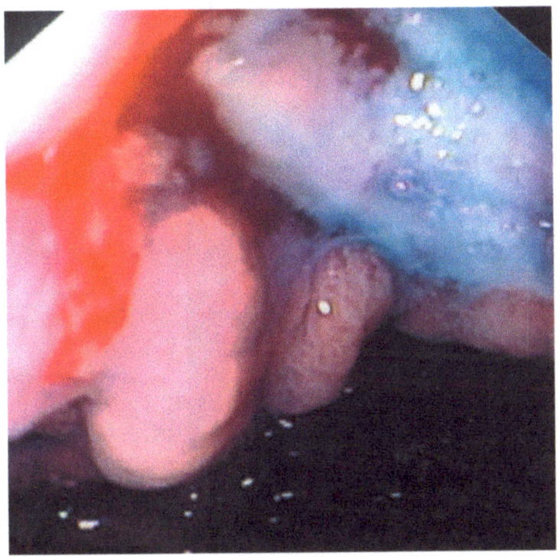

Fig. 3.38. Chromo-endoscopy of a malignant ulcer at the gastric body. Note the thick folds ending at a short distance from the ulcer edge with irregular mucosa in between. Some minimal bleeding is present

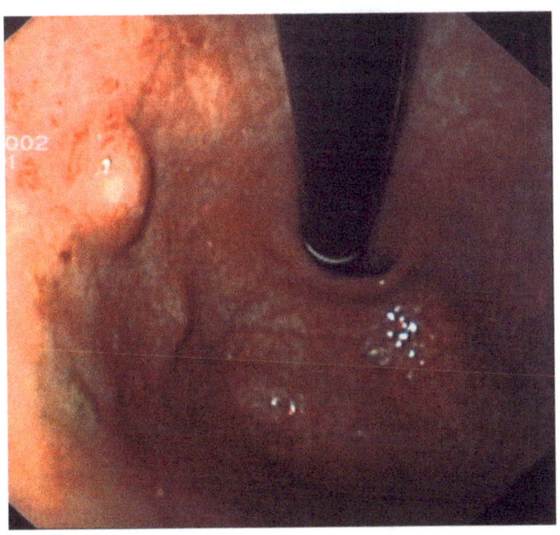

Fig. 3.39. Non-Hodgkin MALT lymphoma as demonstrated by a polypoid lesion in the gastric body

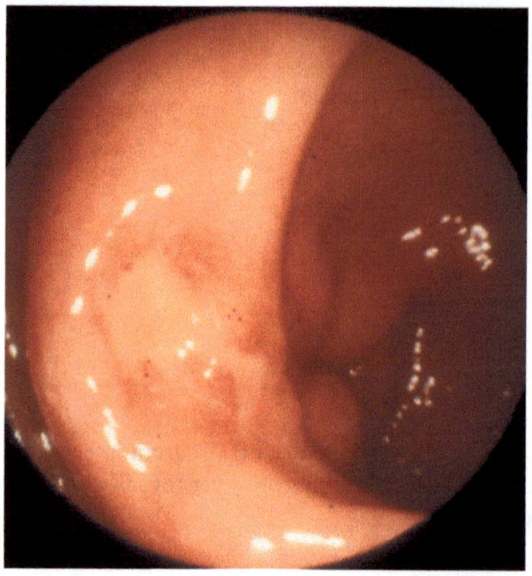

Fig. 3.40. Depressed ulcers in the gastric body with a dendritic interconnection in primary gastric lymphoma

a

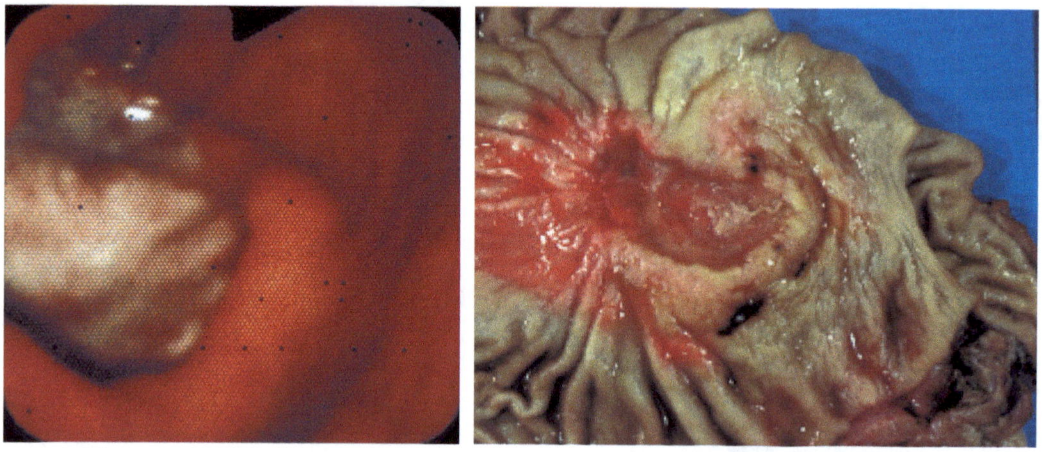

b

Fig. 3.41a,b. An old case with an operated giant ulcer that turned out to represent a primary gastric lymphoma. Gastroscopy demonstrates the so called "volcano crater" (a) confirmed on the surgical specimen (b)

a

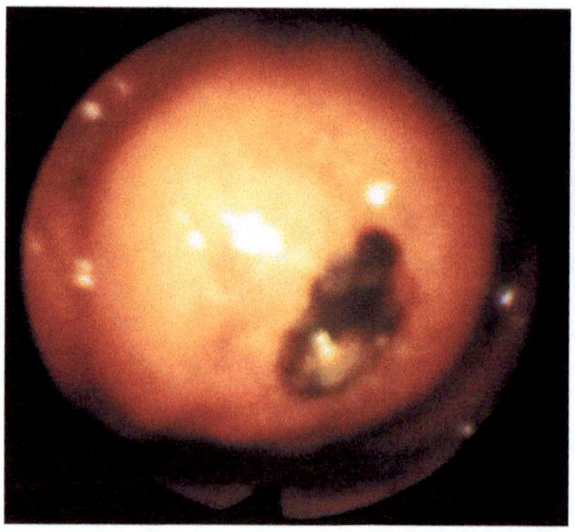

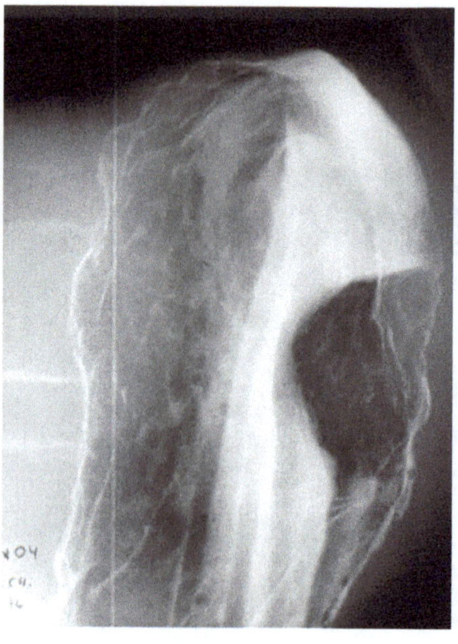

b

Fig. 3.42a,b. A 25-mm leiomyoma with an ulcer containing old blood clot (a). The location and tumour size are obvious on the barium meal (b)

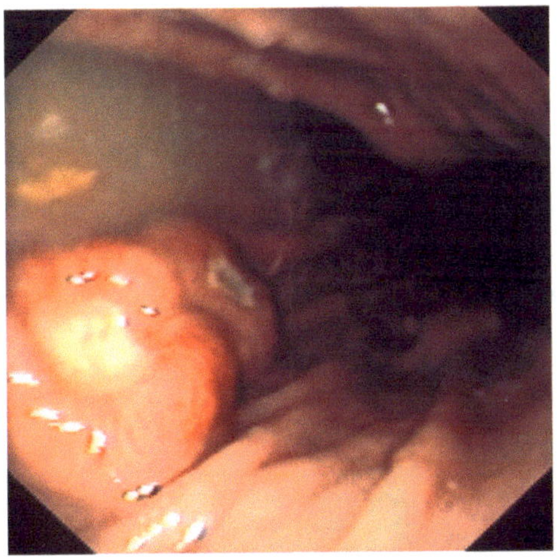

Fig. 3.43. Metastases of a neuro-endocrine carcinoma to the gastric body. Note the "bulls eye"-type lesions which are similar to nonpigmented melanoma deposits

a 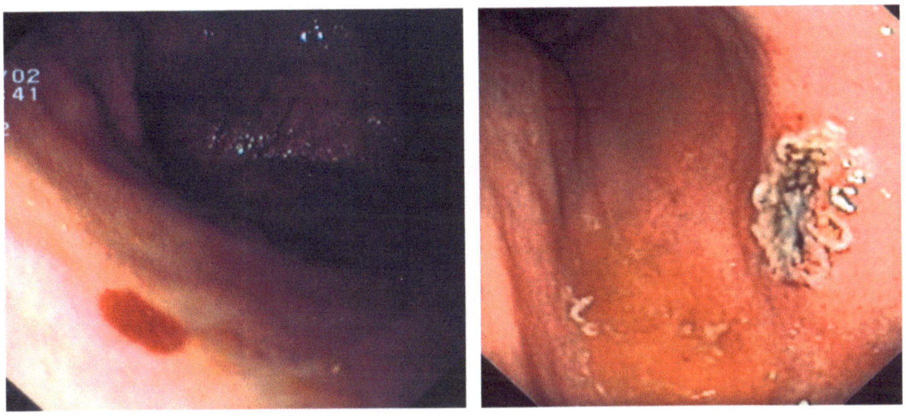 b

Fig. 3.44a,b. Gastric haemangioma shown as a typically well defined, bright red 4-mm lesion (**a**). The same lesion was coagulated with argon plasma beam (**b**)

a 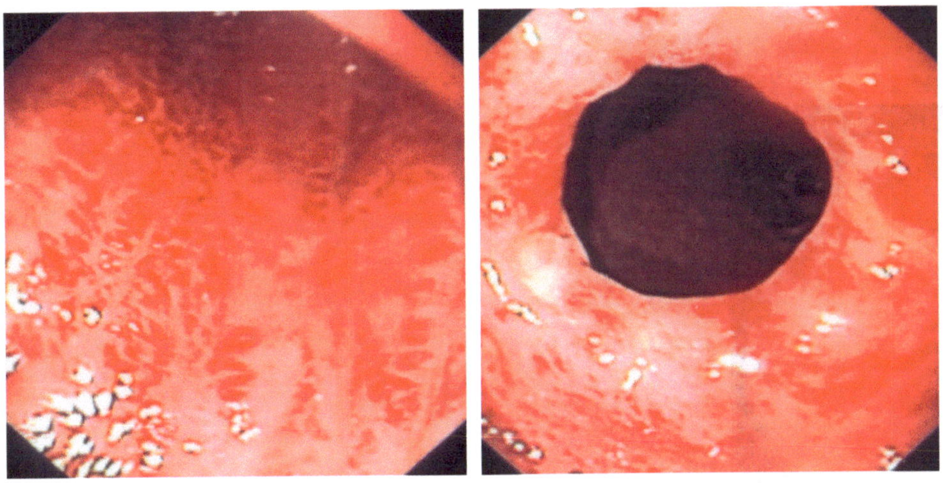 b

Fig. 3.45a,b. Gastric antral vascular ectasia, GAVE, or watermelon stomach as demonstrated by tortuous and widened vessels in the distal body (**a**) Pre-pyloric view of the same case (**b**)

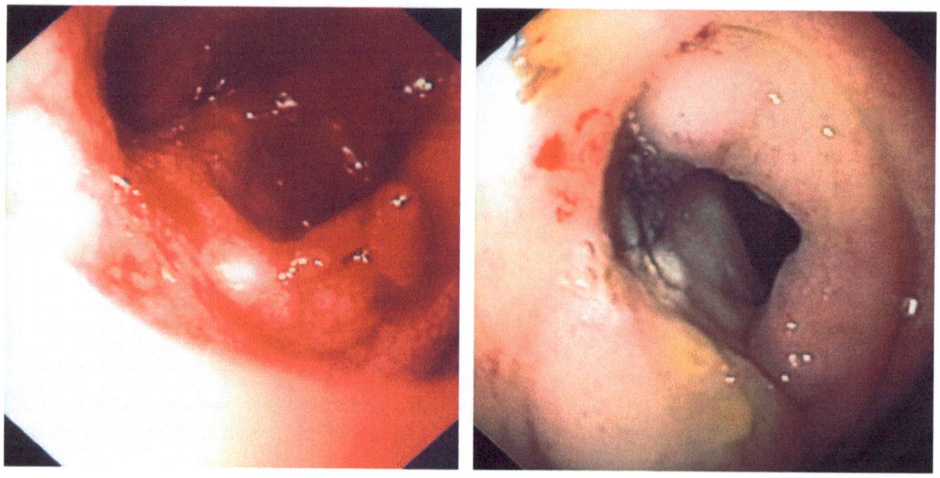

a b

Fig. 3.46a,b. A pulsating bright red bleeding source identified in the duodenal cap at 3 o'clock, (**a**). After injection treatment with 10 ml of dilute adrenalin in multiple aliquots around the ulcer, bleeding ceases, as the mucosa blanches and turns oedematous (**b**)

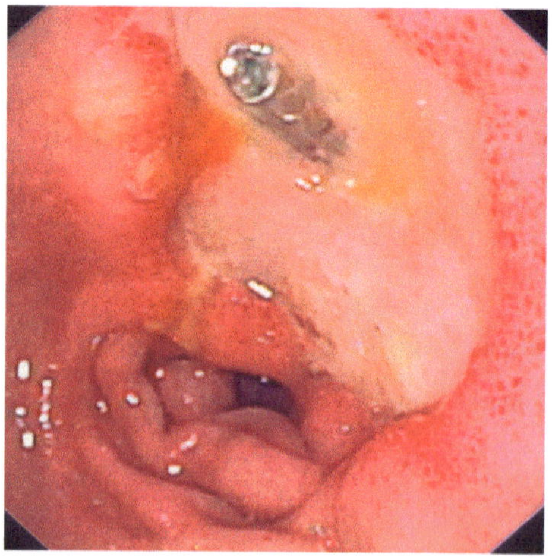

Fig. 3.47. Benign gastric ulcer. The earlier bleeding has been treated with a metallic clip

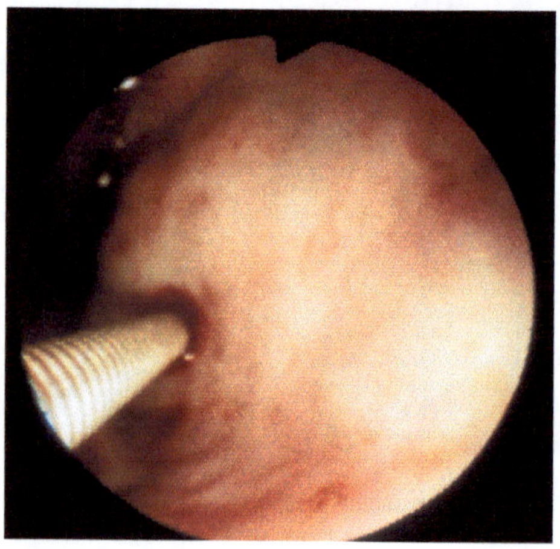

Fig. 3.48. Injection treatment of oesophageal varices. The local swelling causes a tamponade

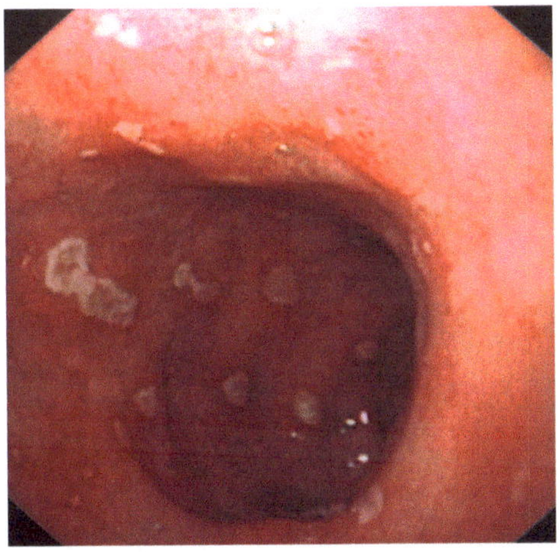

Fig. 3.49. Widespread erosive duodenitis associated with NSAID medication

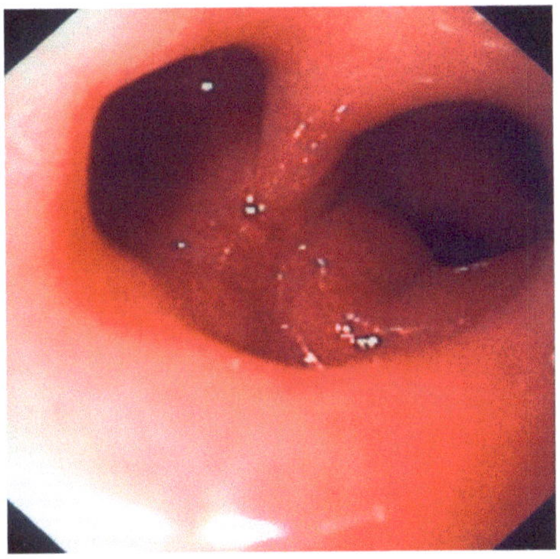

Fig. 3.50. A deformed duodenal cap with pseudodiverticulum and a small ulcer. A little bleeding is present

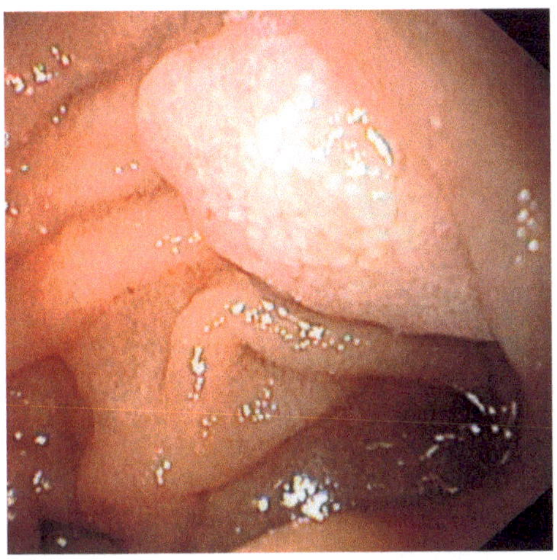

Fig. 3.51. Tubular adenoma in the duodenum as demonstrated by a pale well-defined lesion

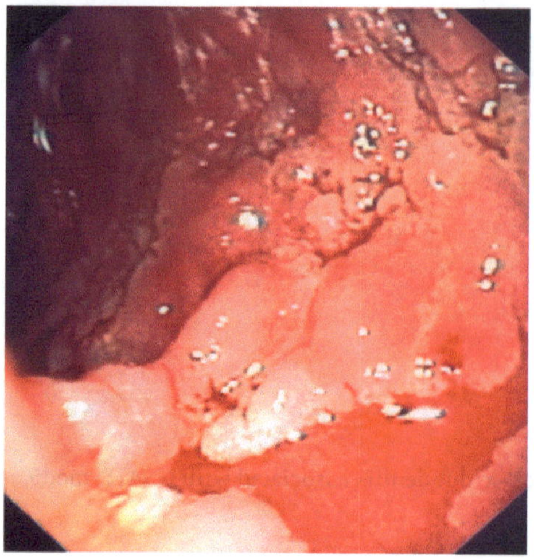

Fig. 3.52. Extensive tubulovillous adenoma in the descending duodenum. Note the considerable lateral spread

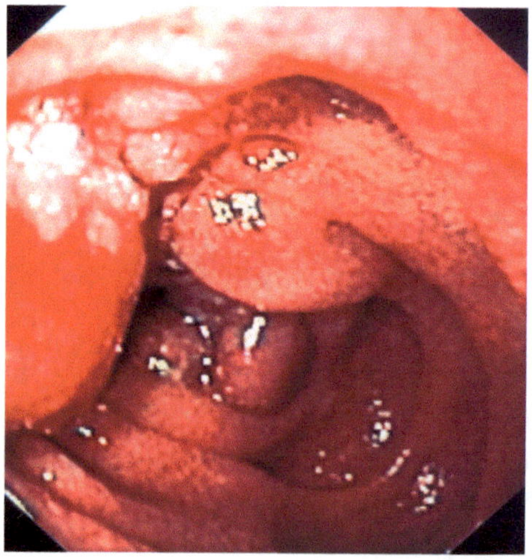

Fig. 3.53. A bleeding adenocarcinoma obstructing the duodenal lumen

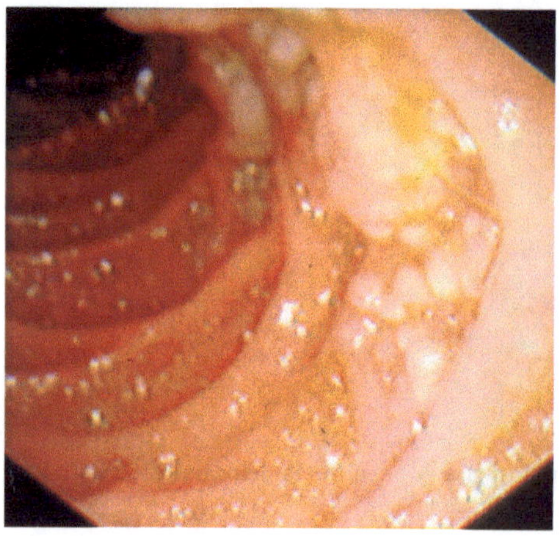

Fig. 3.54. Lymphoma of the duodenum demonstrated by confluent polypoidal protrusions and submucosal spread

References

Aisenberg J, Cohen L, Lewis BS (1991) Marked endoscopic gastrostomy tubes permit one-pass Ponsky-technique. Gastrointest Endosc 37:552–553

Blaser MJ (1999) Hypothesis: The changing relationships of *Helicobacter pylori* and humans: implications for health and disease. J Infect Dis 179:1523–30

Ciociola AA, McSorley DJ, Turner K et al (1999) *Helicobacter pylori* infection rates in duodenal ulcer patients in the United States may be lower than previously estimated. Am J Gastroenterol 94:1834–1840

Cohne H, Rose S, Lewin DN et al (1999) Accuracy of four commercial available serologic tests, including two office-based tests and commercially available 13C urea breath test for diagnosis of *Helicobacter pylori*. Helicobacter 4:49–53

Fork F-T, Ekberg O, Haglund U (1984) Radiology in primary gastric lymphoma. Acta Radiol. Diagn 25:481–488

Fork F-T, Haglund U, Högström H, Wehlin L (1985) Primary gastric lymphoma versus gastric cancer. An endoscopic and radiographic study of differential diagnostic possibilities. Endoscopy 17:5–7

Forrest JAH, Finlayson NDC, Shearman DJC (1976) Endoscopy of upper gastrointestinal bleeding. Lancet 85–87

Fraser AG, Schreuder V, Chua LE, Moore L (1998) Follow-up after successful eradication of *Helicobacter pylori*: symptoms and reinfection. J Gastroenterol Hepatol 13:555–559

Gispert JP, Pajares JM, Garcia-Valriberas R et al (1998) Recurrence of *Helicobacter pylori* infection after eradication: incidence and variables influencing it. Scand J Gastroenterol 33:1144–1151

Grant JP (1993) Percutaneous endoscopic gastrostomy. Initial placement by single endoscopic technique and long-term follow-up. Ann Surg 217:168–167

Gur G, Boyacioglu S, Demirhan B et al (1998) The importance of increasing the number of gastric biopsies in the diagnosis of *Helicobacter pylori*. Hepatogastroenterology 45:2219–2223

Hasselgren G, Carlsson J, Lind T et al (1998) Risk factors for rebleeding and fatal outcome in elderly patients with acute peptic ulcer bleeding. Eur J Gastroenterol Hepatol 10:667–672

Hasselgren G, Lind T, Lundell L et al (1997) Continuous intravenous infusion of omeprazole in elderly patients with peptic ulcer bleeding. Scand J Gastroenterol 32:328–333

Hogan RB, Demarro DC, Hamilton JK et al (1986) Percutaneous endoscopic gastrostomy: To push or to pull: a prospective randomized trial. Gastrointest Endosc 32:253–258

Hui WM, Ng MMT, Lok ASF et al (1991) A randomized comparative study of laser photocoagulation, heater probe, and bipolar electrocoagulation in the treatment of actively bleeding ulcers. Gastrointest Endosc 7:29–304

Johnston JH, Jensen DM, Auth D (1987) Experimental comparison of endoscopic YAG laser, electrosurgery, and heater probe for canine gut arterial coagulation: importance of compression and avoidance of erosion. Gastroenterol 92:1101–1108

Kozarec RA, Ball TJ, Patterson DJ (1986) Prophylactic antibiotics in percutaneous endoscopic gastrostomy (PEG): need or nuisance. Gastrointest Endosc 32:147–148

Kubba KA, Murphy W, Palmer KR (1996) Endoscopic injection for bleeding peptic ulcer: a comparison of epinephrine alone with epinephrine plus human thrombin. Gastroenterol 111:623–628

Laine L, Peterson W (1994) Bleeding peptic ulcer. N Engl J Med 331:717–727

Lau JYW, Chung SS (2000) Practical management of non-variceal upper gastrointestinal bleeding. In: *Practice of therapeutic Endoscopy*. Eds: GNJ Tytgat, M Classen, JD Way and S Nakazawa. 2nd ed., pp 1–11, WB Saunders 2000.

Lau JYW, Sung JJY, Chan ACW et al (1997) Stigmata of haemorrhage in bleeding peptic ulcers: an inter-observer agreement study among international experts. Gastrointest Endosc 46:33–36

Lee KJ, Kim JH, Hahm KB et al (2000) Randomized trial of N-Butyl-2-Cyanoacrylate compared with injection of hypertonic saline-epinephrine in endoscopic treatment of bleeding peptic ulcers. Endoscopy 32:505–511

Lin CK, Lai KH, Lo GH et al (1996) The value of second-look endoscopy after endoscopic injection therapy for bleeding peptic ulcer. Gastroenterology 110:A-117

Lind T, Mégraud F, Unge P et al (1999) The MACH2 study: role of omeprazole in eradication of *Helicobacter pylori* with 1-week triple therapies. Gastroenterology 116:248–253

Lundell L, Dent J, Bennett JR et al (1999) Endoscopic assessment of oesophagitis: clinical and functional correlates and further validation of the Los Angeles classification. Gut 45:172–180

Macri G, Milani S, Surrenti E et al (1998) Eradication of *Helicobacter pylori* reduces the rate of duodenal ulcer rebleeding: a long term follow-up study. Am J Gastroenterol 93:925–927

Mathus-Vliegen EMH (2000) Gastrostomy and enterostomy. In: *Practice of Therapeutic Endoscopy*, 2nd ed., eds.: NGJ Tytgat et al., 16:277–300, WB Saunders

Mendis RE, Gerdes H, Lightdale CJ, Botet JF (1994) Large gastric folds: a diagnostic approach using endoscopic ultrasonography. Gastrointest Endosc 4:437–441

Messmann H, Schaller P, Gross V et al (1996) Can an early second-look endoscopy reduce recurrent bleeding of gastric or duodenal ulcers? Gastrointest Endosc 43:A-354

Norton B, Homer-Ward M, Donnelly MT et al (1996) A randomised prospective comparison of percutaneous endoscopic gastrostomy and nasogastric tube feeding after acute dysphagic stroke. Br Med J 312:13–16

Park RHR, Allison MC, Lang J et al (1992) Randomised comparison of percutaneous endoscopic gastrostomy and nasogastric tube feeding in patients with persisting neurological dysphagia. Br Med J 304:1406–1409

Patel AS. DeRidder PH (1990) Endoscopic appearance and significance of functional lymphangiectasia of the duodenal mucosa. Gastrointestinal Endosc 136:376–368

Petersen TI, Kruse A (1997) Complications of percutaneous endoscopic gastrostomy. Eur J Surg 163:351–356

Ponsky JL, Gauderer MWL (1989) Percutaneous endoscopic gastrostomy: indications, limitations, techniques, and results. World J Surg 13:165–170

Rabeneck L, McCullough LB, Wray NP (1997) Ethically justified, clinically comprehensive guidelines for percuta-

neous endoscopic gastrostomy tube placement. Lancet 349:496–498
Rockall TA, Logan RF, Devlin HB, Northfield TC (1995) Incidence of and mortality from acute upper gastrointestinal haemorrhage in the United Kingdom. Steering Committee and members of the National Audit of Acute Gastrointestinal Haemorrhage. Br Med J 311:222–226
Russell TR, Brotman M, Norris F (1984) Percutaneous gastrostomy: a new simplified and cost effective technique. Am J Surg 148:132–137
Rutgeerts P, Rauws E, Wara P et al (1997) Randomised trial of single and repeated fibrin glue compared with injection of polidocanol in treatment of bleeding peptic ulcer. Lancet 350:692–696
Sabat M, Villanueva J, Ortiz J et al (1998) Final results of a prospective and randomized trial evaluating endoscopic hemoclip for bleeding peptic ulcer. Gastroenterol A-3304
Schaffalitzky de Muckadell OB, Havelund T, Harling H et al (1997) Effect of omeprazole on the outcome of endoscopically treated bleeding peptic ulcers. Scand J Gastroenterol 32:320–327
Soehendra N, Binmoeller KF, Seifert H, Schreiber HW (1998) Therapeutic Endoscopy. 7:74–89, Thieme Stuttgart, New York
Soehendra N, Binmoeller KF, Seifert H, Schreiber HW (1998) Therapeutic endoscopy. 4:34–47, Thieme, Stuttgart
Stal P, Lindberg G, Ost A et al (1999) Gastroesophageal reflux in healthy subjects: significance of endoscopic findings, histology, age and sex. Scand J Gastroenterol 34:121–128
Stolte M, Sticht T, Eidt S et al (1994) Frequency, location, and age and sex distribution of various types of gastric polyps. Endoscopy 26:659–665
Sung JY, Chung SC, Low JM et al (1993) Systemic absorption of Epinephrine after endoscopic submucosal injection in patients with bleeding peptic ulcers. Gastrointest Endosc 39:20–22
Treiber G, Lambert JR (1998) The impact of *Helicobacter pylori* eradication on peptic ulcer healing. Am J Gastroenterol 93:1080–1084
Tytgat GNJ (2000) Ulcers and gastritis. State-of-the-art review. Endoscopy 32:108–117
Villanueva C, Balanzo J, Torras X et al (1994) Value of a second look endoscopy after injection therapy for bleeding peptic ulcer: a prospective and randomized trial. Gastrointest Endosc 40:34–39
Yasunaga Y, Shinomura Y, Kanyama S et al (1994) Improved fold width and increased acid secretion after eradication of the organism in *Helicobacter pylori*-associated enlarged fold gastritis. Gut 35:1571–1574

Problems and Pitfalls of Gastrointestinal Endoscopy. Is There Still a Role for the Barium Meal?

4

PHILIP JOHN SHORVON

CONTENTS

4.1 Introduction

Prior to the development of endoscopy, a barium meal was the sole mechanism for the investigation of upper gastrointestinal disease. Barium meals were mainly performed as single contrast studies, and the lack of competition resulted in few studies of accuracy or efficacy. The onset of endoscopy acted as a spur to the development of more sophisticated techniques, particularly double contrast or multiphasic studies, and at the same time contrast studies in general became subject to evaluation of their accuracy. Endoscopy with direct vision and the ability to take biopsies soon became the accepted gold standard, and barium studies were inevitably found wanting, though in fact there are surprisingly few good comparative studies considering the many hundreds of thousands of endoscopic and radiological studies performed each year. However, in view of the reduction in the number of barium examinations it is unlikely that such studies will be performed in the future, or will indeed have much relevance. It should be remembered that whilst endoscopy and barium studies are often performed for similar clinical indications, the spectra of their potential diagnostic performance overlap, rather than coincide (LEVINE and LAUFER 1993). The whole issue is further compounded by advances in cross-sectional imaging.

Endoscopic techniques are now the first-line investigations for imaging of the oesophagus, stomach, duodenum, and colon in most clinical situations. This is deservedly so, but there is a danger that the shortcomings of this approach are unappreciated. This is particularly the case with younger physicians who are endoscopically trained and have had little exposure to barium studies. However it is important to understand that endoscopy is fallible, and to appreciate the reasons for this. The purpose of this chapter is to point out potential problems for upper gastrointestinal endoscopy and to discuss the reasons behind these. Endoscopy may give a tunnel view, but it is important that this does not result in the endoscopist having tunnel vision.

Endoscopy provides excellent views of the *mucosa*, and of course facilitates mucosal biopsy. However, there is little information available to the endoscopist as to what lies beneath the mucosa, though endoscopic ultrasound (EUS) to some extent circumvents this limitation. At present EUS is still a relatively specialised technique used mainly in the area of cancer staging and does not routinely overcome other endoscopic limitations. To problem solve, the endoscopist must first identify that there is a problem. The following account illustrates the situations in which problems occur, but are not always appreciated.

4.2 Classification of Limitations (Table 4.1)

The limitations of endoscopy may be classified broadly into eight categories that indicate situations

P. J. SHORVON, MA, FRCP, FRCR
Consultant Radiologist, Department of Radiology, North West London Hospitals NHS Trust, Central Middlesex Hospital, Acton Lane, London, NW10 7NS, UK

Table 4.1. Classification of endoscopic limitations in upper gastrointestinal disease diagnosis

Category	Reason	Example
1) Sites of poor visualisation	Usually at sites of poor distension/steep angulation/ beyond easy reach of endoscope	Just beyond cricopharangeus/2nd part duodenum
2) Motility disorders	Endoscopy poorly assesses motility	Achalasia
3) Subtle strictures	Requires good distension and can be difficult to visualise	Webs and rings
4) Fistulae	No ability to see where fistulae extend and orifices can be small and difficult to see	TB of oesophagus
5) Positional abnormalities	Lack of external landmarks makes identification of location in space difficult for endoscopist	Organ herniations
6) Submucosal and extrinsic disease	If the mucosa is uninterrupted then appreciation and diagnosis are difficult	Leiomyomas, pseudodiverticulosis of the oesophagus
7) Mucosal patterns	Barium outlines crevices and folds not readily appreciated visually, and difficult for endoscopist to obtain overview	Distortions of the areae gastricae
8) Large lesions	Small field of view can make 'big picture' difficult to appreciate	Fibrovascular polyp of oesophagus

where endoscopy *may* miss the diagnosis. If these limitations are kept in mind, then a negative endoscopy in some clinical scenarios will not be seen as the definitive investigation. Indeed in other scenarios the gastroenterologist may even see endoscopy as a second-line investigation.

4.2.1 Sites of Poor Visualisation

During intubation, the endoscopist has to overcome the upper oesophageal sphincter. This is usually achieved with a sudden 'give', and the endoscopist does not have visualisation as this occurs. The upper oesophagus remains collapsed for most of the time, and distension is difficult to maintain. Thus upper oesophageal webs are frequently overlooked and may in fact be inadvertently dilated by the endoscopist (Fig. 4.1). As a consequence they will not be visible as the endoscope is withdrawn at the end of the study (visual review at this point of the examination is always an important part of endoscopy). For the same reason the presence of ectopic gastric mucosa (Fig. 4.2) in the upper oesophagus is rarely seen at endoscopy despite a quoted incidence of up to 10%, but in everyday endoscopic practice it is much lower than this (Berkelhammer et al. 1997). Endoscopists are likely to miss a Zenker's diverticulum (Fig. 4.3) unless these are inadvertently intubated. This is not without danger, as they can be easily perforated by the endoscope due to the fact that they are only lined by mucosa. These diverticula are often associated with incomplete relaxation of the cricopharyngeus muscle or a cricopharyngeal bar (Fig. 4.1). It is worth noting that cricopharyngeal muscle incoordination is also part of the wider spectrum of dysfunction at the level of the pharyngo-oesophageal segment; in this situation the diagnosis

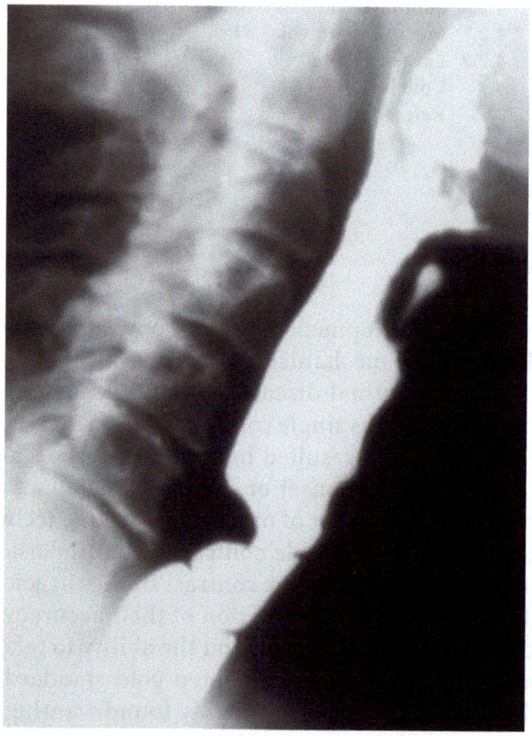

Fig. 4.1. Oesophageal web. Lateral view of the upper oesophagus demonstrating a tight web just below a prominent cricopharyngeal muscle impression. The web was not identified on endoscopy

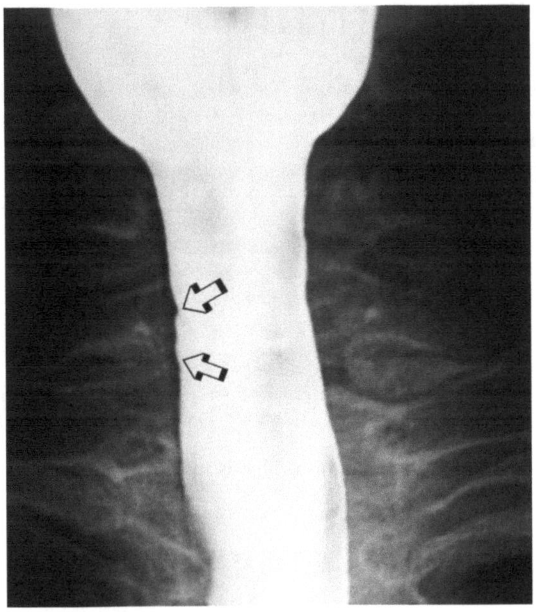

Fig. 4.2. Ectopic gastric mucosa. This is demonstrated as a mucosal irregularity on the right lateral aspect of the upper oesophagus (*arrows*); this was only confirmed on a repeat endoscopy

is better appreciated by barium studies, particularly using videofluoroscopy.

As the stomach is entered, views of the cardia may be limited (Fig. 4.4). These are best achieved by good retroversion, but this is not always possible. This is particularly the case in a patient who has poor compliance of the stomach wall, as the ability to distend the stomach is reduced (Fig. 4.5). Similar problems are encountered in a small stomach remnant following Polya gastrectomy. Fluid, particularly blood in a patient with upper tract bleeding, can accumulate in the fundus and obscure lesions.

Gastric diverticula (Fig. 4.6) are usually situated close to the cardia and normally are of no clinical significance. However, as with other diverticula elsewhere they can be a cause of diverticulitis and may harbour tumours. Again they are poorly diagnosed by endoscopy. The body of the stomach is usually well visualised, but even here lesions may be missed if they are obscured by luxuriant or oedematous folds surrounding large ulcers (Fig. 4.7a,b).

In the duodenal cap, endoscopy is undoubtedly a more sensitive technique than radiography for ero-

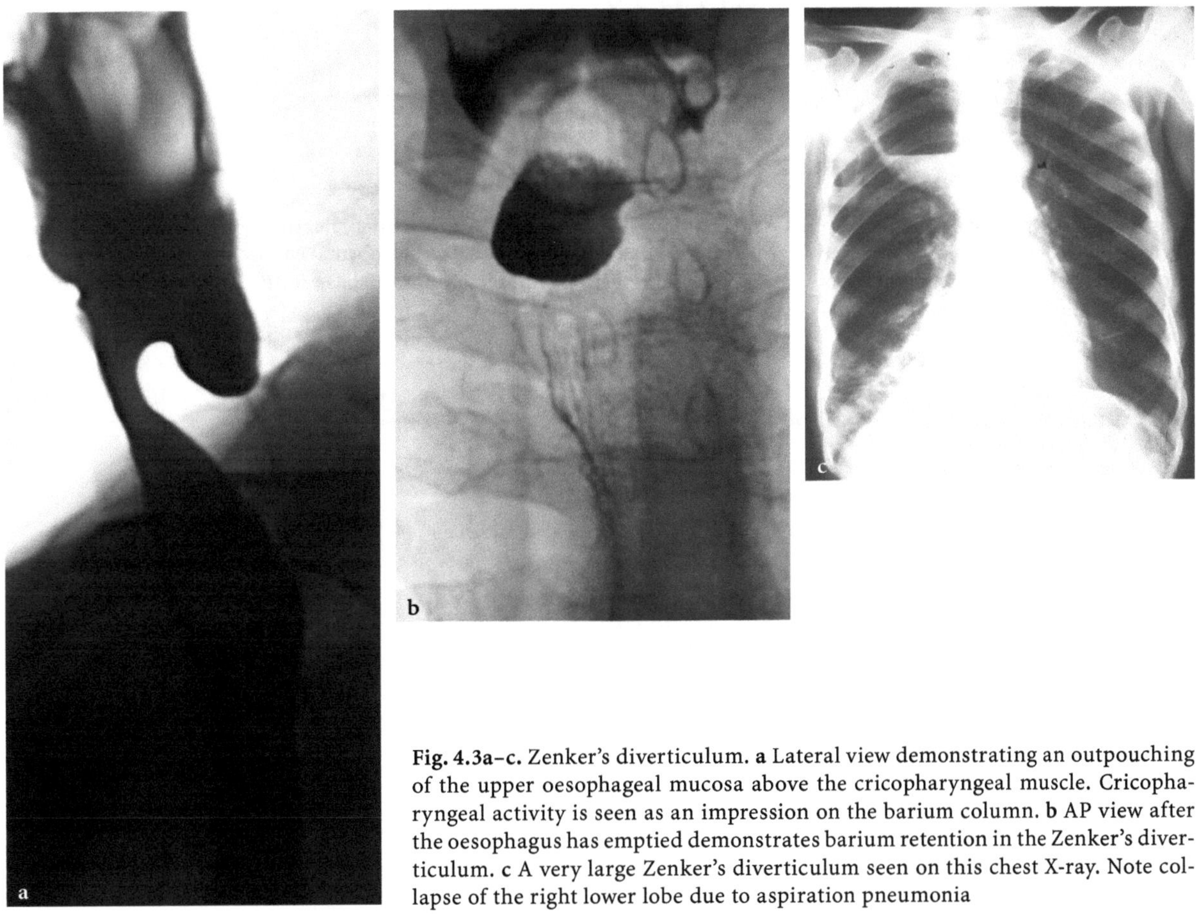

Fig. 4.3a–c. Zenker's diverticulum. **a** Lateral view demonstrating an outpouching of the upper oesophageal mucosa above the cricopharyngeal muscle. Cricopharyngeal activity is seen as an impression on the barium column. **b** AP view after the oesophagus has emptied demonstrates barium retention in the Zenker's diverticulum. **c** A very large Zenker's diverticulum seen on this chest X-ray. Note collapse of the right lower lobe due to aspiration pneumonia

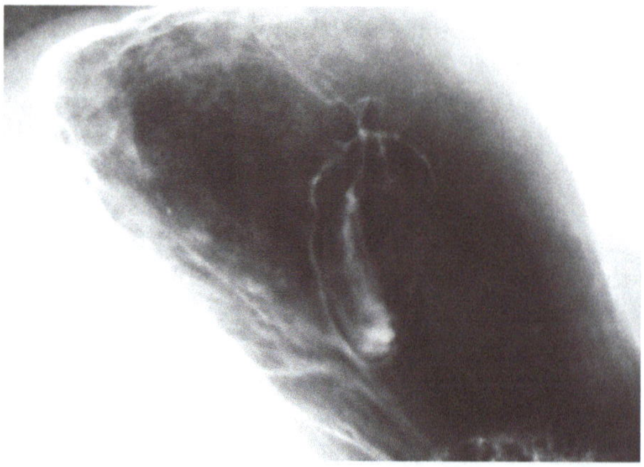

Fig. 4.4. Plaque-like tumour. This was missed at endoscopy probably because a poor retroverted view of the cardiac area failed to appreciate the subtle elevation of the mucosa

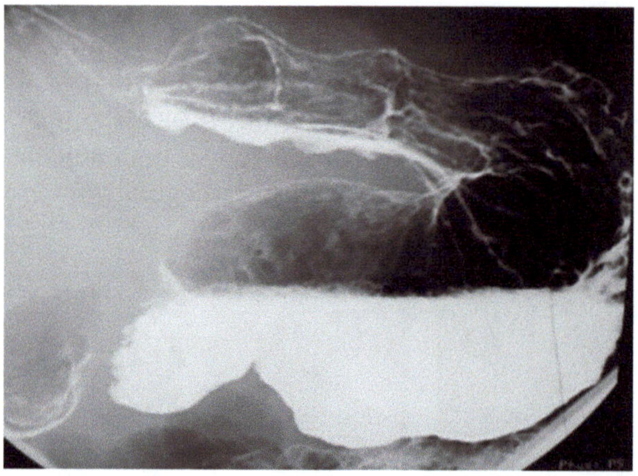

Fig. 4.5. Linitis plastica. This patient had a normal but difficult endoscopy in which distension of the stomach was problematical. He had symptoms of dyspepsia, early satiety, and weight loss, and the barium study clearly shows a linitis pattern in the fundus

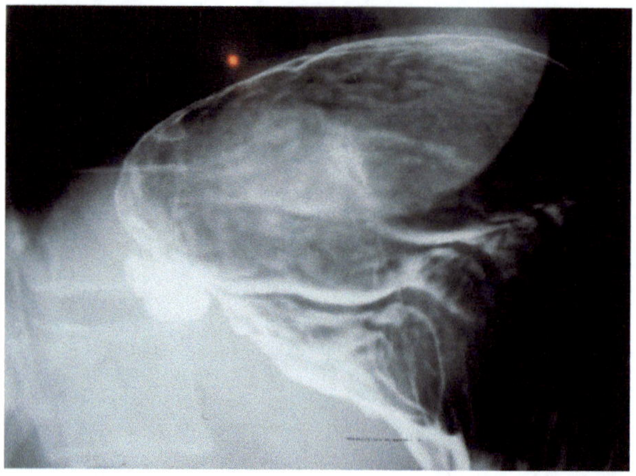

Fig. 4.7. Gastric diverticulum. This is in the typical location

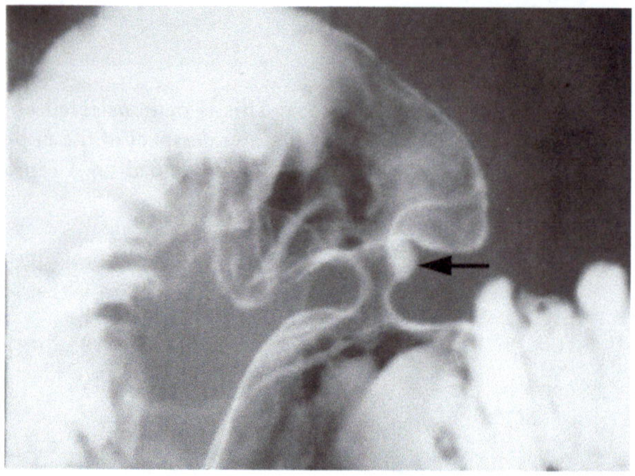

Fig. 4.8. Pyloric canal ulcer. A small ulcer in the distal pyloric canal with a normal endoscopy (*arrow*). There is also an impression on the base of the superior duodenal fornix due to oedema

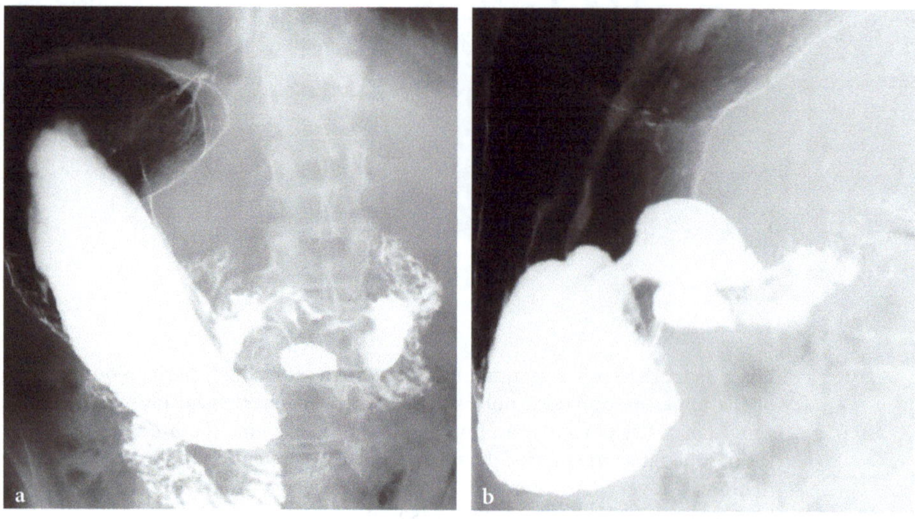

Fig. 4.6a,b. Antral ulcer. This large deep antral gastric ulcer was not observed at endoscopy because the ulcer crater was obscured by luxuriant inflamed gastric folds

sions and ulceration. However, ulcers can be missed, particularly at the base of the duodenal bulb, as the duodenal fornices are a blind area to the endoscope passing through the pylorus (Fig. 4.8). The duodenum just beyond the superior duodenal angle may also be difficult to visualise, and sometimes routine forward viewing of the second part of the duodenum is suboptimal (Fig. 4.9a–d). The third and fourth parts of the duodenum are not routinely examined at an upper GI examination.

In the situation of upper gastrointestinal haemorrhage, endoscopic sensitivity is over 90%, and in expert hands less than 2% of cases of acute upper gastrointestinal haemorrhage are left undiagnosed (Chung et al. 2000). However, lesions in the relative 'blind spots' described above are occasionally missed, and others may still be within the duodenum but beyond the normal range of the upper gastrointestinal endoscope. Interestingly, it has been demonstrated that in patients with occult upper gastrointestinal bleeding and a negative endoscopy, the causative lesion has been shown on subsequent enteroscopy to be within the range of a standard endoscope in 10% of cases (Descamps et al. 1999).

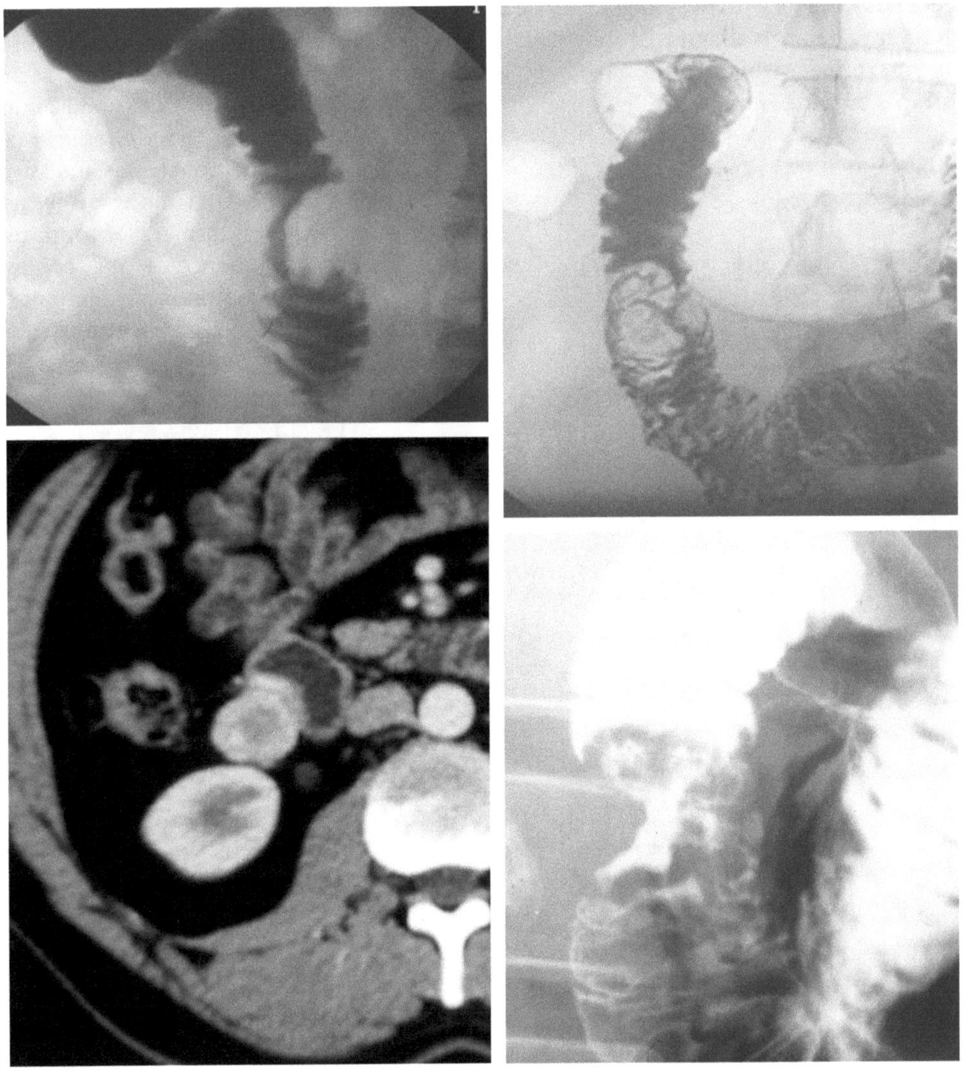

a b c d

Fig. 4.9a–d. Tumours in the second part of the duodenum. Case A. Two separate barium studies demonstrated a mass in the descending duodenum (**a**, **b**). Endoscopies performed before and after the second barium meal were negative, and it was presumed that the barium studies were false. However CT confirmed the enhancing mass (**c**). This proved to be a neurogenic tumour, and the reason for the negative endoscopies was likely to be the position of the mass (low second part of duodenum) and its submucosal position. Case B. A carcinoma of the second part of the duodenum (**d**), not visualised at endoscopy because of a failure to negotiate into the descending duodenum

4.2.2 Motility Assessment

Endoscopy cannot assess motility adequately. An oesophagus may appear dilated and amotile, but formal assessment is not possible as the primary wave progression cannot be followed, and the presence of the endoscope may interfere with function. Endoscopists are of course fully aware of this limitation and would not attempt a definitive motility diagnosis. However, some motility disorders will present with symptoms similar to those caused by structural lesions, and a motility cause may be overlooked. Patients with dysphagia may be investigated for years before a diagnosis of achalasia (Fig. 4.10) is entertained, which could have been achieved by simple barium swallow.

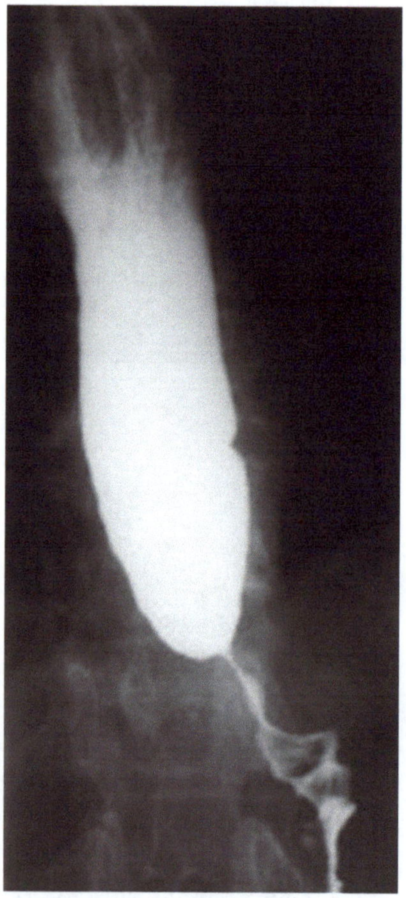

Fig. 4.10. Achalasia of the cardia. Typical appearances with mild dilatation of the oesophagus and 'rat tail' configuration of the lower oesophageal sphincter. This and the lack of any normal peristaltic activity in the lower oesophagus indicated the diagnosis immediately, although the patient had suffered dysphagia without diagnosis for three years and had undergone three endoscopies

Barium studies are accurate at assessing oesophageal motility if performed in a dedicated manner, and this assessment should be considered in patients with oesophageal symptoms, especially dysphagia. Comparisons have been made with manometry and show reasonable concordance, and some centres perform combined fluoroscopic screening and manometry studies. Achalasia is diagnosed accurately by barium studies, which also provide a good technique for follow-up after balloon dilatation or Heller's myotomy. Other motility disorders are also well demonstrated including diffuse oesophageal spasm (Fig. 4.11) and scleroderma. The 'feline' oesophagus (Fig. 4.12) is thought to be due to transient contraction of the muscularis mucosae, often secondary to reflux, and is commonly seen during barium studies but rarely described endoscopically. There are limitations to radiological assessment of motility; it only demonstrates motility in a relatively short 'snapshot' in time and does not give much accuracy in the assessment of amplitude of contraction. As a consequence of this, conditions such as the 'nut cracker oesophagus' cannot be made by radiology with confidence (Chobanian et al. 1986).

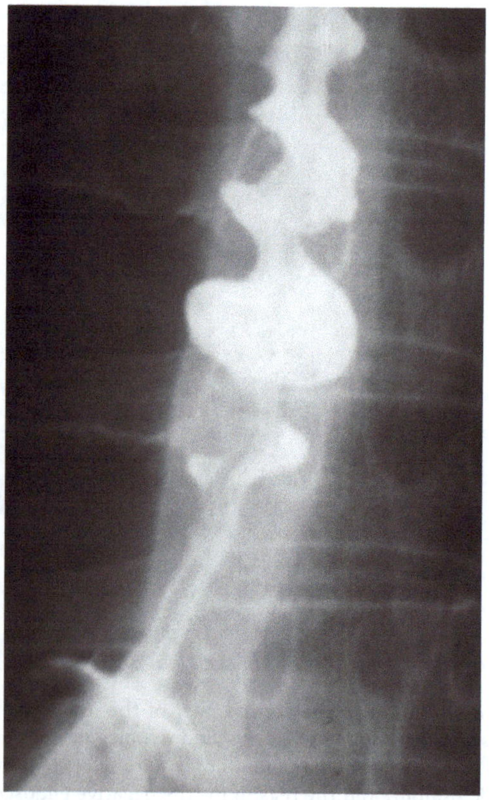

Fig. 4.11. Diffuse oesophageal spasm. This is characterised by the typical 'corkscrew' appearance

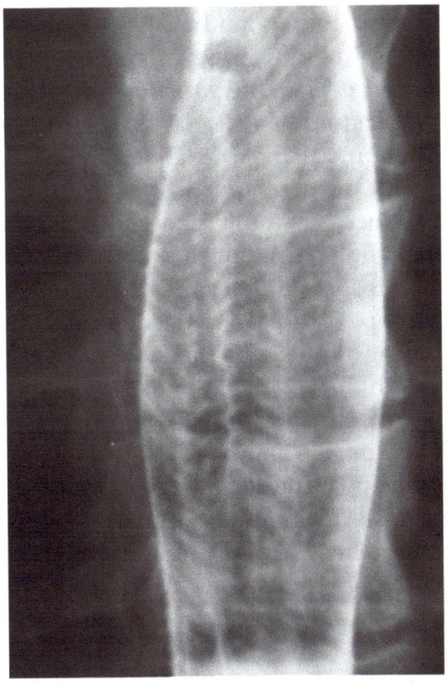

Fig. 4.12. Feline oesophagus. The characteristic 'herring bone'pattern of the feline oesophagus in a patient with gastro-oesophageal reflux

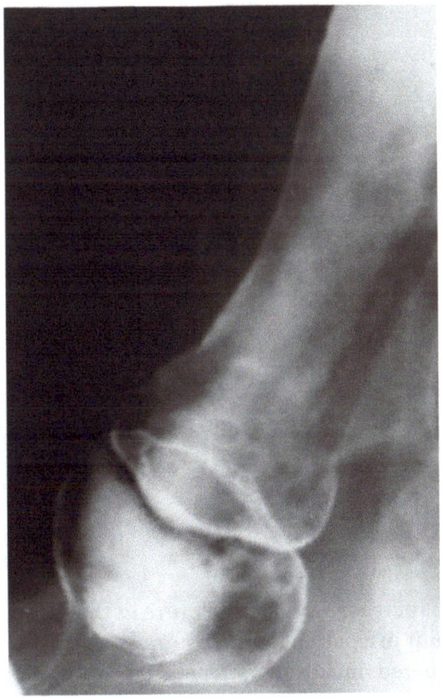

Fig. 4.13. Schatzki ring. These are best demonstrated with maximum distension of the hiatus hernia and oesophagus in the prone position. This was not seen at endoscopy

4.2.3 Subtle Strictures

To fully appreciate a subtle stricture, a well distended gut lumen is needed both above and below the stricture. This can be difficult for both endoscopy and barium studies, but is less of a problem for the latter as distension is an essential part of the technique (Marks and Shukla 1996). This is important in a number of scenarios. Subtle strictures, webs, and Schatzki rings (Fig. 4.13) (Ott et al. 1986) can all be missed on endoscopy yet still be symptomatic. Confirmation of the significance of a subtle stricture seen during a barium swallow may be achieved by the addition of a solid bolus to the study (e.g., a marshmallow). If the marshmallow impacts at the stricture and reproduces the feeling of dysphagia, the diagnosis is confirmed (van Westen and Ekberg 1993; Somers et al. 1986). This test can also be used to evaluate the dysphagia, which may occasionally be caused by vascular structures impressing the oesophagus (Fig. 414) (Mittal et al. 1986). Strictures are more likely to be overlooked by the endoscopist if the mucosa looks healthy and intact, such as the case of an annular pancreas presenting in adulthood. Barium studies will show a 'waisting' of the second part of the duodenum with

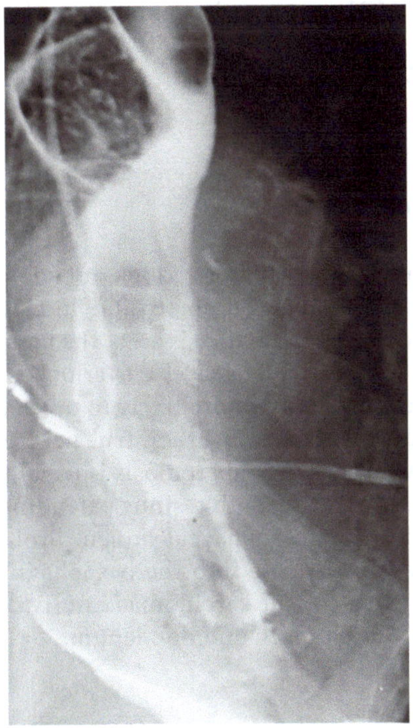

Fig. 4.14. Extrinsic vascular compression. Endoscopy did not demonstrate a cause for dysphagia in this patient with congestive cardiac failure and mitral regurgitation. A marshmallow swallow demonstrated hold-up of the marshmallow above an indentation of the oesophagus caused by an enlarged left atrium. The marshmallow reproduced the sensation of dysphagia

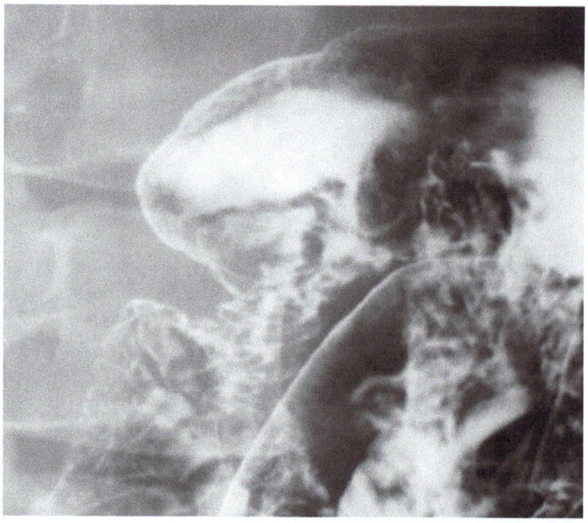

Fig. 4.15. Annular pancreas. A typical stricture in the second part of the duodenum in a patient with an annular pancreas. Note the uninterrupted mucosal pattern explaining why endoscopy is often negative

normal appearing mucosa (Fig. 4.15), although a definitive diagnosis requires either cross-sectional imaging (CT or MRI) or an endoscopic retrograde cholangiopancreatography (ERCP) (Jadvar and Mindelzun 1999).

4.2.4 Fistulae and Sinuses

Fistulae and sinuses are easy to overlook at endoscopy as their orifices may be small and hidden within folds, and even if the orifice is seen, the presence of an underlying fistula may be overlooked. Contrast studies however are more likely to outline fistulas and sinus tracts, revealing their true nature. Oesophageal involvement by tuberculosis is usually secondary to nodal disease, with a sinus extending from the node into the oesophageal lumen. Bronchial neoplasms can fistulate into the oesophagus and vice versa, whilst colonic carcinomas can fistulate directly into the stomach and duodenum.

4.2.5 Positional Abnormalities

At endoscopy, the precise position and spatial relationships of the organ under investigation are difficult to assess. This is because only the mucosa of the upper gastrointestinal tract is visualised, without reference to other landmarks. Although the diaphragmatic hiatus can be inferred by the indentation produced when the patient sniffs, there are few other indicators of external anatomy. For example, before puncturing the abdominal wall during placement of percutaneous gastrostomy (PEG) tubes, reliance has to be made on the glow of the endoscopic light through the surface of the abdomen in order to locate the stomach. It is notable that when endoscopic difficulty is encountered, for example in finding the exit of the stomach or in identifying the light for PEG placement, the reason is often because of some positional abnormality of the stomach. The stomach may have an almost complete intrathoracic position in what is effectively a massive sliding or rolling hiatus hernia. In these situations the stomach has often undergone a volvulus (Fig. 4.16a,b), although this can occur in a normally situated stomach as well. These positional abnormalities and various types of volvulus (organo-axial, vertical, and horizontal) are demonstrated by barium studies. Severe intermittent symptoms of vomiting and abdominal distension may predate a gastric volvulus and its potential complication of gastric necrosis, necessitating prompt diagnosis. Likewise, the diagnosis of internal hernias and hernias involving abdominal wall defects are also difficult to make at endoscopy (Fig. 4.17), as are problems with rotation, e.g. the reversed duodenal loop (Fig. 4.18) and situs inversus. These may be suspected but are difficult to prove without recourse to radiology. There is some evidence that duodenal rotational anomalies are associated with dyspeptic symptoms and delayed gastric emptying (Thommesen 1988).

4.2.6 Submucosal or Extrinsic Disease

The endoscopist can only visualise the mucosa from within and must infer submucosal and extrinsic abnormalities from changes in contour, stricturing, and lack of distensibility. Radiological images also supply some mucosal detail, but in addition give a two-dimensional representation of a three-dimensional organ. Therefore abnormalities of shape, stricturing, mucosal contour, and extrinsic compressions are easier to detect. Double contrast studies may have a particular advantage over endoscopy when dealing with so-called scirrhous carcinomas which infiltrate submucosally and where endoscopic inspection may not arouse suspicion of a tumour

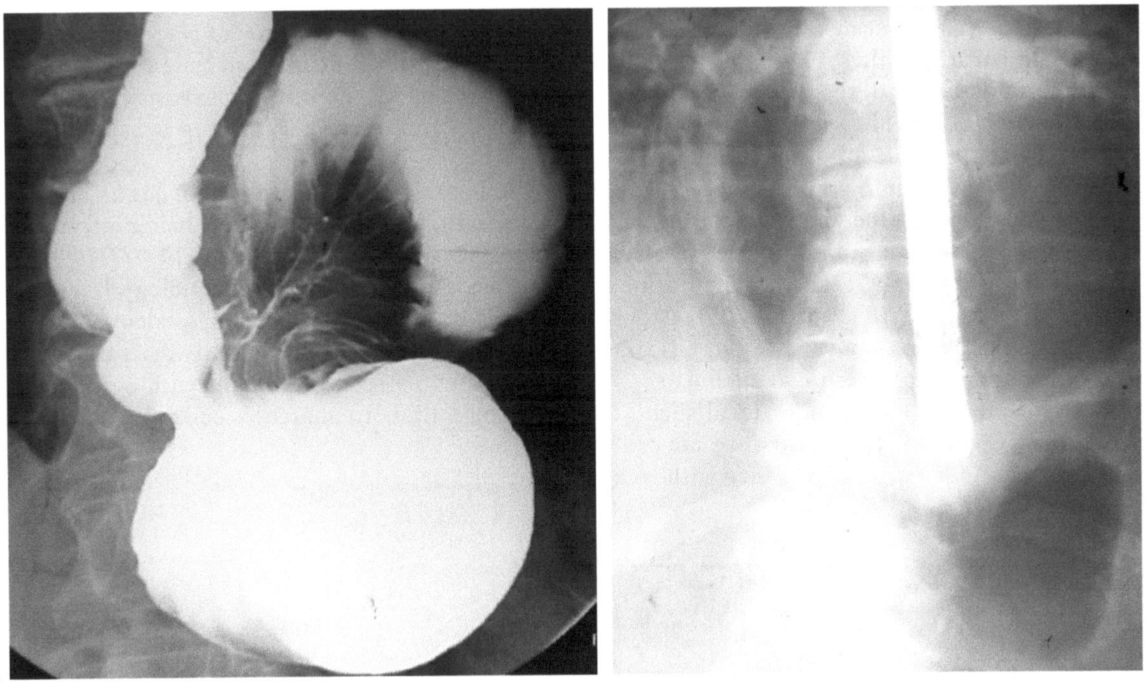

a b

Fig. 4.16a,b. Mesentero-axial volvulus (a) barium study and (b) endoscopy. The antrum of the stomach has herniated into the chest alongside the oesophagus. Endoscopy was described as difficult and could not be completed, but the cause of the problems encountered was not understood

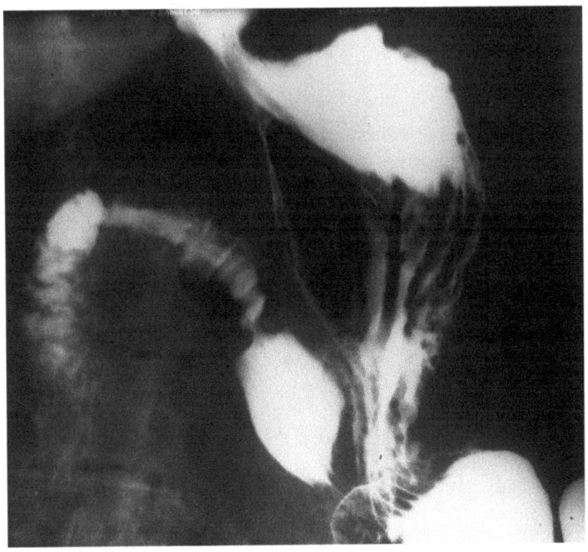

Fig. 4.17. Anterior abdominal wall hernia. This obese patient had epigastric discomfort after meals. Endoscopy was normal but the barium study demonstrated the stomach herniating through a large defect in the anterior abdominal wall

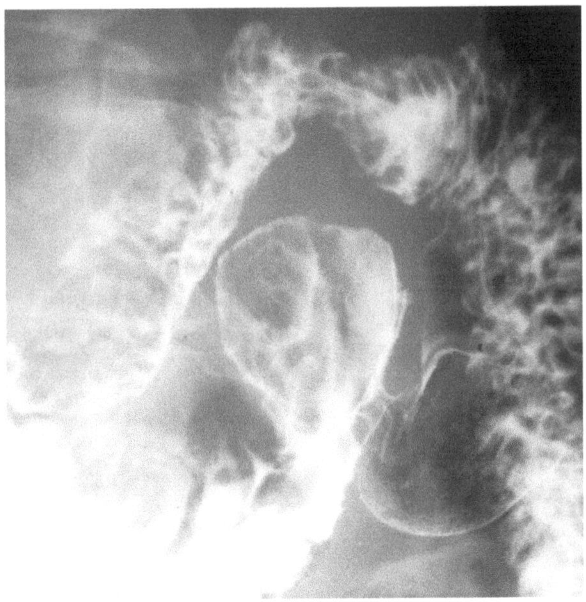

Fig. 4.18. Reversed duodenal loop. Anomalies such as the reversed duodenal loop are easy to appreciate with a barium meal, but the cause of difficulty at endoscopy is often not appreciated

(Figs. 4.19, 4.20). This is because rigidity is easier to recognise on barium studies, often aided by fold thickening and nodularity of the mucosa. Japanese experience suggests that these are the commonest malignancies that may be missed on endoscopy but demonstrated on barium studies (Levine and Laufer 1993). Even quite large submucosal tumours like gastrointestinal stromal tumours (GISTs) may be overlooked at endoscopy because of the normal mucosa on their surface (Figs. 4.23, 4.24). Other nontumorouss conditions may have significant submucosal components; widespread such as eosinophilic gastroenteritis (Fig. 4.23), or focal such as a pancreatic rest (Fig. 4.24). Serosal disease can produce a characteristic serrated appearance with lack of distension on barium images (Fig. 4.25a–c), but again may be difficult to appreciate at endoscopy. When submucosal, serosal, or extrinsic disease is suspected, cross-sectional imaging is usually indicated to assess its nature.

Submucosal lesions in the oesophagus are also encountered, a relatively rare one being intramural pseudodiverticulosis (Flora et al. 1997) (Fig. 4.26). This is a condition of unknown aetiology, but which has an association with diabetes, alcohol abuse, reflux disease, and oesophageal strictures. It is more commonly seen in patients with oesophageal carcinomas than in matched controls, and there

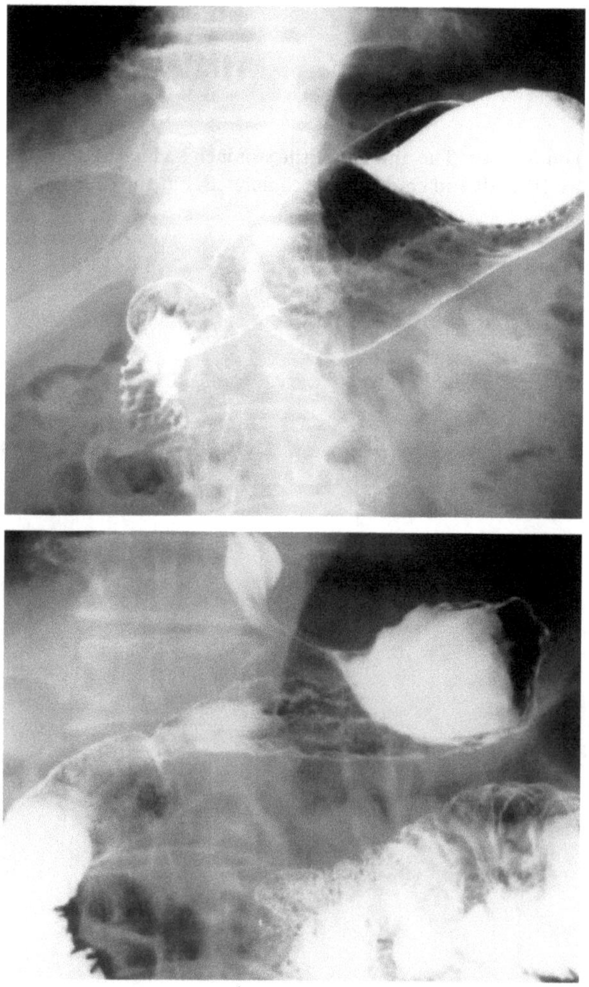

a

b

Fig. 4.19a,b. Linitis plastica. In this patient with pernicious anaemia and gastric atrophy, an infiltrating, scirrhous carcinoma had developed which was not appreciated at endoscopy. The examinations (**a**) and (**b**) were separated by two years. Note the nodular, nondistensible stomach in (**b**)

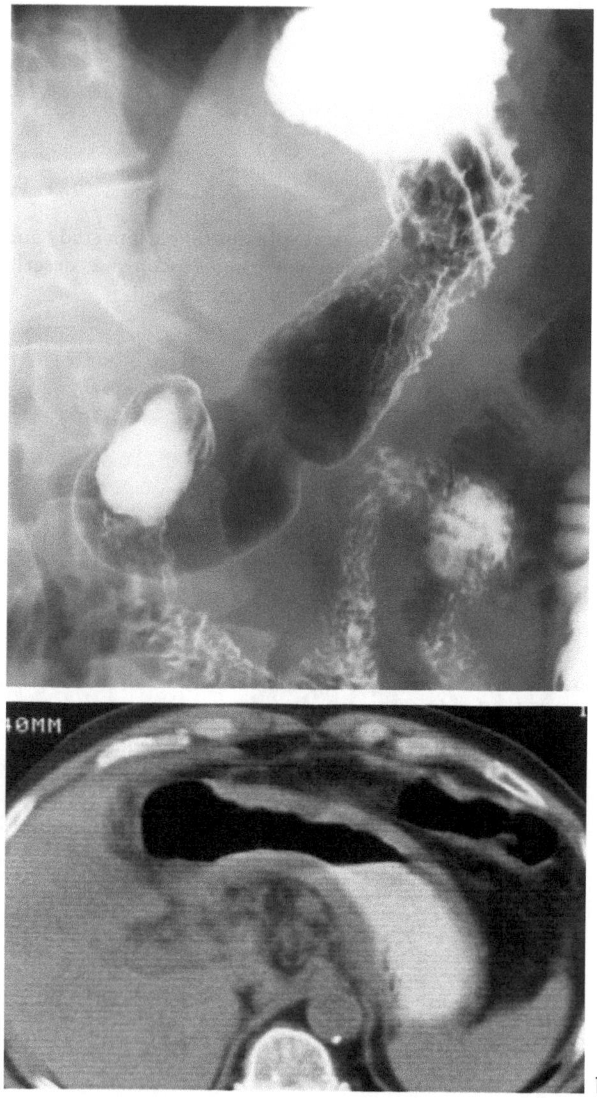

a

b

Fig. 4.20a,b. Linitis plastica. Another example of a scirrhous carcinoma with linitis plastica appearance undiagnosed by endoscopy. Poor distensibility of the stomach is shown on the barium study (**a**) and wall thickening confirmed by CT (**b**)

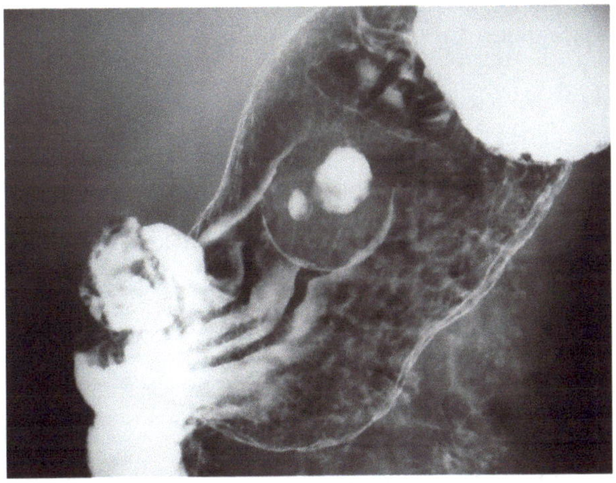

Fig. 4.21. A benign gastric ulcer was diagnosed endoscopically but failed to heal. The barium study clearly shows the large associated mass with typical appearances of a GIST

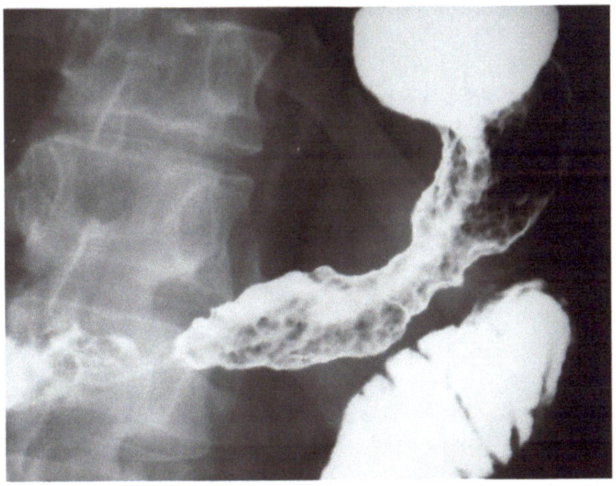

Fig. 4.23. Eosinophilic gastroenteritis. Linitis plastica appearance caused by eosinophilic gastroenteritis. The clue to the diagnosis relates to the infiltration extending into the duodenum, although this was not appreciated at endoscopy

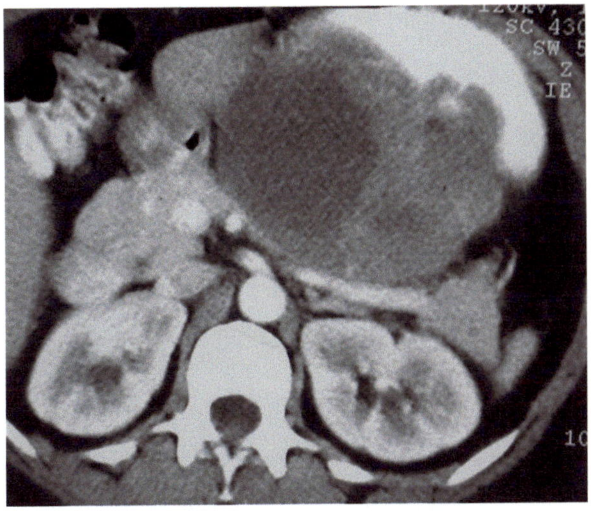

Fig. 4.22. This huge gastric mass prevented good distension of the stomach. Gastritis was diagnosed but because of poor vision, a CT was arranged, confirming the presence of a large GIST arising from the posterior gastric wall

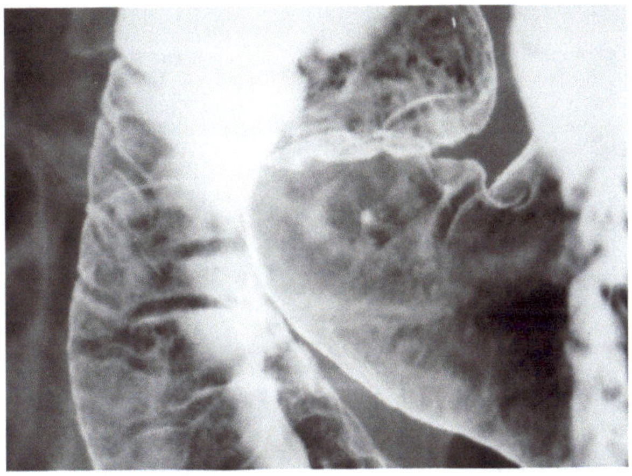

Fig. 4.24. Pancreatic rest. The typical position in the gastric antrum and the small pit due to the rudimentary duct gave the clue to the diagnosis

is an association with saprophytic colonisation by *Candida*. The diagnosis is easily made radiologically with a characteristic appearance of multiple small club-like sinuses extending into the oesophageal wall. Endoscopically the diagnosis is commonly missed (in about 80% of cases) as the only visible abnormalities are tiny pin-size pits in the mucosa. Occasionally a yellowish exudate may be observed. Postmortem studies have shown that these lesions represent cystic dilatation of the submucosal gland ducts.

4.2.7 Mucosal Patterns

The areae gastricae (Fig. 4.27) represent a network of fine crevices around gastric glandular structures. They require excellent barium coating of the surface of the stomach, as demonstration and distortion of these patterns may be seen in disease processes. In Japan in particular, this is used in the analysis of gastric lesions to assess their malignant potential (Fig. 4.28). The areae gastricae are accentuated in

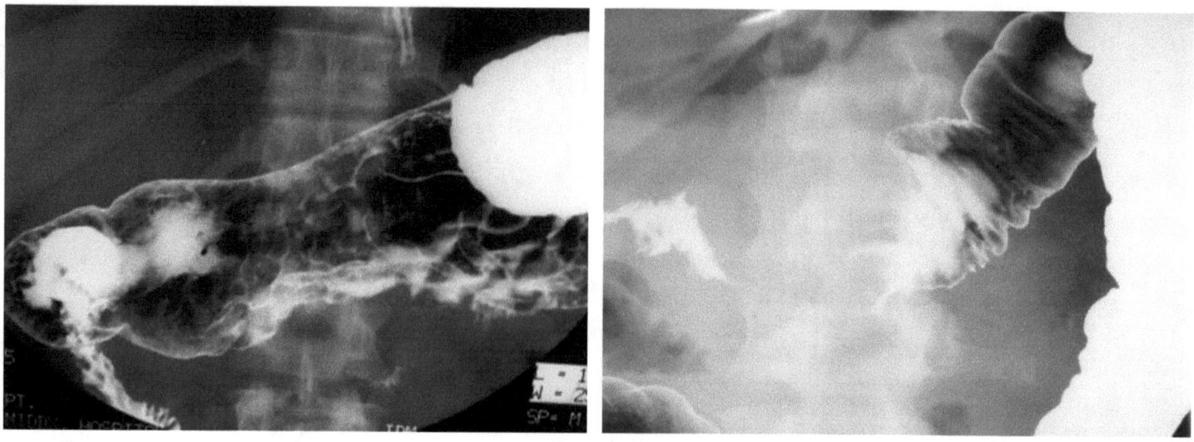

a b

Fig. 4.25a,b. Extrinsic involvement of the stomach. In this patient with weight loss and anaemia, endoscopy was reported as showing gastritis with biopsy confirmation of this. A barium meal demonstrated an abnormal greater curve (a), and serosal malignant involvement was suspected. Barium enema demonstrated the primary tumour arising from the transverse colon (b)

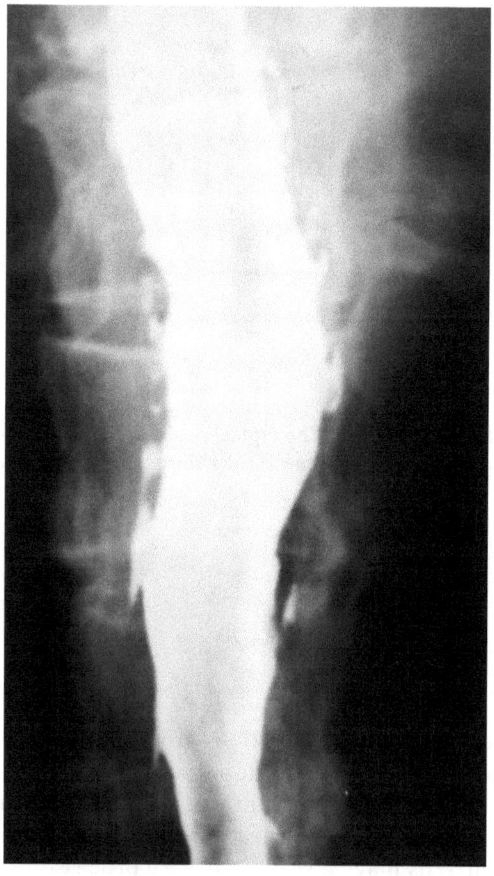

Fig. 4.26. Intramural pseudodiverticulosis. Typical and striking appearances of oesophageal pseudodiverticulosis that was not noted at endoscopy

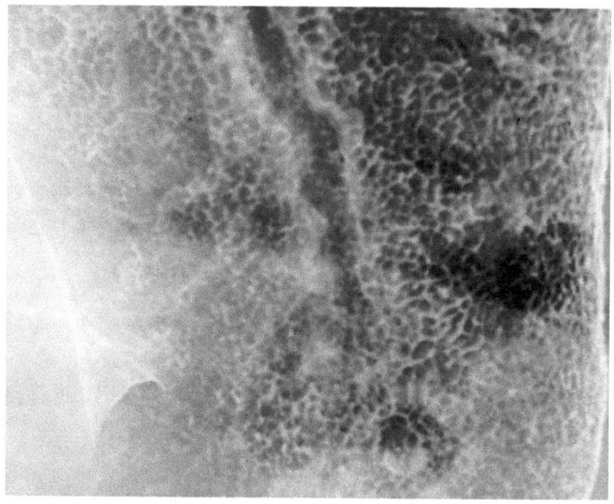

Fig. 4.27. Areae gastricae. The normal pattern seen with a well-coated gastric mucosa at barium meal

hypersecretory states and are absent in atrophic gastritis. However, they are not easily seen at endoscopy and are better appreciated during barium studies, because the radiological image gives a 'distant' overview rather than a small area viewed through the endoscope. A variety of radiological patterns of folds around gastric ulcers (Figs. 4.29, 4.30) have been described, which enable distinction of benign from malignant. It has been shown that a confident diagnosis of both benign and malignant ulcers on

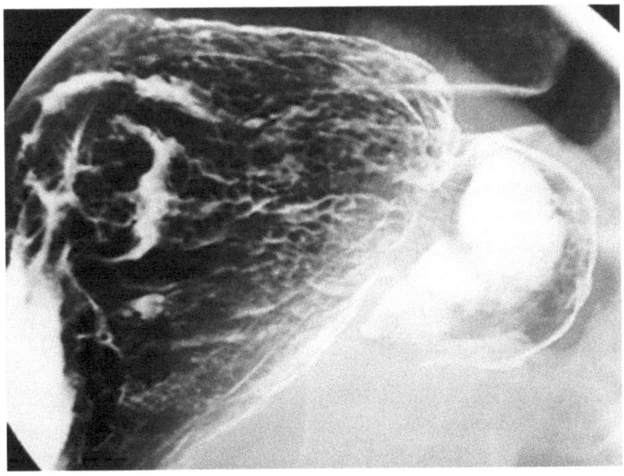

Fig. 4.28. Abnormal areae gastricae. The pattern is disturbed in this patient with a carcinoma of the fundus not noted at endoscopy (also note the gastric diverticulum)

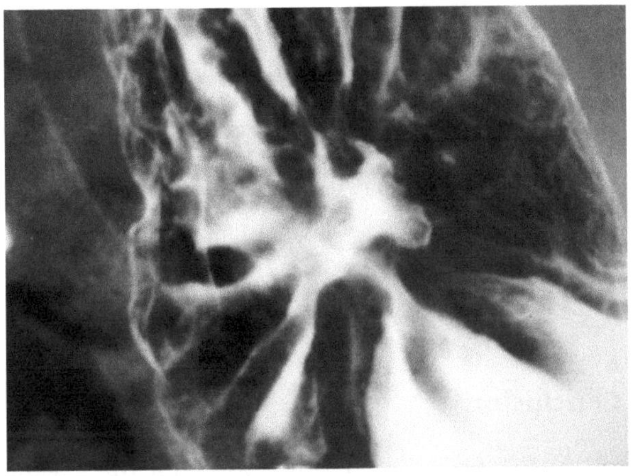

Fig. 4.29. Malignant gastric ulcer. Note the clubbing and fusion of some folds

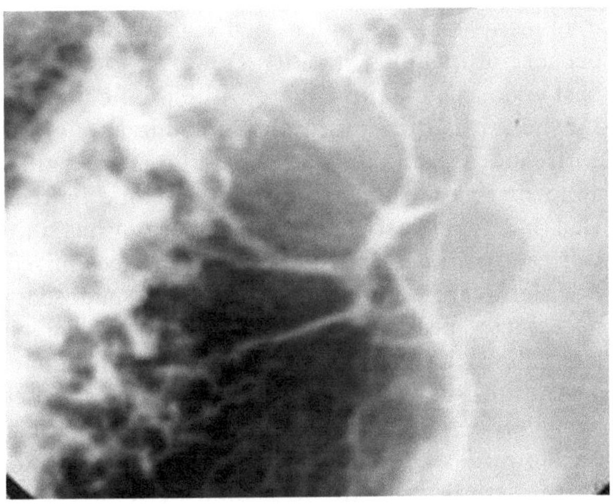

Fig. 4.30. Benign gastric ulcer with scarring. Note the linear scars extending right to the ulcer edge and the lack of distortion of the areae gastricae

barium studies is safe, though with the caveat that this approach requires that 'equivocal' ulcers need to be treated as potentially malignant (Levine et al. 1987; Thompson et al. 1983). Although endoscopic biopsy is the gold standard it is not infallible, and in a study of 51 patients with endoscopically diagnosed benign gastric ulcers, two patients (4%) died within 2 years of gastric cancer (Mulliwah et al. 1996).

There is also evidence to suggest that the visual appearances of lymphoid hyperplasia, gastric metaplasia, and Brunner's gland hyperplasia (Fig. 4.31a,b) are easier to differentiate with barium radiology than at endoscopy without biopsy.

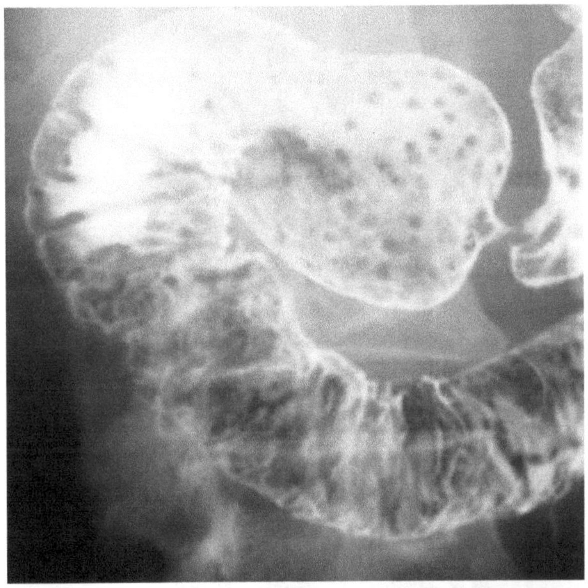

a

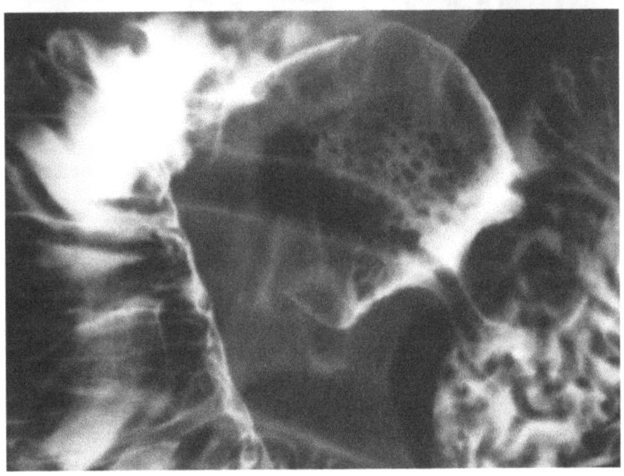

b

Fig. 4.31a,b. Duodenal nodules. The different causes all show very distinct patterns that are easy to confuse at endoscopy. **a** Follicular lymphoid hyperplasia, **b** gastric metaplasia ('spilling out of the pylorus')

4.2.8
Large Lesions

Paradoxically, very large lesions can be difficult to assess at endoscopy. This is particularly true if surrounded by normal mucosa, for example a giant fibrovascular polyp of the oesophagus (Fig. 4.32), which is often missed at endoscopic examination. Other large and unusual conditions which may cause endoscopic confusion include Bouveret syndrome, when the nature of the obstructing lesion seen at endoscopy only becomes apparent as an eroding gallstone on contrast examination (Fig. 4.33) (Khan et al. 2002). Again the ability of radiology to view a large field and thus give a wider overview offers an advantage with large and unusual lesions.

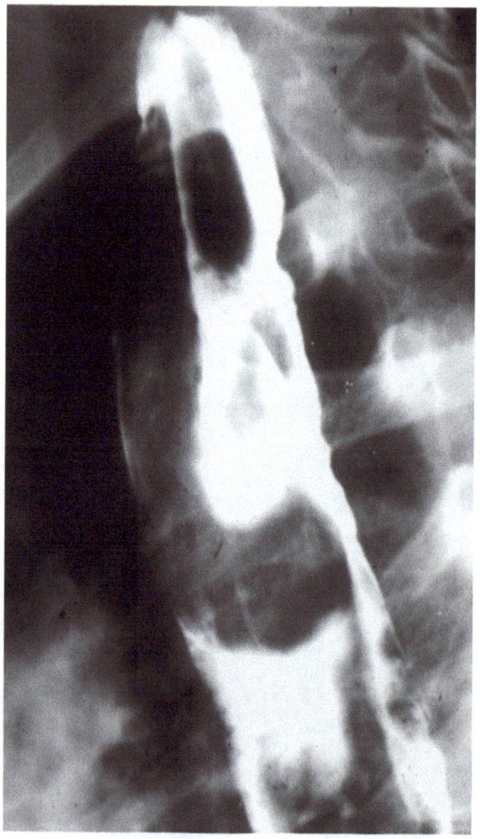

Fig. 4.32. Fibrovascular polyp. The patient complained of increasing dysphagia and occasional regurgitation of a large fleshy mass, which she then had to swallow again. There is a very large mass in the lumen of the oesophagus. The mucosa of the mass was normal, and the original endoscopy reported no abnormality as the endoscope ran alongside this huge polyp. The history and appearance are typical of giant fibrovascular polyps of the oesophagus. These patients are at danger of asphyxiation

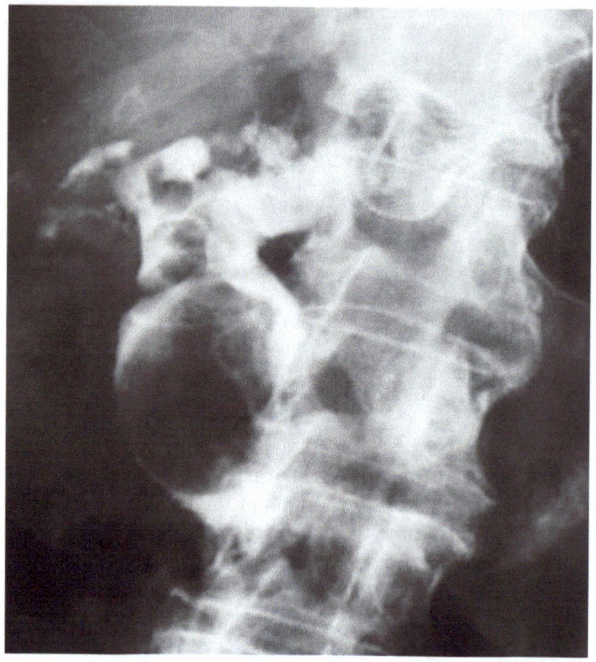

Fig. 4.33. 'Bouveret syndrome': A large gall bladder stone has eroded into the second part of the duodenum, causing pain, fever, and symptoms of gastric outlet obstruction

4.3
Conclusion

Upper gastrointestinal endoscopy and the barium meal should not be seen as rival examinations but rather as complimentary forms of imaging. Endoscopy has a pre-eminent place as the definitive diagnostic tool for mucosal disease, particularly because of its biopsy facility. However, even in the best endoscopic hands, there will be some patients in whom it is difficult to obtain good views of the entire mucosa, and there may be failure to recognise abnormal patterns. Furthermore it should be realised that upper gastrointestinal endoscopy has some inherent weaknesses which need to be recognised, in order to avoid the belief that a normal endoscopy necessarily means a normal upper GI tract. This is particularly important as most patients with upper gastrointestinal symptoms will usually be assessed by gastroenterologists, who may have a natural bias towards endoscopy, thus reducing requests for barium studies. Finally, it should be remembered that endoscopy has a small but significant complication rate, particularly related to cardiovascular events (Quine et al. 1995).

References

Berkelhammer C, Bhagavan M, Templeton A, Raines R, Wallock J (1997) Gastric Inlet Patch containing submucosally infiltrating adenocarcinoma. J Clin Gastroenterol 25:678–681

Chobanian SJ, Curtis DJ, Benjamin SB, Cattau EL (1986) Radiology of the nutcracker esophagus. J Clin Gastroenterol 8:230–232

Chung YFA, Wong WK, Soo KC (2000) Diagnostic failures in endoscopy for acute upper gastrointestinal haemorrhage. Br J Surg 87:614–617

Descamps C, Schmit A, van Gossum A (1999) "Missed" upper gastrointestinal lesions may explain "occult" bleeding. Endoscopy 31:452–545

Flora KD, Gordon MD, Lieberman D, Schmidt W (1997) Esophageal intramural pseudodiverticulosis. Dig Dis 15:113–119

Jadvar H, Mindelzun RE (1999) Annular pancreas in adults: imaging features in seven patients. Abdominal Imaging 24:174–177

Khan AZ, Escofet X, Miles WF, Singh KK (2002) The Bouveret syndrome: an unusual complication of gallstone disease. J R Soc Health 122:125–126

Levine MS, Laufer I (1993) The upper gastrointestinal series at a crossroads. AJR 161:1131–1137

Levine MS, Creteur V, Kressel HY, Laufer I, Herlinger H (1987) Benign gastric ulcers: diagnosis and follow-up with double contrast radiography. Radiology 164:9–13

Marks RD, Shukla M (1996) Diagnosis and management of peptic esophageal strictures. Gastroenterologist 4:223–227

Mittal RK, Siskind BN, Hongo M, Flye W, Mccallum RW (1986) Dysphagia aortica. Clinical , radiological and manometric findings. Dig Dis Sci 31:379–384

Mulliwah JA, Tabaqchali M, Watson J, Venables CW (1996) An audit of the outcome of peptic ulcer disease diagnosed 10-20 years previously. Gut 38:812–815

Ott DJ, Chen YM, Wu WC, Gelfand DW, Munitz HA(1986) Radiographic and endoscopic sensitivity in detecting lower esophageal mucosal ring. AJR 147:261–265

Quine MA, Bell GD, McCloy RF, Charlton JE, Devlin HB, Hopkins A (1995) Safety of endoscopy in the UK. Gut 36:462–467

Somers S , Stevenson GW, Thompson G (1986) Comparison of endoscopy and barium swallow with marshmallow in dysphagia. J Can Assoc Radiol 37:73–75

Thommesen P (1988) The shape of the duodenal loop. Radiological, physiological and clinical aspects in patients with X-Ray negative dyspepsia. Dan Med Bull 35:537–549

Thompson G, Somers S, Stevenson GW (1983) Benign gastric ulcer: a reliable radiologic diagnosis? AJR 141:331–333

Van Westen D, Ekberg O (1993) Solid bolus swallowing in the radiologic evaluation of dysphagia. Acta Radiol 34:372–375

Conventional Radiology of the Stomach and Duodenum

5

Evis Sala and Alan H. Freeman

CONTENTS

E. Sala, MD, PhD, FRCR
Univerity Lecturer/Honorary Consultant Radiologist, Department of Radiology, Addenbrooke's Hospital, Box 219, Hills Road, Cambridge, CB2 2QQ, UK
A. H. Freeman, MB, BS, FRCR
Consultant Radiologist, Department of Radiology, Addenbrooke's Hospital, Box 219, Hills Road, Cambridge, CB2 2QQ, UK

5.1 Basic Principle of Conventional Radiology of Stomach and Duodenum

The widespread use of cross-sectional imaging has significantly diminished the role of conventional radiographic techniques (plain radiography and contrast X-ray examinations) in the diagnosis of diseases of the stomach and duodenum. Currently, the plain abdominal radiograph remains a first-line investigation in the acute setting; although there is a clear move towards cross-sectional techniques such as US and CT as part of the initial patient assessment. In the non-acute situation, plain abdominal radiography offers little information and is now almost obsolete.

Although largely replaced by endoscopy, X-ray contrast studies remain the basic radiological technique for investigation of diseases of the oesophagus, stomach, and duodenum (Levine and Laufer 1993; Levine 1995; Levine et al. 2002). These are comprised of a barium swallow and meal with barium sulphate acting as a contrast agent. A barium swallow implies examination of the oesophagus alone, whereas a barium meal is used for examination of the lower oesophagus, stomach, and duodenum. Double-contrast techniques provide excellent detail of the mucosal surface of the stomach and duodenum as evidenced by the demonstration of area gastricae (Fig. 5.1) (Evers and Kressel 1982; Levine et al. 1988, 2002; Charagundla et al. 2001).

Adequate mucosal coating is achieved by the use of a high-density barium suspension. The type of barium used significantly affects the quality of the examination, as mucosal coating depends on the physical and chemical properties of the barium sulphate suspension. The best results are achieved using either high-density barium (200% wt/vol – i.e. E-Z-HD) or intermediate density (100% wt/vol) barium such as Baritop. Gaseous distension is required in order to distend normal folds and properly visualise the mucosa (Levine et al. 1988).

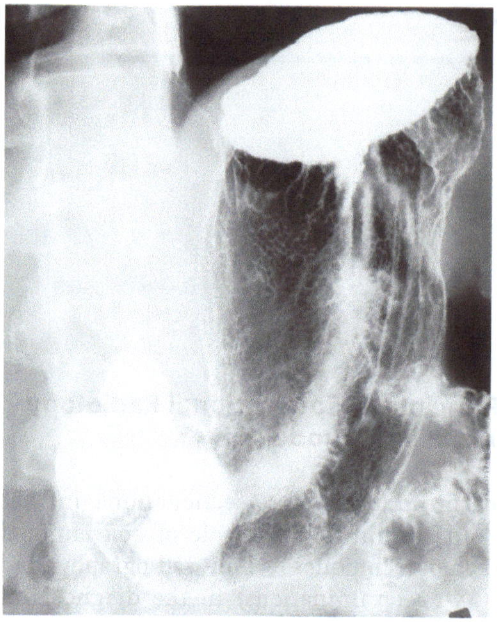

Fig. 5.1. Area gastricae: double-contrast barium meal study providing excellent detail of the mucosal surface of the stomach as evidenced by elegant demonstration of area gastricae

Spasmolytic drugs used during the double-contrast barium meal include glucagon and Buscopan (hyoscine N-butyl bromide). Glucagon produces gastric hypotonia within 45 s of the injection. It also tends to delay gastric emptying, allowing better views of the antrum and the body of the stomach. Contraindications to glucagon include pheochromocytoma and insulinoma. Buscopan produces transient hypotonia of stomach and duodenum. In addition, it causes pyloric relaxation, allowing excellent double-contrast views of the duodenum. It is contraindicated in patients with glaucoma, although its potential cardiovascular side effects are more significant (Fink and Aylward 1995).

A barium meal should be performed with reasonable speed to avoid impaired visualisation of stomach and duodenum by overlying small bowel loops. Continuous repositioning of the patient is required in order to manipulate the barium and obtain good mucosal coating before each exposure. Spot radiographs are obtained with the patient in different positions in order to assess the different portions of the stomach and duodenum. Prone compression views should always be obtained to assess anterior wall lesions of the stomach (Levine et al. 1988).

An important issue is the choice of contrast media in case of suspected gastrointestinal perforation. Barium in the mediastinal or peritoneal cavity is harmful and may cause mediastinal or peritoneal fibrosis, and the latter is particularly dangerous. Water-soluble non-ionic contrast media such as iopamidol are safer, although they lack the anatomical definition of barium. Similarly, if aspiration is suspected or likely, water-soluble, non-ionic (low osmolar) contrast media should always be used first, followed by barium if there is no obvious leak. An ionic, water-soluble contrast medium such as Gastrografin must be avoided as it can cause severe pulmonary oedema if aspirated.

In this chapter we describe conditions affecting the stomach and duodenum, the diagnosis of which can be reliably made using conventional double-contrast techniques.

5.2 Gastric Erosions and Peptic Ulceration

Gastric erosions are aphthous ulcers that do not penetrate the muscularis mucosa. They are most often related to *H. pylori* infection (Levine and Rubesin 1995). Other causative agents include alcohol, salicylates, and nonsteroidal anti-inflammatory drugs (NSAIDs). They are also seen in critically ill patients due to multiple trauma, sepsis, shock, etc. At double-contrast barium studies, gastric erosions appear as shallow small, 1–2-mm-diameter collections of barium surrounded by a radiolucent rim of oedema; an appearance mirrored at endoscopy with a haemorrhagic centre and oedematous rim (Fig. 5.2a,b) (Levine and Rubesin 1995; Sohn et al. 1995; Dheer et al. 2002). *H. pylori* infection is also related to the presence of lymphoid follicular hyperplasia, which is commonly present in patients with peptic ulcer disease (Fig. 5.3a,b) (Torigian et al. 2001).

Peptic ulcers may be found in the stomach or duodenum, and indeed lower oesophageal ulcers from gastro-oesophageal reflux disease are part of the spectrum. The majority are related to *H. pylori* infection, and the remainder due to NSAID and alcohol abuse (Levine and Rubesin 1995; Pattison et al. 1997; Gore et al. 1999). Other contributing factors include steroids, smoking, coffee, Zollinger-Ellison syndrome, delayed gastric emptying, bile reflux, and blood group O. Most gastric ulcers are benign. They are usually situated in the lesser curve and occur more commonly on the posterior wall of the antrum and body of the stomach (Fig. 5.4a–d).

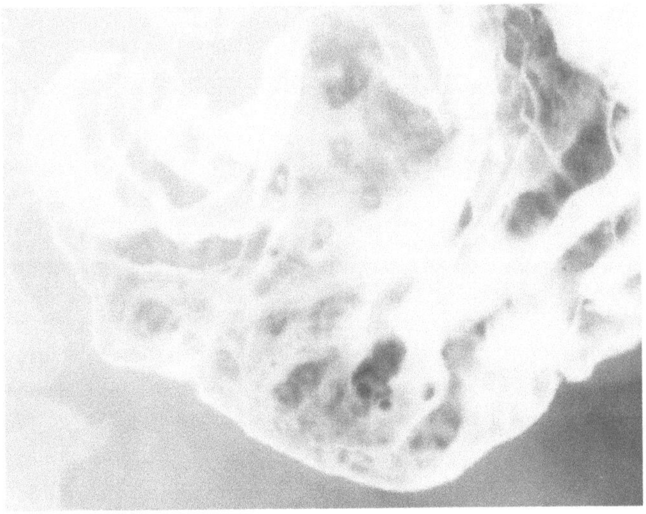

a

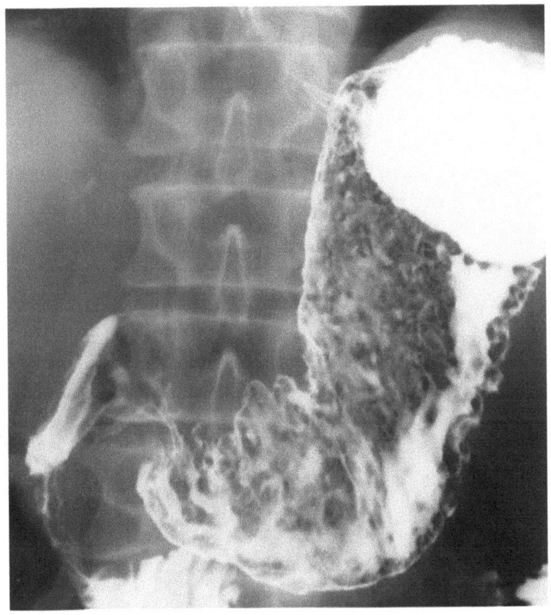

b

Fig. 5.2a,b. Erosive gastritis: double-contrast barium meal studies in two different patients demonstrating erosive gastritis involving the antrum (**a**) and the entire stomach (**b**)

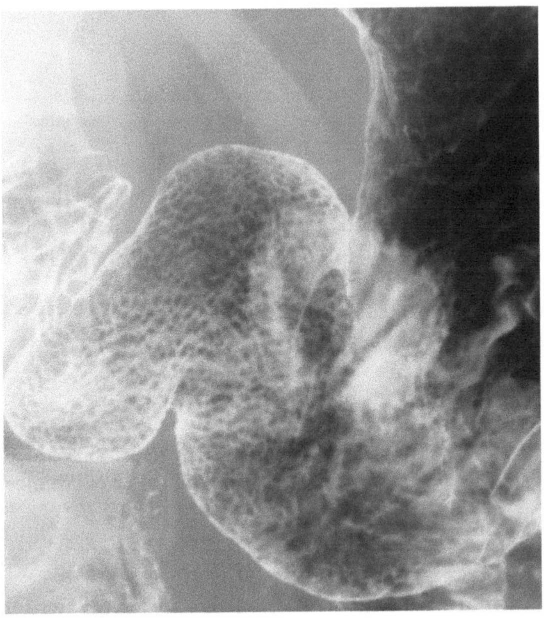

a

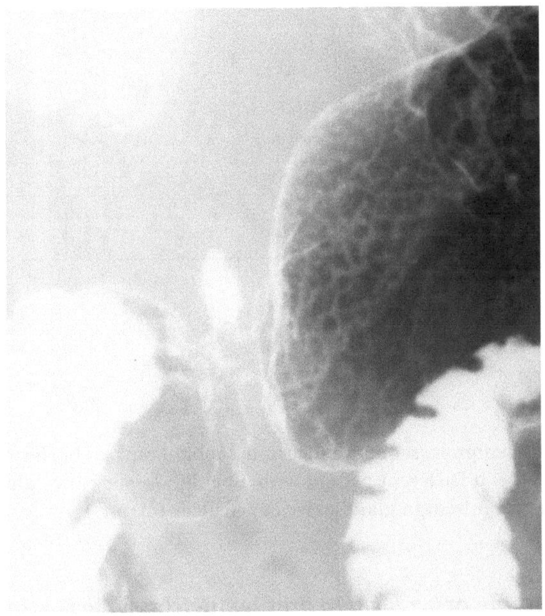

b

Fig. 5.3a,b. Follicular lymphoid hyperplasia: **a** double-contrast barium meal study shows follicular lymphoid hyperplasia involving the antrum. **b** A second patient shows antral follicular lymphoid hyperplasia with an associated pyloric ulcer

Ulcers occurring in the proximal half of the greater curve are more likely to be malignant, and those in the fundus are always so. Gastric ulcers related to NSAID and alcohol are usually seen on the greater curve of the antrum. Gastric ulcers at any location can result in major haemorrhage due to high vascularity of the stomach wall, typically from erosion of the left gastric artery in the case of lesser curve ulceration.

Whilst the majority of the peptic ulcers are diagnosed by endoscopy, they also exhibit classic appearances on double-contrast barium studies (Levine and Rubesin 1995; Pattison et al. 1997). The appearance depends on whether the ulcer is

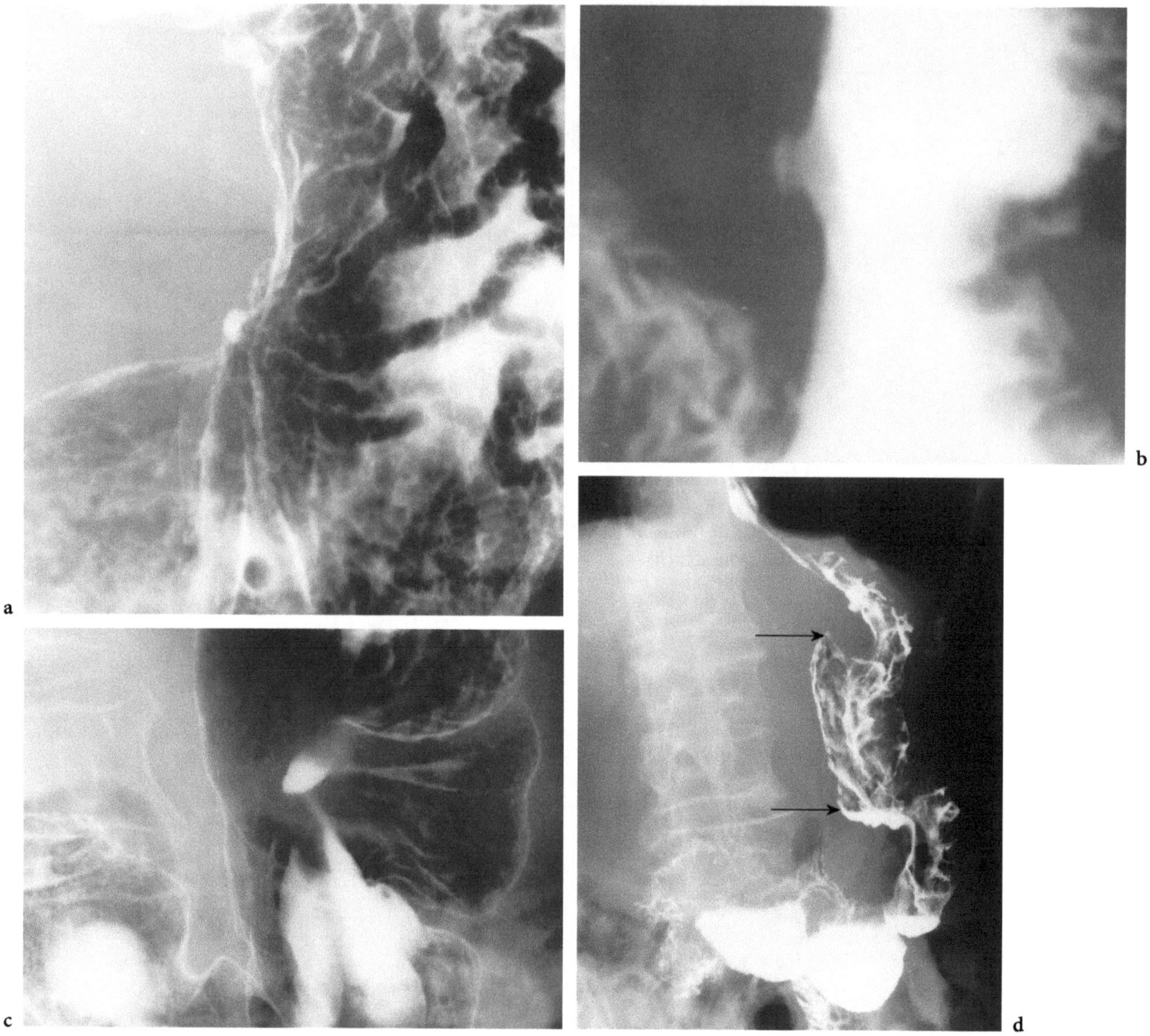

Fig. 5.4a–d. Benign lesser curve ulcers: **a** double-contrast barium meal study shows a benign penetrating lesser curve ulcer seen in profile. **b** Different patient with a benign lesser curve ulcer shows the Hampton line. **c** A benign lesser curve ulcer seen *en face*. **d** A benign giant lesser curve ulcer (*arrows*)

seen *in profile* or *en face*. *In profile*, the classic feature of a benign ulcer is the sign of penetration, i.e. the ulcer crater projects through the wall of the stomach. It may demonstrate a thin lucent line representing intact mucosa (Hampton line), or oedema around the margin may cause the so-called ulcer collar. Sometimes the oedema may be so prominent that it results in an ulcer mound which projects into the lumen of the stomach. Seen *en face* the ulcer is demonstrated as a collection of barium with folds radiating to it, and these usually fade gently as they reach the edge of the ulcer. Enlarged areae gastricae in the adjacent mucosa represent oedema and inflammation. Features in this situation which suggest a malignant gastric ulcer are an irregular ulcer crater with nodular and amputated radiating mucosal folds indicating infiltration (Fig. 5.5a). The ulcer does not project beyond gastric wall (seen *in profile*) and usually forms an acute angle with it. Rarely, a "Carman meniscus" sign is seen, which represents the ulcer crater with an associated elevated border (Fig. 5.5b).

Duodenal ulcers are virtually always benign and are three times more frequent than gastric ulcers. They are almost always (95%–100%) related to *H. pylori* infection. The majority (95%) of the duo-

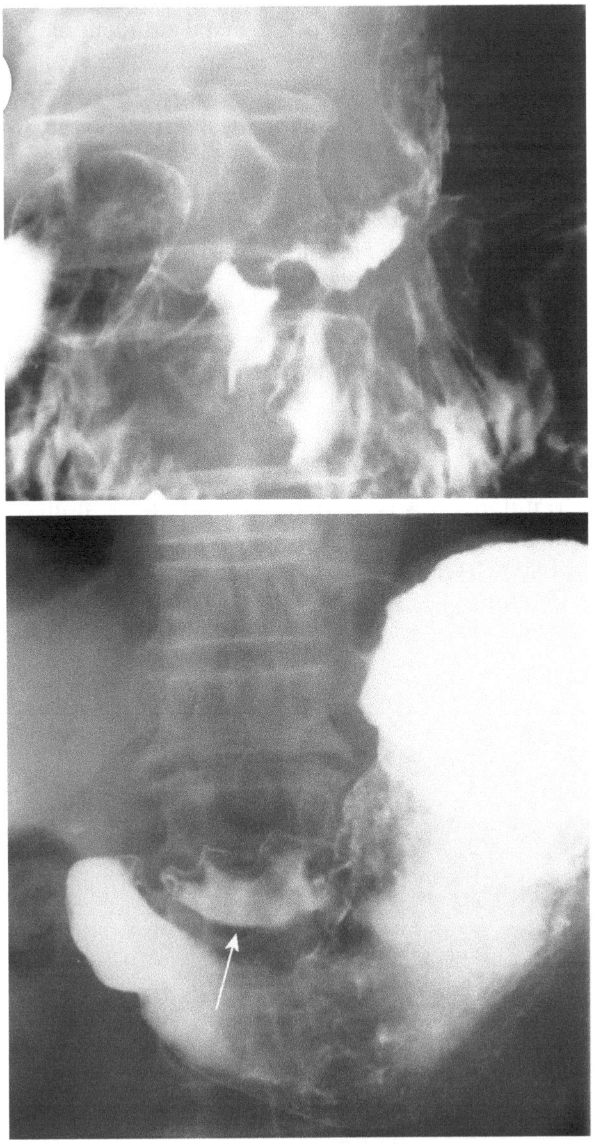
a

b

Fig. 5.5a,b. Malignant lesser curve ulcers: **a** double-contrast barium meal study shows a malignant lesser curve ulcer. Note the nodular margin and amputated radiating mucosal folds. **b** "Carman meniscus" sign (*arrow*) in a different patient with malignant lesser curve ulcer

denal ulcers occur in the duodenal bulb, 5% being postbulbar. Most bleeding duodenal ulcers are situated in the posterior wall of the duodenal bulb, where they erode the gastroduodenal artery. Duodenal ulcers may cause minimal or significant deformity to the duodenal bulb due to oedema and scarring later in the disease process (Fig. 5.6) (Levine et al. 1987; Levine and Rubesin 1995; Pattison et al. 1997; Levine et al. 2002). Giant duodenal ulcers appear as a round or ovoid collection of barium larger than 2 cm in transverse diameter. They are always located in the duodenal bulb and can replace virtually the entire bulb. Their diagnosis is often missed simply because a large ulcer can be mistaken for a normal or perhaps eccentric duodenal bulb that is not deformed and thus simulates a normal duodenal bulb contour (Fig. 5.7).

Recurrent anastomotic ulcers when they occur are usually found on the jejunal side of the anastomosis (Fig. 5.8a). In patients who present with persistent or complex duodenal or anastomotic ulcer, especially if associated with diarrhoea, weight loss, and liver metastasis, Zollinger-Ellison syndrome should be suspected. The syndrome consists of recurrent intractable peptic ulcers caused by hypergastrinaemia produced by gastrin-secreting tumours of the pancreas (75%) or duodenum (15%) (Hirschowitz 1997). Tumour localisation is critical to aid in the identification of patients with potentially respectable disease (Berg and Wolfe 1991). Twenty percent of patients have multiple endocrine neoplasia type I which includes parathyroid, pituitary, and adrenal tumours.

The barium meal may demonstrate a solitary ulcer in the duodenal bulb (90%), but atypical forms of ulceration should suggest this diagnosis.

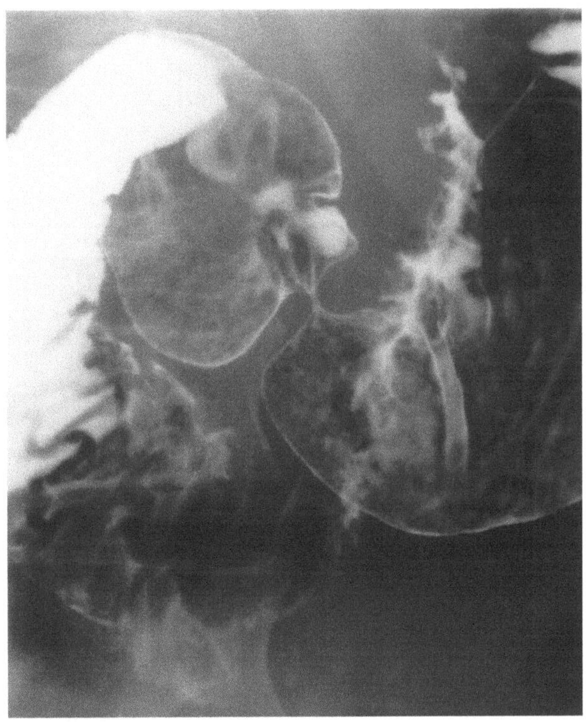

Fig. 5.6. Duodenal bulb ulcer: double-contrast barium meal study shows an ulcer at the base of the bulb with associated deformity of the superior fornix

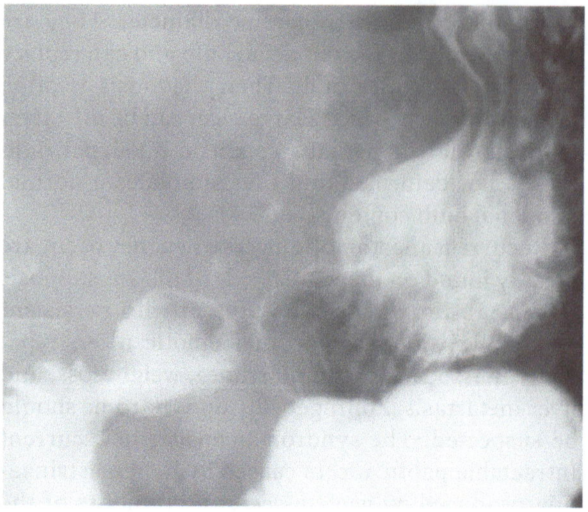

Fig. 5.7. Giant duodenal ulcer: double-contrast barium meal study shows a giant duodenal ulcer which has virtually replaced the entire duodenal bulb

These include ulcers in the distal duodenum, the presence of a double pyloric canal (Fig. 5.8b,c), or multiple recurrent anastomotic ulcers. Other findings include a non-dilated non-obstructed stomach filled with diluted barium due to hypersecretion, dilatation of the duodenum and proximal small bowel, sluggish gastric peristalsis, and thickening of gastric and duodenal folds (Berg and Wolfe 1991; Hirschowitz 1997).

5.3 Granulomatous Diseases

Granulomatous conditions that affect the stomach and duodenum include Crohn's disease and very rarely, tuberculosis, sarcoidosis, syphilis, and fungal infections.

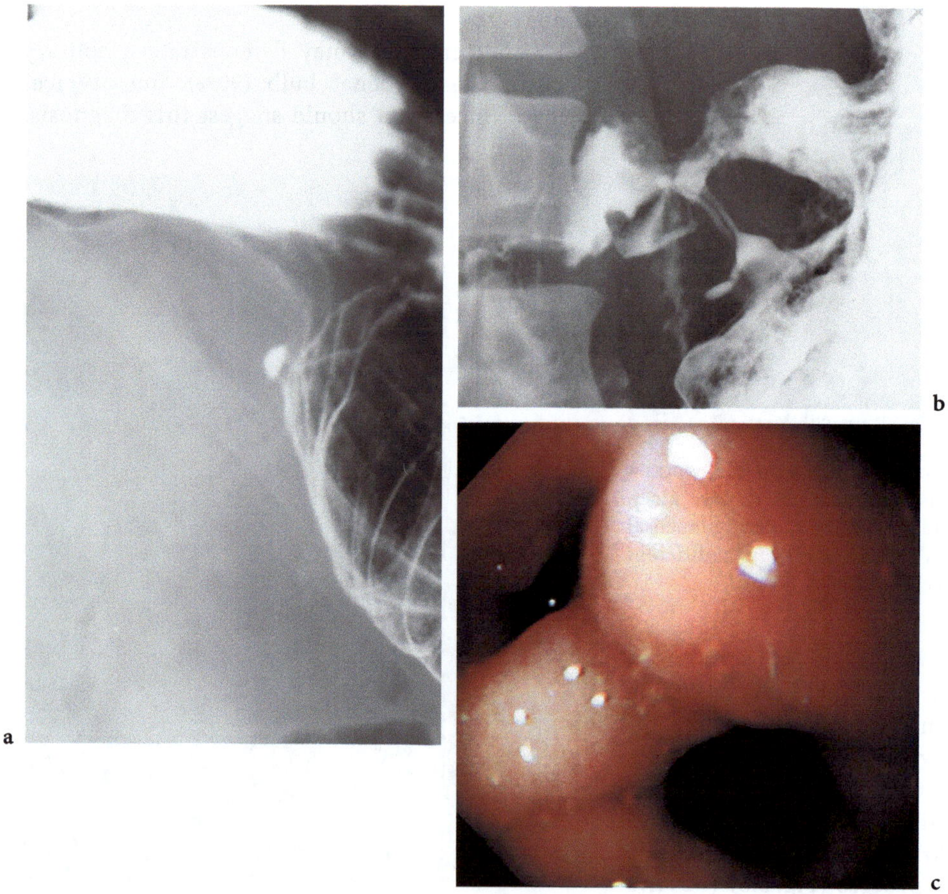

Fig. 5.8a–c. Other benign gastroduodenal ulcers: a Recurrent anastomotic ulcer in a patient with previous gastroenterostomy. Note that the ulcer is just on the jejunal side of the anastomosis. b Double pyloric canal on a double contrast barium meal in a patient with Zollinger-Ellison syndrome and c endoscopic view of a double pyloric canal (separate patient)

Crohn's disease is a chronic granulomatous inflammatory disease which can occur anywhere in the gastrointestinal tract from the mouth to the anus. The incidence of gastroduodenal involvement is between 2% and 10%, and whilst both structures are usually involved there may be solitary involvement (Fielding et al. 1970; Levine 1987). In this situation, involvement of the duodenum is more common than that of the stomach, but usually both stomach and duodenum are simultaneously involved in cases of upper gastrointestinal tract Crohn's disease (Fielding et al. 1970; Legge et al. 1970).

The antrum and/or distal body of the stomach are almost always involved in cases of gastric Crohn's disease. Endoscopy and barium meal are complementary in the diagnosis of the disease (Rutgeerts et al. 1980). Endoscopy allows better visualisation of mucosal abnormalities, whereas diminished stomach expansion and contiguity of the lesions are better demonstrated by barium meal. Aphthoid ulcers represented as punctate barium collections surrounded by a halo (Fig. 5.9a), and fissuring ulcers (Fig. 5.9b) are commonly seen during the early course of the disease. Asymmetrical thickening of the wall is another important feature and is due to a combination of inflammation and fibrosis. A cobblestone pattern is usually attributed to a combination of longitudinal and transverse ulcers and is frequently encountered in the early non-stenotic phase (Cohen 1967; Fielding et al. 1970; Legge et al. 1970; Levine 1987; Hizawa et al. 1994). Narrowing of the gastric antrum and pylorus and foreshortening of the stomach caused by scarring and fibrosis represent the late, stenotic phase of the disease (Fig. 5.9c,d). Appearances can be indistinguishable from those of scirrhous carcinoma of the stomach (Cohen 1967).

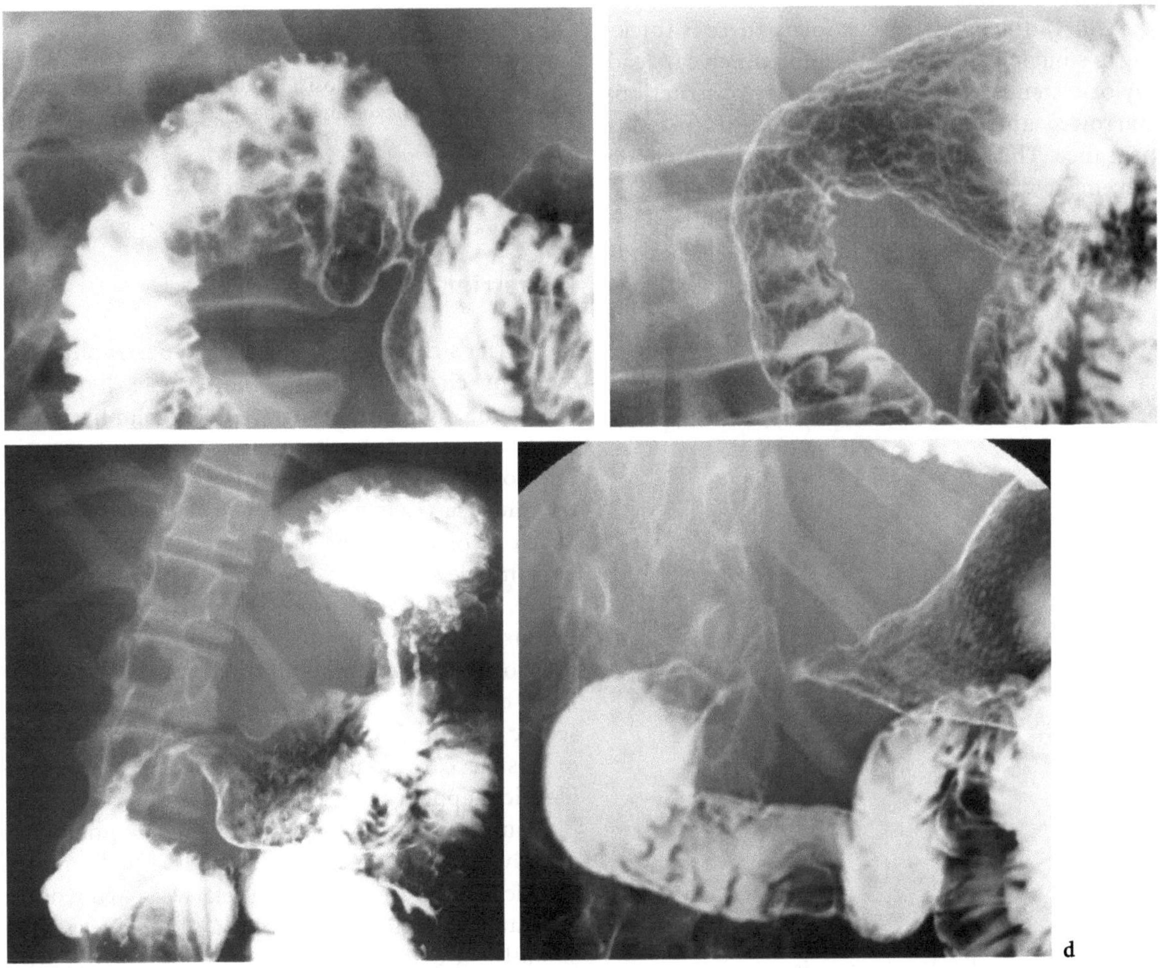

a b c d

Fig. 5.9a–d. Different stages of Crohn's disease: **a** Aphthoid ulcers. **b** Interlacing ulcers involving first and second part of the duodenum producing a cobblestone appearance. **c, d** Two different patients showing stenotic phase with narrowing of the gastric antrum and pylorus

The radiological findings of Crohn's disease of the distal duodenum are similar to those of the rest of the small bowel and terminal ileum, with skip lesions, cobble stoning, asymmetry, and in the more advanced stage of the disease, strictures causing eccentric narrowing. Other features of Crohn's disease such as sinuses, fistulas, sacculations, and inflammatory pseudopolyps are uncommon in the duodenum (Fielding et al. 1970; Levine 1987; Hizawa et al. 1994).

Primary tuberculosis of stomach and duodenum is very rare and usually develops secondary to pulmonary tuberculosis. Simultaneous involvement of the duodenum occurs in 10% of patients. There is increased incidence in patients with AIDS. The radiological appearances are classified as predominantly ulcerative or hypertrophic type (Tishler 1979; Agrawal et al. 1999). The ulcerative form is more frequent and consists of multiple large and deep ulcerations, sometimes with antral fistulas (Fig. 5.10). In the hypertrophic form, there is thickening of stomach and duodenal folds which can lead to pyloric stenosis and gastric outlet obstruction. A narrowed antrum can mimic a linitis plastica appearance. There is usually extensive lymph node involvement in the adjacent areas (Tishler 1979; Agrawal et al. 1999). Sarcoidosis and syphilis have identical appearances on conventional barium studies, both ulcerative and hypertrophic (Fig. 5.11).

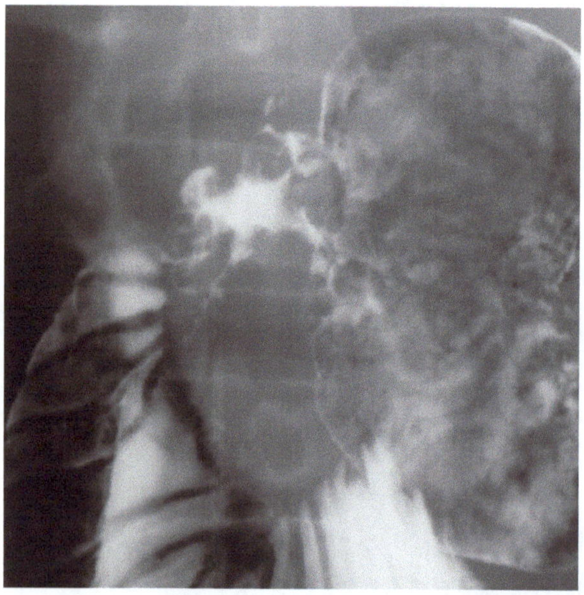

Fig. 5.10. Gastroduodenal tuberculosis: Double-contrast barium meal showing destruction of the pre-pyloric region, pylorus, and first part of the duodenum due to intramural ulcers and fibrosis

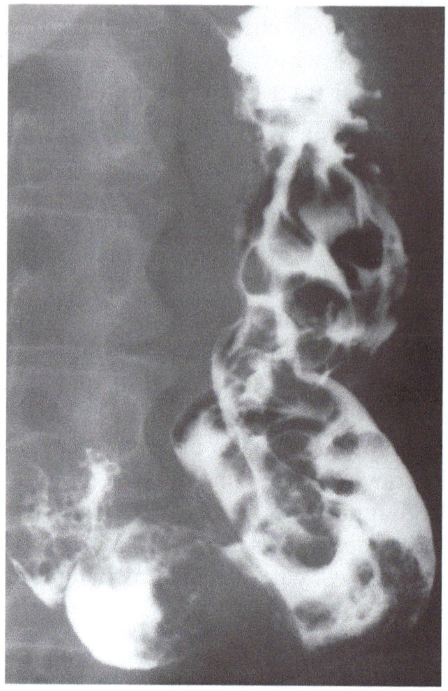

Fig. 5.11. Gastric sarcoidosis: Double-contrast barium meal shows nodular thickening of the gastric rugae in a patient with sarcoidosis

5.4 Menetrier's Disease

Menetrier's disease is a form of hypertrophic gastropathy characterised by giant rugae, hypoalbuminaemia, hypochlorhydria, and foveolar hyperplasia. Some patients have a protein-losing enteropathy due to loss of protein from the hyperplastic gastric mucosa (Reese et al. 1962). Gastric carcinoma develops in about 10% of patients. Double-contrast barium meal is the recommended imaging technique, but the diagnosis is often suggested at CT. Extensive mucus production may cause barium dilution and lead to suboptimal mucosal coating. Final diagnosis of this condition is made by endoscopic full-thickness biopsy to exclude lymphoma or gastric carcinoma, both of which can produce identical appearances on barium studies.

Double-contrast barium meal demonstrates grossly thickened, lobulated folds involving the gastric fundus and body with relative sparing of the antrum (Fig. 5.12) (Wolfsen et al. 1993). Very occasionally the disease may affect the antrum and proximal duodenum (Wu et al. 1997). Sometimes a focal area of giant rugal hypertrophy may be seen along the greater curve of the stomach which assumes a configuration of a mass-like elevation of the stomach folds, and this in particular may be mistaken for a polypoid gastric carcinoma. However, the stomach remains pliable and distensible, which helps to differentiate from the infiltrative form of gastric carcinoma.

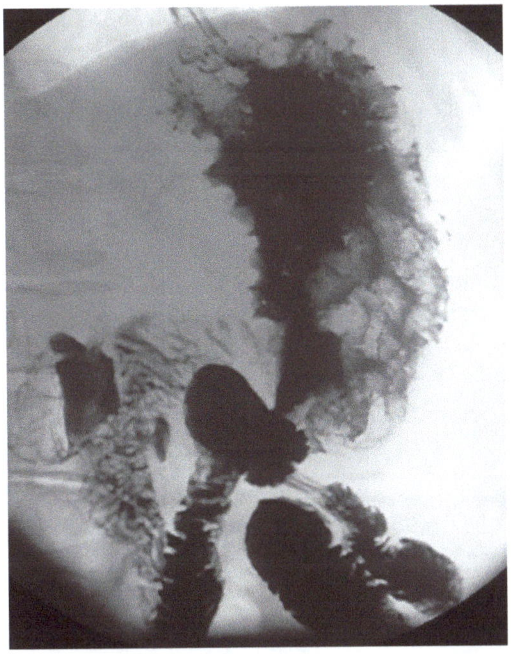

Fig. 5.12. Menetrier's disease: Giant gastric rugae in a patient with Menetrier's disease

5.5 Eosinophilic Gastroenteritis

Eosinophilic gastroenteritis is characterised by high eosinophilic count and diffuse or focal infiltration of the gastrointestinal wall by eosinophils (Wehut et al. 1976; Lee et al. 1993). The correct diagnosis is vital because of the benign nature of the disease and good response to medical therapy. The entire gastrointestinal tract may be affected, with the stomach being the most common location. Eosinophilic gastritis is almost always limited to the antrum. It may affect all the layers of the stomach wall (the muscular type) or just the mucosa (the mucosal type) (Wehut et al. 1976; Balfe 1989; Lee et al. 1993). The muscular type is characterised by thickened, rigid wall of the antrum and pylorus which can lead to pyloric obstruction, and the appearances may again mimic a scirrhous gastric cancer. The mucosal type is characterised by nodules and polyps but ulcers are rare (Wehut et al. 1976; Balfe 1989; MacCarty and Talley 1990).

Duodenal involvement is demonstrated by thickening and straightening of the mucosal folds (Fig. 13a,b).

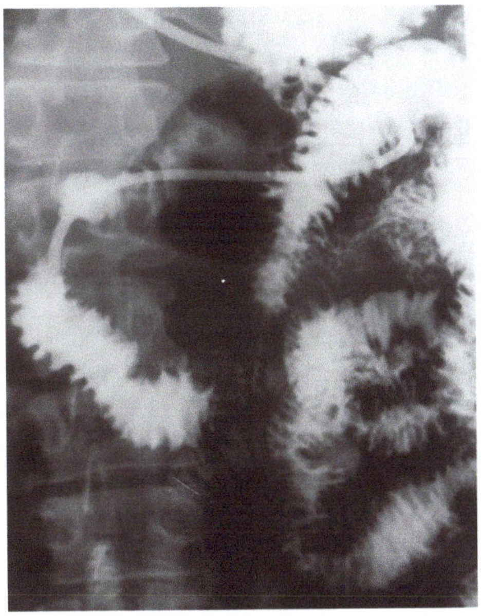

a

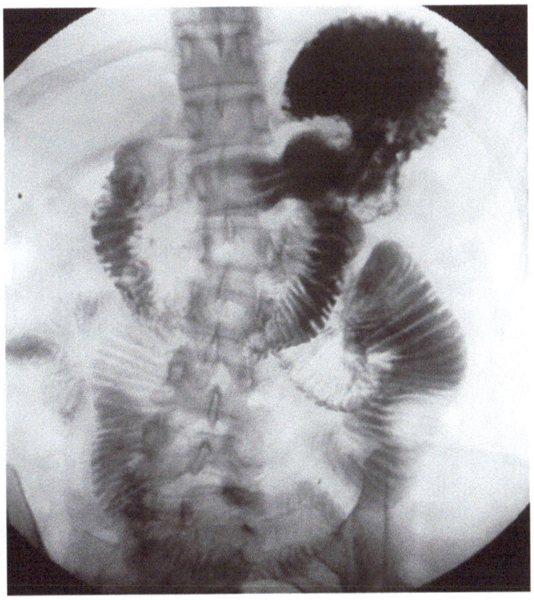

b

Fig. 5.13a,b. Eosinophilic gastroenteritis: **a** Note thickening and straightening of the folds of the descending duodenum together with jejunal involvement. **b** More prominent involvement of the distal duodenum and jejunum (different patient)

5.6 Amyloidosis

Amyloidosis is caused by interstitial deposition of a protein-polysaccharide in various organs. It can be primary (idiopathic) or secondary, associated with prolonged infections and inflammatory processes. Gastrointestinal involvement is more common in primary amyloidosis, with the stomach being affected in approximately 40% of cases. On barium meal examination, the diffuse form is characterised by a thick-walled rigid stomach with diminished or absent peristalsis simulating linitis plastica (Carlson and Breen 1986; Tada et al. 1990). The localised form mainly affects the antrum, which is irregularly narrowed due to the thickened rugae with superficial ulcerations. Very rarely, a well-defined submucosal mass which represents an amyloidoma may be demonstrated on barium meal (Carlson and Breen 1986). Changes in the duodenum are similar to those found in the rest of the small bowel with diffuse thickening of the valvulae conniventes (Fig. 5.14).

5.7 Systemic Mastocytosis

Mastocytosis is a systemic disease characterised by proliferation of mast cells in the skin and reticulo-endothelial system. The severity of the disease varies from indolent mastocytosis (most common) to aggressive lymphadenopathic mastocytosis and very rare mast cell leukaemia. Barium studies demonstrate irregular thickening of the gastric rugae and valvulae conniventes (Fig. 5.15a). Other features include small mucosal nodules or urticaria-like

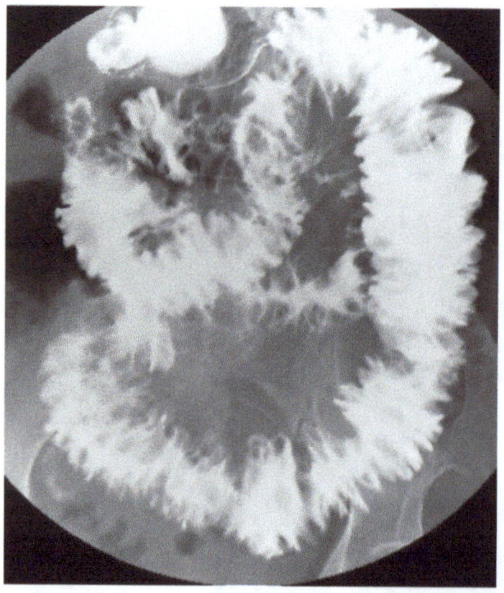

Fig. 5.14 Amyloidosis: Small bowel barium follow-through shows marked irregular thickening of the entire duodenum and jejunum

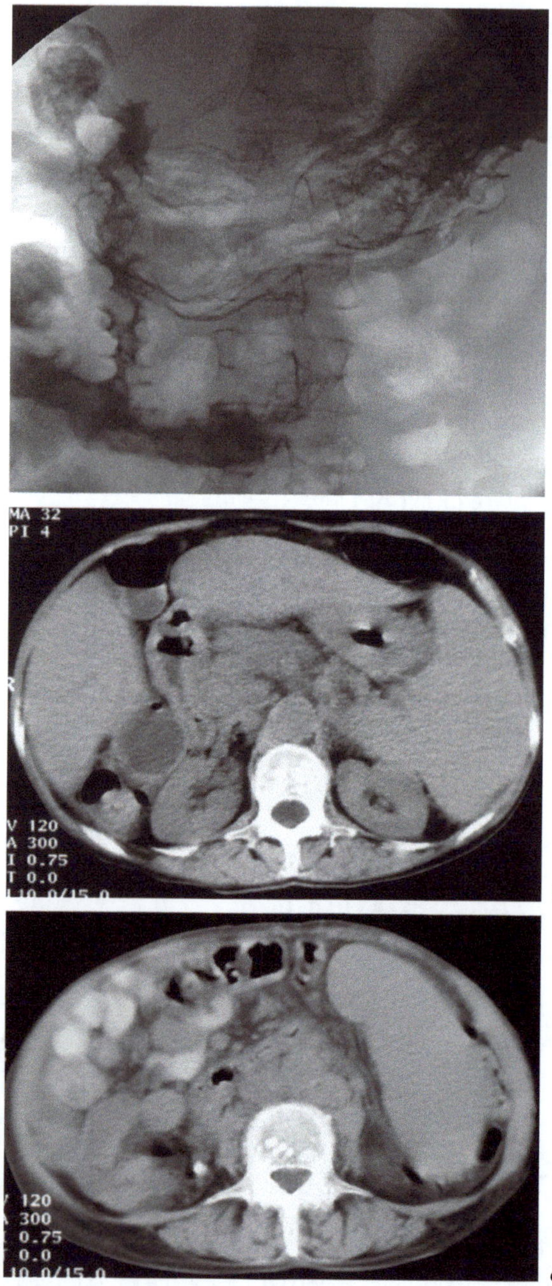

Fig. 5.15a–c. Systemic mastocytosis: **a** Small bowel barium follow-through shows marked thickening of stomach and proximal duodenal wall; **b, c** CT confirms marked thickening of the stomach and small bowel together with associated para-aortic lymphadenopathy, splenomegaly, and sclerotic vertebral lesions

lesions of gastric and intestinal mucosa. Peptic ulcer may complicate the disease due to release of histamine from the mast cells. Other associated imaging findings are hepatosplenomegaly, lymphadenopathy, and sclerotic bone lesions (Fig.5.15b,c) (Huang et al. 1987; Nguyen 2002).

5.8 Coeliac Disease

This condition is caused by an allergy to gluten, a protein found in wheat germ. Radiology does not play a role in the initial diagnosis, and in fact most small bowel series will be normal. However it is a disease with protean manifestations not necessarily related to the classic features of diarrhoea, pale stools, and weight loss. An anaemia without any other symptoms is a common presentation, as are bone lesions from osteomalacia. Patients may even present with neuropsychiatric symptoms. The radiologist needs to be aware of the small bowel changes as he may be the first to suspect the disease in an atypical presentation. Although the proximal jejunum is the area of small bowel which usually demonstrates changes, in severe cases they are often seen in the duodenum as well. Indeed distal duodenal biopsy is now regarded as a perfectly acceptable area from which the definitive diagnosis can be made. Radiological changes seen here mirror those seen in the jejunum, from loss of fold pattern to reduced number of folds (Fig. 5.16a) In

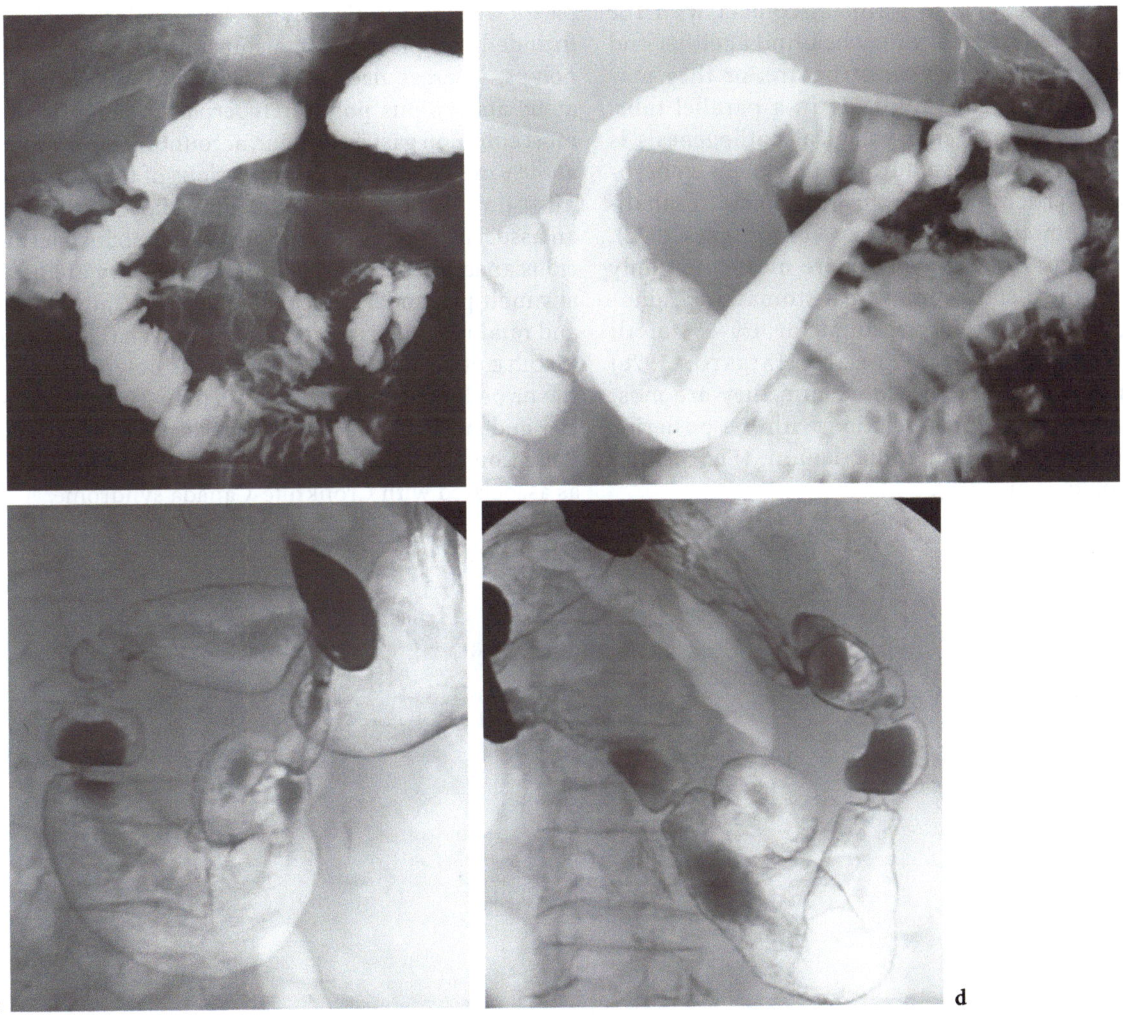

a b c d

Fig. 5.16a–d. Coeliac disease: **a** Small bowel barium follow-through shows loss of fold pattern and reduced number of folds in a patient with celiac disease. **b** Enteroclysis showing a completely featureless duodenum, so called Moulage sign. **c,d** Multiple strictures involving duodenum and jejunum in supine (**c**) and prone (**d**) position in a patient with advanced celiac disease. Images (**c**) and (**d**) courtesy of Dr. Peter Preston severe states the fold pattern may be completely lost, leading to a completely featureless duodenum sometimes referred to as the "moulage" effect (Burrows and Toye 1974) (Fig. 5.16b) Acute ulcerative jejunoileitis is a rare but serious complication of celiac disease which is thought to be a harbinger of T-cell lymphoma. It results in multiple ulcerations probably related to a vascular phenomenon. As the ulcers heal they may cause multiple strictures in the duodenum and jejunum (Fig. 5.16c,d) (Biagi et al. 1998).

5.9 Duplication Cysts

Duplication cysts can be defined as tubular or cystic structures which lie in intimate contact with the bowel wall. As such they may be blind at either end and thus result in a cystic structure, or they may be open at both ends resulting in a parallel tube. Although the exact embryological pathogenesis is unknown they may result from a persistent embryological diverticulum or from incomplete recanalisation of bowel (Gray and Skandalalakis 1972). Duplication cysts of the bowel are most commonly found in the distal ileum, whilst stomach and duodenal duplications only account for 4%–5% of all intestinal duplications (Taft and Hairston 1976) When they occur in the duodenum they are most commonly found in association with the posterior wall of the descending duodenum (Fig. 5.17a,b) (Leenders et al. 1970).

5.10 Tumours of the Stomach and Duodenum

The differentiation of many neoplastic condition affecting stomach and duodenum can be often difficult because of the overlap of radiological findings on conventional barium studies. However some tumours may exhibit characteristic radiological features pointing towards a specific diagnosis.

5.10.1 Benign Tumours of the Stomach and Duodenum

Gastric polyps are the most common benign gastric tumours. They can be broadly divided into non-neoplastic and neoplastic polyps. Non-neoplastic polyps include hyperplastic, hamartomatous, and retention polyps, whereas neoplastic polyps include adenomatous and villous polyps. Hyperplastic polyp is the most common gastric tumour, accounting for as much as 90% of all benign polypoid lesions of the stomach. They do not have malignant potential but there is an association with chronic atrophic gastritis, pernicious anaemia, and gastric carcinoma. They are usually multiple, under 1 cm in diameter, typically sessile and randomly distributed within stomach (Fig. 18a,b) (Stolte et al. 1994). Hamartomatous polyps are sessile or pedunculated, usually less than 2 cm in diameter and are associated with Peutz-Jeghers syndrome. Retention or inflammatory polyps are very rare such as associated with Cronkhite-Canada syndrome.

a

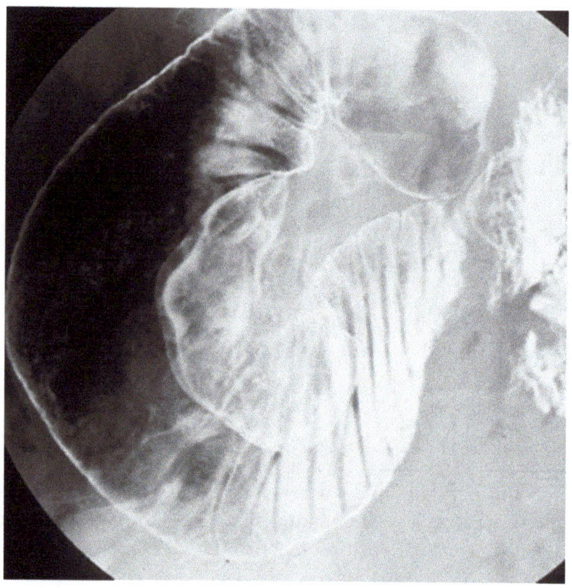

b

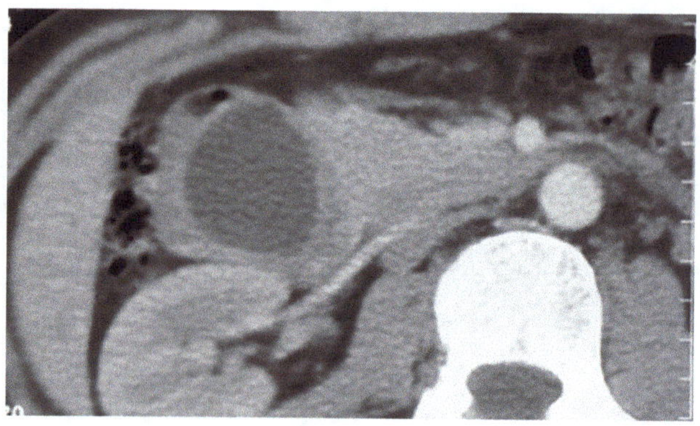

Fig. 5.17a,b. Duodenal duplication cyst: **a** Barium study showing a relatively smooth impression arising from the medial wall of the descending duodenum extending around the inferior duodenal flexure. **b** CT of the same patient confirms the fluid nature of the cyst

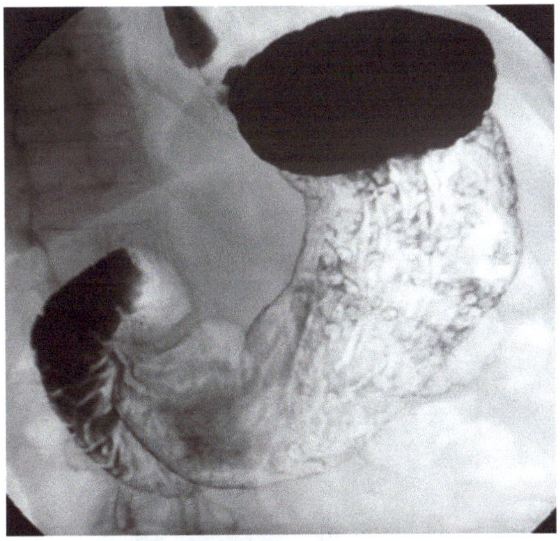

a

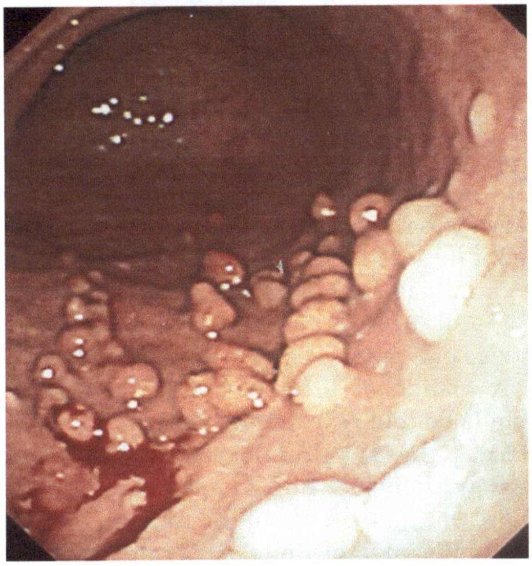

b

Fig. 5.18a,b. Multiple gastric polyps: **a** Double-contrast barium meal showing multiple filling defects in the stomach due to hyperplastic polyps and (**b**) endoscopic view of hyperplastic polyps in a different patient

Adenomatous and villous polyps are important due to their potential for malignant transformation. Adenomatous polyps coexist with gastric carcinoma in 35% of cases and malignancy is detected histologically in 50% of adenomas larger than 2 cm (Tomasulo 1971). Adenomas are usually solitary, can be broad base or pedunculate and have a lobulated appearance with a smooth or irregular contour. They are most commonly found in the antrum. On double-contrast barium meal they have smooth circular outline, with the stalk seen *en face* overlying the head of the polyp – the "Mexican hat sign" (Fig. 5.19) (Ming 1976; Gordon et al. 1980). Villous polyps carry a very high risk for malignancy. They are characterised by numerous frond-like projections which give them a typical bubbly appearance on double-contrast barium meal.

Gastric lipoma is rare and usually appears as a smooth submucosal mass (Fig. 5.20) (Maderal et al. 1984). Brunner gland hamartomas are typically found in the first part of the duodenum and at barium study produce a characteristic "cobblestone" appearance due to multiple small nodules. They can also act as a lead point for intussusception (Fig. 5.21a,b) (Park et al. 1999).

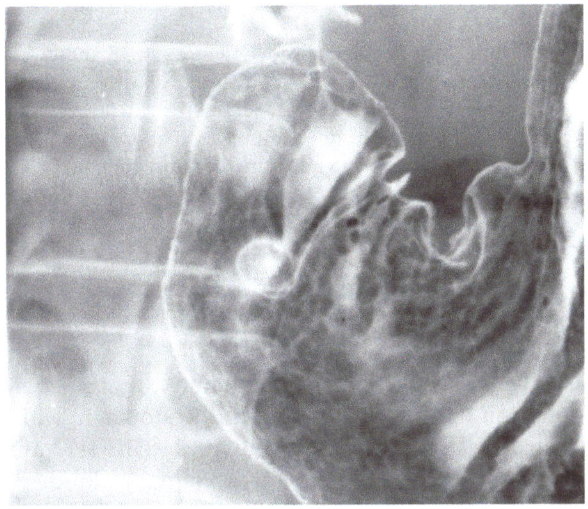

Fig. 5.19. Gastric adenoma: Double-contrast barium meal shows an adenoma as seen *en face* – "Mexican hat sign"

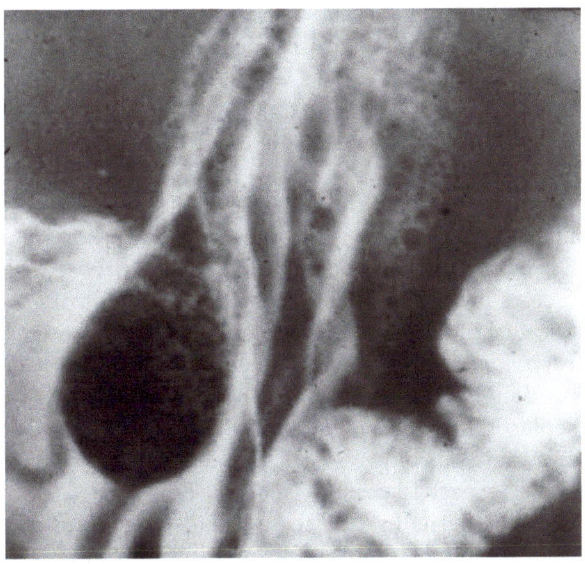

Fig. 5.20. Gastric lipoma: Double-contrast barium meal shows a perfectly smooth submucosal mass due to a lipoma

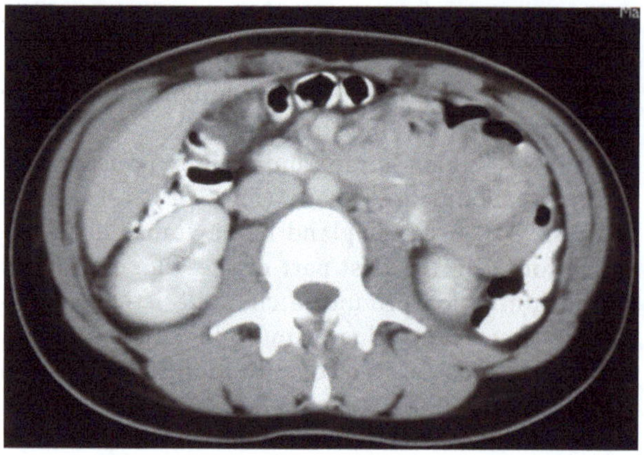
a

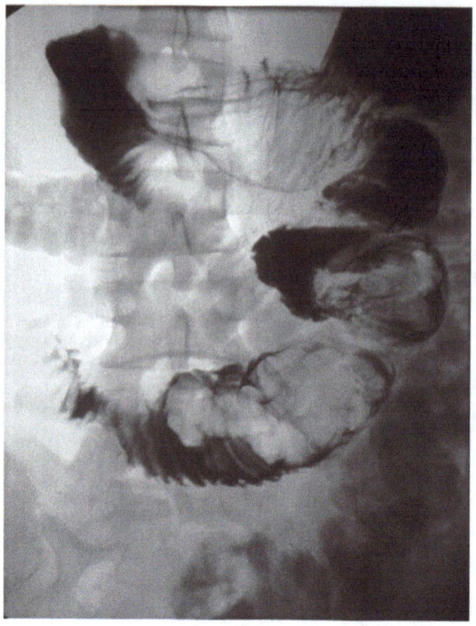
b

Fig. 5.21a,b. Brunner's gland adenoma: **a** CECT shows an intussusception in the distal duodenum. **b** Barium follow-through performed later shows a large filling defect arising from the first part of the duodenum which at operation was confirmed as being due to a Brunner's gland adenoma

5.10.2 Malignant Tumours of the Stomach and Duodenum

Gastric carcinoma and lymphoma are the most common malignant tumours of the stomach, while gastrointestinal stromal tumours (GISTs) and metastasis are relatively rare. Primary duodenal neoplasms are rare, carcinoma being the most frequent. The duodenum may be invaded by carcinomas from other adjacent organs such as colon, pancreas, right kidney, etc. Each of these entities has a variable appearance with some overlap of radiographic signs at barium studies.

5.10.2.1 Gastric Carcinoma

Gastric adenocarcinoma is the most common primary gastric tumour and the third most common GI malignancy. Exposure to environmental risk factors has a major role in the development of gastric carcinoma. There is a positive association with *H. pylori* and pernicious anaemia. The diagnosis by double-contrast barium meal has been largely replaced by endoscopy with the added advantage of simultaneous biopsy.

Early gastric cancer is defined as gastric carcinoma that is limited to the mucosa and submucosa with or without associated lymphadenopathy (Gore et al. 1997). At double-contrast barium meal early gastric cancer appears as an elevated polypoid lesion (type I), superficial plaque-like lesion (type II), or shallow irregular ulcer with adjacent nodular mucosa and associated amputation of radiating folds (type III) (Gold et al. 1984).

Advanced gastric cancer has a number of different appearances on barium studies. It may be ulcerative, polypoid, or infiltrative (Gore et al. 1997). A malignant ulcer has irregular borders with lobulated folds converging towards the crater (Fig. 5.5a). Malignant ulcers located on the anterior wall appear as double ring shadows with the outer ring representing the edge of the tumour, and the inner ring the edge of the ulcer. Prone compression views show filling of the ulcer crater within a discrete tumour. In profile, the ulcer often has an intraluminal location and demonstrates an abrupt acute angle at its margin with normal mucosa. Malignant ulcers located along the lesser curve of antrum or body appear as broad flat lesions with central ulceration and elevated margins – Carman-Kirkland meniscus complex (Fig. 5.5b). Polypoid cancer shows as a smooth or lobulated filling defect (Fig. 5.22a). If this is located in the antrum it can prolapse into the duodenum. The infiltrative form (5%–15%) usually arises near the pylorus and extends upwards. It appears as thickened irregular folds with increased nodularity and spiculations with or without ulceration. Sometimes, the stomach can be diffusely infiltrated by a scirrhous tumour resulting in a linitis plastica or "leather bottle" appearance (Fig. 5.22b) (Low et al. 1994; Gore et al. 1997).

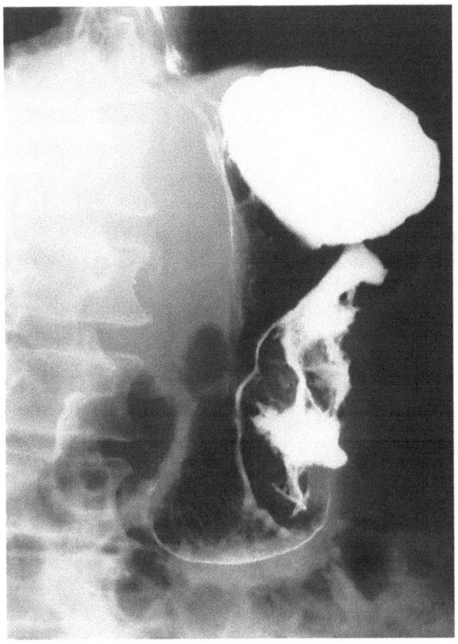

a

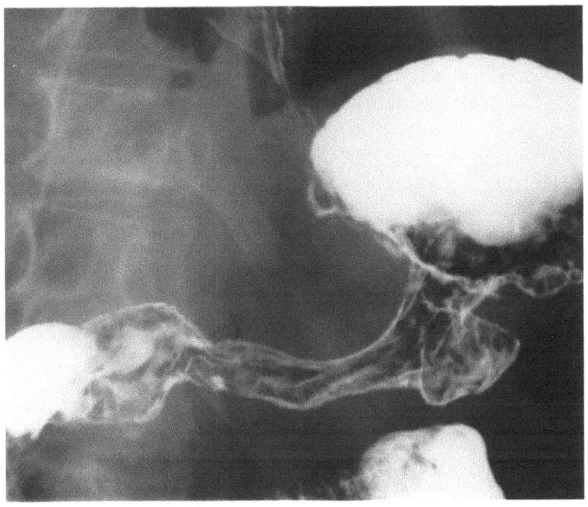

b

Fig. 5.22 Gastric carcinoma: **a** Double-contrast barium meal shows an ulcerated, polypoid greater curve tumour. **b** Infiltrative gastric carcinoma producing a linitis plastica or "leather bottle appearance"

5.10.2.2
Gastric Lymphoma

Gastric lymphoma accounts for 1%–5% of all gastric malignancies and 50% of all gastrointestinal lymphomas (Park et al. 1999). Primary gastric lymphoma occurs in 10% of cases. They are mostly non-Hodgkin lymphomas with histiocytic cell type, but the stomach is the most common site of extra-nodal Hodgkin disease. There is no anatomic predilection but when the antrum is involved duodenum is often affected. Gastric involvement may also be secondary to direct extension from involved adjacent lymph nodes or organs such as pancreas, spleen, etc.

At double-contrast barium meal gastric lymphoma may demonstrate an infiltrative appearance with thickened broad tortuous mucosal folds, a circumscribed mass growing inside or outside the lumen of the stomach, or large irregular ulcers (Sherrick et al. 1965; Menuck 1976). It may appear identical to gastric carcinoma, although some radiologic features such as preservation of flexibility of gastric wall and infrequent luminal narrowing would favour the diagnosis of lymphoma (Fig. 5.23a–c) (Park et al. 1999). The stomach wall thickening is more significant and homogeneous in lymphoma than in adenocarcinoma.

Low-grade gastric mucosa-associated lymphoid tissue (MALT) lymphoma accounts for the majority of primary gastric lymphomas (50%–72%) (Yoo et al. 1998). They are associated with *H. pylori* infection and are shown to regress completely following appropriate treatment for *H. pylori* infection. Double-contrast upper gastrointestinal studies demonstrate rounded, often confluent nodules of varying size which can be difficult to distinguish from gastritis or leukaemic infiltration (Levine et al. 1996; Yoo et al. 1998; Brown et al. 2000). Depressed lesions and thickened fold may also be seen (see Chapter 6.1 for illustrations).

5.10.2.3
Gastrointestinal Stromal Tumour

Gastrointestinal stromal tumour (GIST) is a submucosal mesenchymal tumour that originates from smooth muscle cells. They may occur anywhere in the GI tract, although the stomach is the most common site. These tumours may ulcerate due to underlying necrosis, resulting in significant bleeding. Double-contrast barium meal demonstrates a round, endophytic submucosal mass with borders forming sharp borders to the adjacent mucosa (Fig. 5.24a–c). Seen *en face*, the preservation of normal area gastrica pattern over the filling defect confirms the presence of normal mucosa and the extramucosal location of the lesion. An ulcer appears as a central collection of barium within a smooth or lobulated mass (Davies 1978; Miettinen et al. 2002). Malignancy should be strongly considered if the mass is greater than 5 cm. When these tumours are primarily exophytic, they may produce bizarre appearances such as cavitating masses which communicate with the bowel lumen (Fig. 5.25a–d) (Beggs and Freeman 1982).

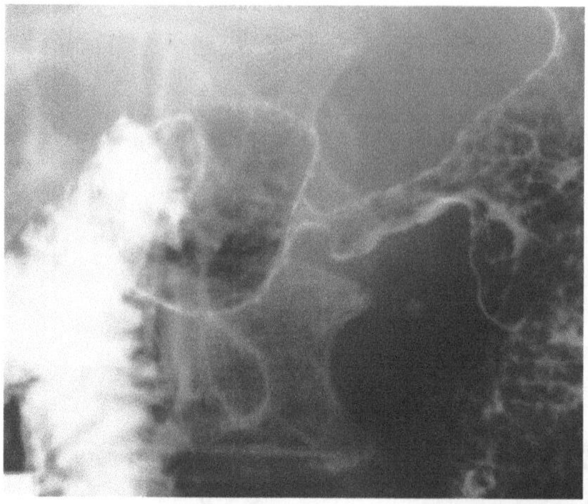
a

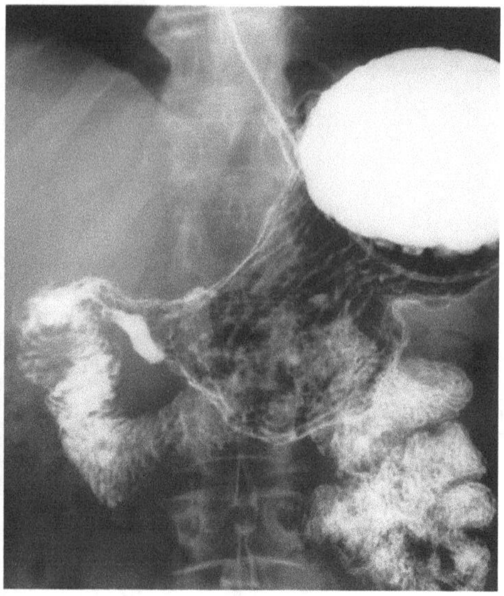
b

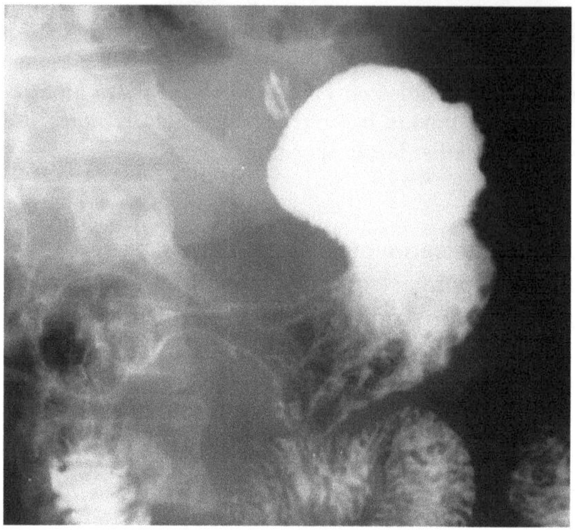
c

Fig. 5.23a–c. Gastric antral infiltration: Double-contrast barium meal in three different patients showing similar appearances of antral and pyloric infiltration due to (**a**) lymphoma, (**b**) primary gastric carcinoma and (**c**) metastasis from invasive lobular carcinoma of the breast. Note in this patient the presence of sclerotic metastasis involving multiple vertebral bodies

5.10.2.4 Metastasis to the Stomach

Gastric metastases are uncommon. They may appear as a solitary mass (50%), multiple nodules (30%), or diffuse infiltrative involvement of the stomach. The most common primary tumours that metastasize to the stomach are malignant melanoma, breast, lung, colon, and secondary lymphomas. At double-contrast barium meal, melanoma metastases appear as multiple umbilicated nodules – "bull's-eye" appearances. Kaposi's sarcoma can produce identical appearances (Dutta and Costa 1979). Metastases from invasive lobular breast carcinoma produce a linitis plastica-type appearance typically involving the antrum (Fig. 5.23c), whereas those from invasive ductal carcinoma tend to be nodular (Harake et al. 2001). Tumours of adjacent organs can produce an extrinsic mass effect on the stomach (Fig. 5.26).

5.10.2.5 Primary Carcinoma of the Duodenum

The commonest duodenal malignancy is adenocarcinoma (75%) followed by leiomyosarcoma, carcinoid, and lymphoma. They are usually located in the second or third part of the duodenum and can be divided into two subgroups: adenocarcinoma of the duodenum which may cause obstruction and bleeding, and ampullary carcinoma which may present with obstructive jaundice. In addition, periampullary tumours occur which may be associated with Peutz-Jeghers and familiar adenomatous polyposis (FAP) syndromes. Non-papillary carcinomas appear as annular (Fig. 5.27), polypoid, or ulcerative lesions on barium studies (Nix 1980), whilst ampullary tumours demonstrate an enlarged papilla with irregular borders and occasional ulcerations (Bradford et al. 2000). Leiomyosarcomas are large

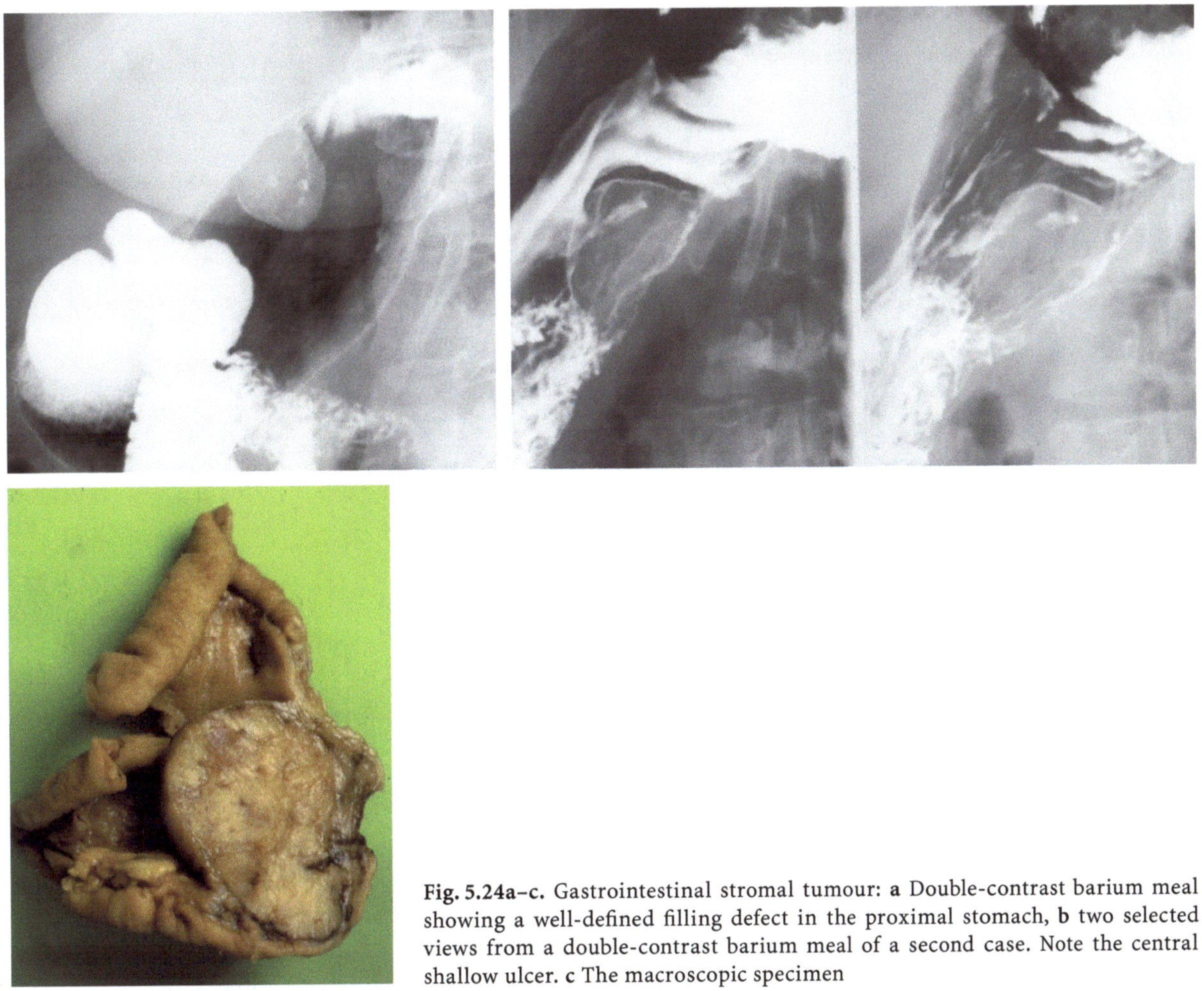

Fig. 5.24a–c. Gastrointestinal stromal tumour: **a** Double-contrast barium meal showing a well-defined filling defect in the proximal stomach, **b** two selected views from a double-contrast barium meal of a second case. Note the central shallow ulcer. **c** The macroscopic specimen

tumours that appear as exo/endophytic ulcerative mass reaching up to 20 cm in diameter. Lymphomas are rare, accounting for 2% of duodenal malignancies. They usually demonstrate marked wall thickening and bulky periduodenal lymphadenopathy.

5.10.2.6
Secondary Involvement of the Duodenum

The duodenum may be involved by direct extension of malignant neoplasms from adjacent organs or be the site of hematogenous metastases. Both gastric lymphoma and carcinoma can spread by direct infiltration through the mucosa or submucosa or less frequently through lymphatic channels via the submucosal layer (Cho et al. 1996). Radiographically detectable spread is seen in 5%–25% of adenocarcinomas and up to 40% of lymphomas, but, if present is more likely to be due to adenocarcinoma as this is much more common than gastric lymphoma (Cho et al. 1996).

Direct invasion from pancreatic head carcinoma causes widening of the duodenal C loop and irregularity of the inner wall of the second part of the duodenum due to serosal infiltration – the reversed "3" sign of Frostberg (Frostberg 1938). Direct invasion may also result in irregular ulceration of the descending duodenum (Fig. 5.28). Carcinoma of the tail of pancreas can occasionally invade the duodenum and may lead to bowel obstruction (Mani et al. 1966). Carcinoma of the transverse colon, especially hepatic flexure, can infiltrate the duodenum. Double-contrast barium meal may show mucosal irregularity, duodenal luminal narrowing, and the presence of duodeno-colic fistulae (Treitel et al. 1970). Less frequently, carcinoma of the right kidney or gallbladder carcinoma can invade the duodenum (Khilnani et al. 1962). Haematogenous metastases to the duodenum are very rare.

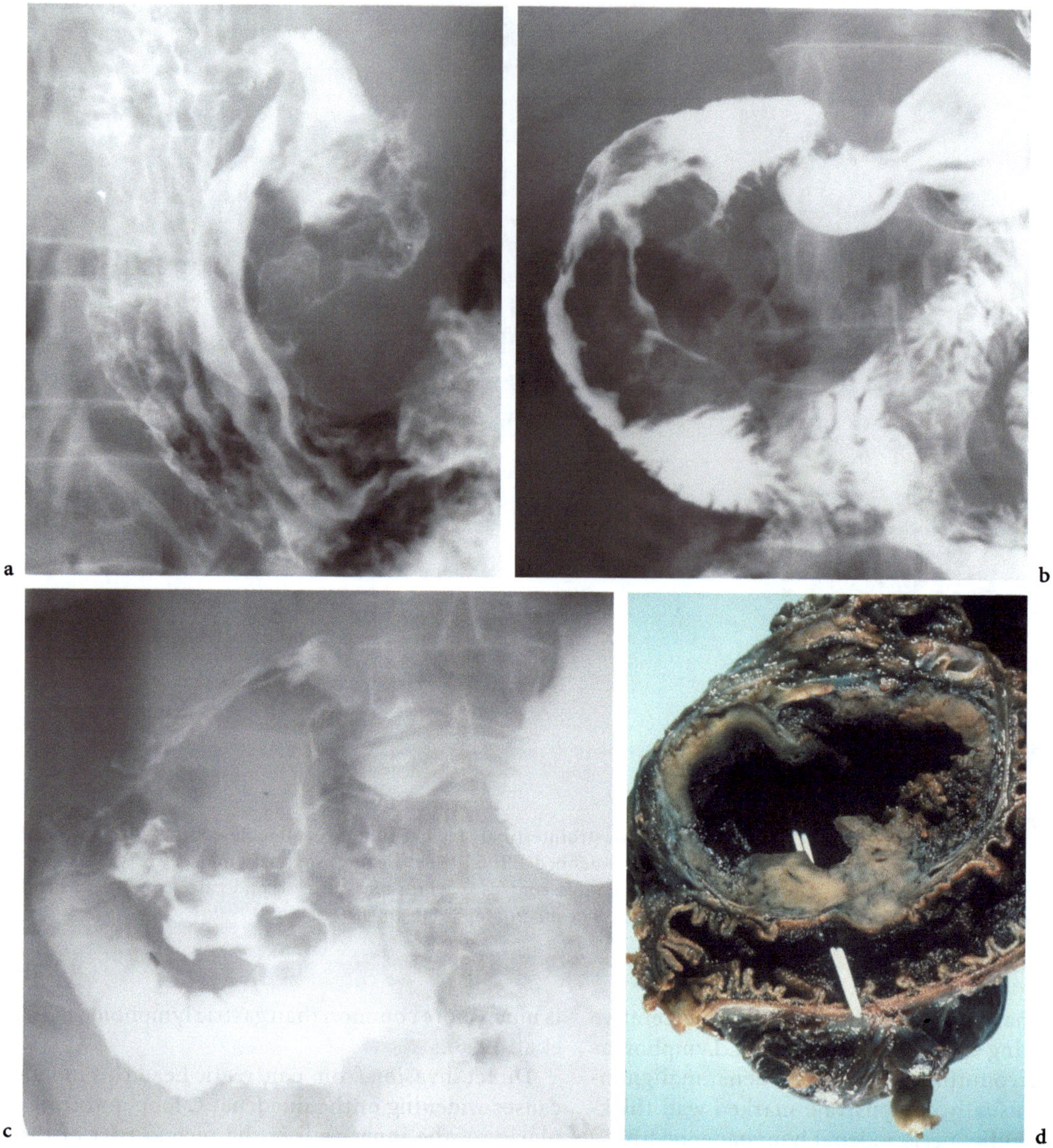

Fig. 5.25a–d. Malignant GIST tumour: **a** Double-contrast barium meal showing a large excavating mass arising from the lesser curve of the stomach. Note the large soft tissue nodules. **b** A large irregular filling defect which is partly cavitating filling the whole of the medial aspect of the duodenum due to a recurrent leiomyosarcoma. **c** A large irregular excavating mass which has filled the whole of the region of the head of the pancreas due to an exophytic GIST, the cavity of which is in communication with the third part of the duodenum. **d** Macroscopic specimen with probes outlining the fistulous tract. (with permission from Beggs and Freeman)

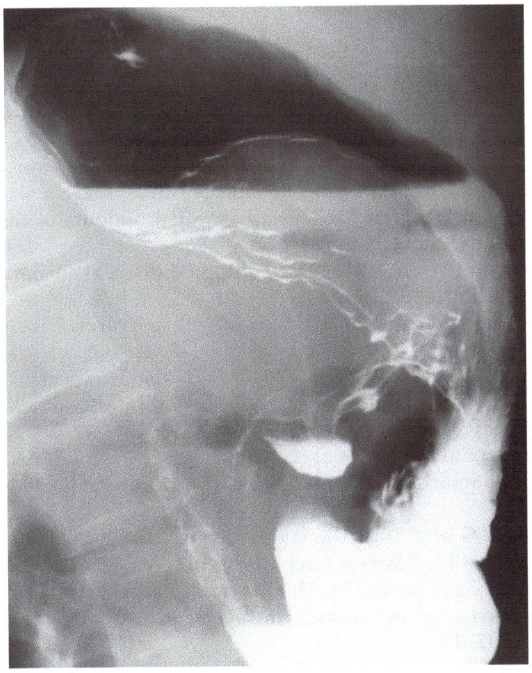

Fig. 5.26 Recurrent left renal carcinoma: Double-contrast barium meal showing extrinsic compression and displacement of the stomach due to recurrent left renal carcinoma

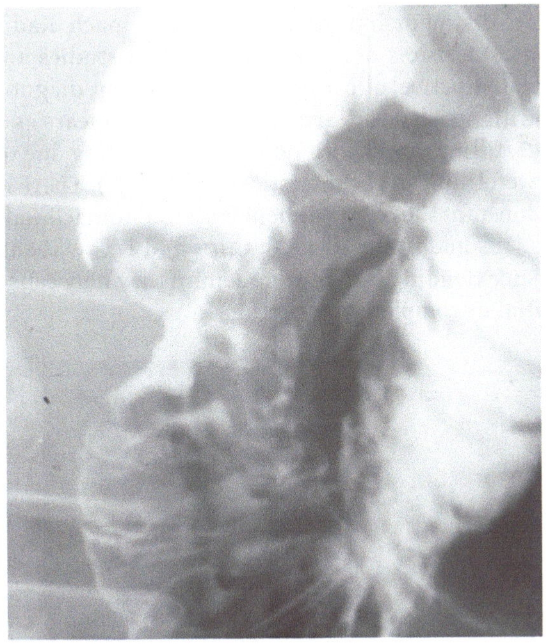

Fig. 5.27 Primary peri-ampullary carcinoma of the duodenum: Double-contrast barium meal shows a peri-ampullary carcinoma of the duodenum showing as an "apple core"-like lesion

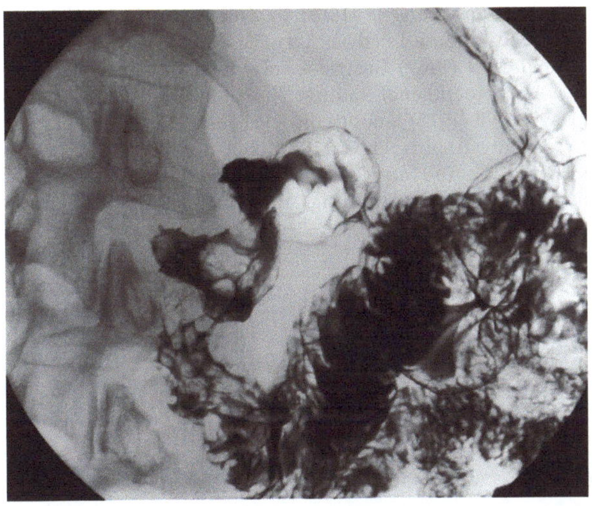

Fig. 5.28 Secondary involvement of the duodenum: Double-contrast barium meal shows malignant infiltration of the second part of the duodenum due to direct extension of pancreatic carcinoma. This has eroded through the wall of the duodenum to produce a malignant-looking ulcer. Note the extensive nodular change around the ulcer due to tumour infiltration

5.11 Bezoars

A bezoar is a mass of foreign matter composed of retained ingested material in the stomach and small bowel. While most bezoars occur in the stomach, they also have been found in the duodenum. They can be classified into two main types: phytobezoars and trichobezoars. Phytobezoars are caused by ingestion of poorly digested fibres, most commonly orange, persimmon skin, and seeds. Predisposing conditions to phytobezoars include previous gastric surgery such as Billroth I and II operations, especially if complemented by a vagotomy procedure (Fig. 5.29) (Szemes and Amberg 1968). These may lead to decreased motility and digestive ability of the remaining portion of the stomach, thus impairing gastric emptying. Trichobezoars consist of large quantity of ingested hair firmly matted together, forming an intraluminal cast in the stomach and frequently extending into the duodenum (Choi and Kang 1988). These are found most commonly in young psychiatric patients, almost exclusively females.

A plain abdominal radiograph demonstrates a mottled pattern in the stomach which can be difficult to distinguish from a food-filled stomach. Radiological features of bezoars on contrast studies are very distinctive, allowing a more confident diagnosis with no need for further imaging. It appears as a large, filling defect with poor barium coating due to uneven filling of the interstices (Fig. 30a,b). There is no constant site of attachment with the stomach wall (Szemes and Amberg 1968; Choi and Kang 1988). When extending into the duodenum they may cause partial or complete obstruction.

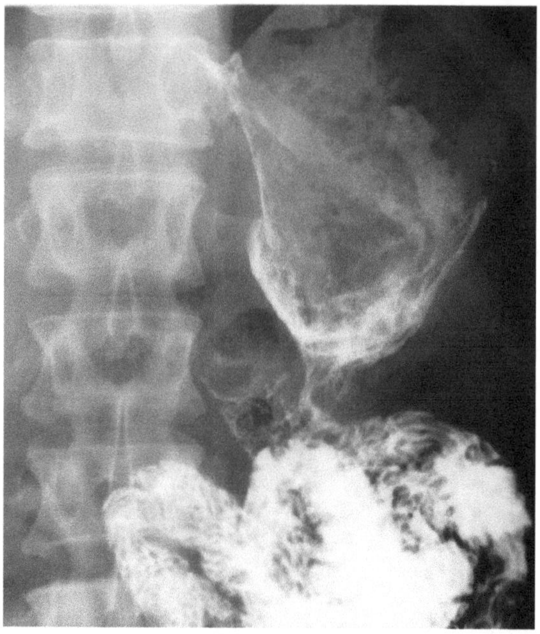

Fig. 5.29 Phytobezoar: double-contrast barium meal shows a phytobezoar in a patient with previous partial gastrectomy

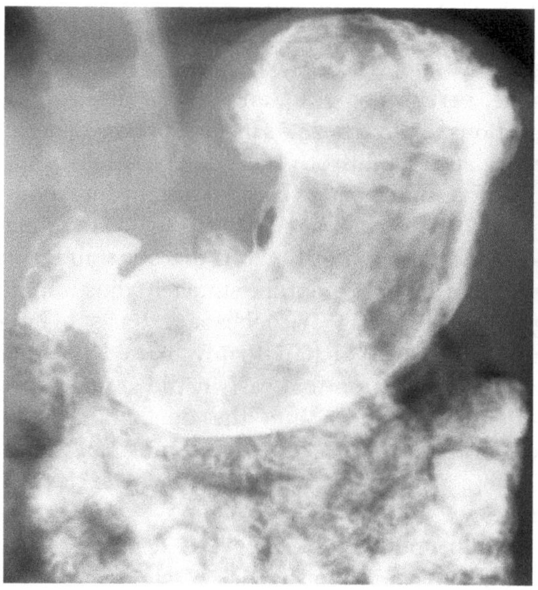

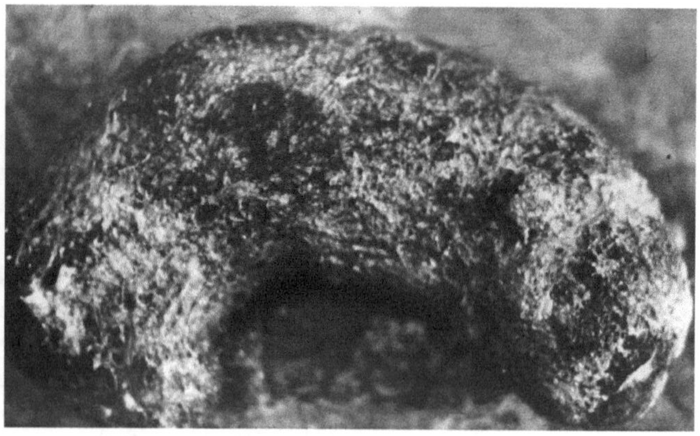

Fig. 5.30a,b. Trichobezoar: **a** double-contrast barium meal showing a large filling defect occupying the whole lumen of the stomach and **b** photograph of the removed trichobezoar

References

Agrawal S, Shetty SV et al (1999) Primary hypertrophic tuberculosis of the pyloroduodenal area: report of 2 cases. J Postgrad Med 45(1):10–12

Balfe DM (1989) General diagnosis case of the day. Eosinophilic gastritis. AJR Am J Roentgenol 152(6):1322

Beggs I and Freeman AH (1982) Excavated tumours of the gut. Clin Radiol 33(5):523–527

Berg CL and Wolfe MM (1991) Zollinger-Ellison syndrome. Med Clin North Am 75(4):903–921

Biagi F, Poggioli G et al (1998) Intestinal strictures. Lancet 352(9131):876

Bradford D, Levine MS et al (2000) Early duodenal cancer: detection on double-contrast upper gastrointestinal radiography. AJR Am J Roentgenol 174(6):1564–1566

Brown JA, Carson BW et al (2000) Low grade gastric MALT Lymphoma: radiographic findings. Clin Radiol 55(5):384–389

Burrows FG and Toye DK (1974) Coeliac disease. Barium studies. Clin Gastroenterol 3(1):91–107

Carlson HC and Breen JF (1986) Amyloidosis and plasma cell dyscrasias: gastrointestinal involvement. Semin Roentgenol 21(2):128–138

Charagundla SR, Levine MS et al (2001) Visualization of areae gastricae on double-contrast upper gastrointestinal radiography: relationship to age of patients. AJR Am J Roentgenol 177(1):61–63

Cho KC, Baker SR et al (1996) Transpyloric spread of gastric tumors: comparison of adenocarcinoma and lymphoma. AJR Am J Roentgenol 167(2):467–469

Choi SO and Kang JS (1988) Gastrointestinal phytobezoars in childhood. J Pediatr Surg 23(4):338–341

Cohen WN (1967) Gastric involvement in Crohn's disease. Am J Roentgenol Radium Ther Nucl Med 101(2):425–430

Davies PM (1978) Smooth muscle tumours of the upper gastrointestinal tract. Clin Radiol 29(4):407–414

Dheer S, Levine MS et al (2002) Radiographically diagnosed antral gastritis: findings in patients with and without

Helicobacter pylori infection. Br J Radiol 75(898):805–811

Dutta SK and Costa BS (1979) Umbilicated gastric polyposis. An indicator of metastatic gastric tumor. Am J Gastroenterol 71(6):598–600

Evers K and Kressel HY (1982) Principles of performance and interpretation of double-contrast gastrointestinal studies. Radiol Clin North Am 20(4):667–685

Fielding JF, Toye DK et al (1970) Crohn's disease of the stomach and duodenum. Gut 11(12):1001–1006

Fink AM and Aylward GW (1995) Buscopan and glaucoma: a survey of current practice. Clin Radiol 50(3):160–164

Frostberg N (1938) Characteristic duodenal deformity in cases of different kinds of perivaterial enlargement of the pancreas. Acta Radiologica 19:164–173

Gold RP, Green PH et al (1984) Early gastric cancer: radiographic experience. Radiology 152(2):283–290

Gordon R, Laufer I et al (1980) Gastric polyps on routine double-contrast examination of the stomach. Radiology 134(1):27–29

Gore RM, Levine MS et al (1999) Drug-induced disorders of the stomach and duodenum. Abdom Imaging 24(1):9–16

Gore RM, Levine MS et al (1997) Gastric cancer. Radiologic diagnosis. Radiol Clin North Am 35(2):311–329

Gray SW and Skandalalakis JE (1972) Embryology for Surgeons:129–136

Harake MD, Maxwell AJ et al (2001) Primary and metastatic lobular carcinoma of the breast. Clin Radiol 56(8):621–630

Hirschowitz BI (1997) Zollinger-Ellison syndrome: pathogenesis, diagnosis, and management. Am J Gastroenterol 92(4 Suppl):44S–48S; discussion 49S–50S

Hizawa K, Iida M et al (1994) Crohn disease: early recognition and progress of aphthous lesions. Radiology 190(2):451–454

Huang TY, Yam LT et al (1987) Radiological features of systemic mast-cell disease. Br J Radiol 60(716):765–770

Khilnani MT, Wolf BS et al (1962) Roentgen features of carcinoma of the gallbladder on barium-meal examination. Radiology 79:264–273

Lee CM, Changchien CS et al (1993) Eosinophilic gastroenteritis: 10 years experience. Am J Gastroenterol 88(1):70–74

Leenders EL, Osman MZ et al (1970) Treatment of duodenal duplication with international review. Am Surg 36(6):368–371

Legge DA, Carlson HC et al (1970) Roentgenologic features of regional enteritis of the upper gastrointestinal tract. Am J Roentgenol Radium Ther Nucl Med 110(2):355–360

Levine MS (1987) Crohn's disease of the upper gastrointestinal tract. Radiol Clin North Am 25(1):79–91

Levine MS (1995) Role of the double-contrast upper gastrointestinal series in the 1990s. Gastroenterol Clin North Am 24(2):289–308

Levine MS, Creteur V et al (1987) Benign gastric ulcers: diagnosis and follow-up with double-contrast radiography. Radiology 164(1):9–13

Levine MS, Elmas N et al (1996) Helicobacter pylori and gastric MALT lymphoma. AJR Am J Roentgenol 166(1):85–86

Levine MS and Laufer I (1993) The upper gastrointestinal series at a crossroads. AJR Am J Roentgenol 161(6):1131–1137

Levine MS and Rubesin SE (1995) The Helicobacter pylori revolution: radiologic perspective. Radiology 195(3):593–596

Levine MS, Rubesin SE et al (1988) Double-contrast upper gastrointestinal examination: technique and interpretation. Radiology 168(3):593–602

Levine MS, Rubesin SE et al (2002) Barium studies. Gastrointest Endosc 55(7 Suppl):S16–24

Low VH, Levine MS et al (1994) Diagnosis of gastric carcinoma: sensitivity of double-contrast barium studies. AJR Am J Roentgenol 162(2):329–334

MacCarty RL and Talley NJ (1990) Barium studies in diffuse eosinophilic gastroenteritis. Gastrointest Radiol 15(3):183–187

Maderal F, Hunter F et al (1984) Gastric lipomas-an update of clinical presentation, diagnosis, and treatment. Am J Gastroenterol 79(12):964–967

Mani JR, Zboralske FF et al (1966) Carcinoma of the body and tail of the pancreas. Am J Roentgenol Radium Ther Nucl Med 96(2):429–446

Menuck LS (1976) Gastric lymphoma, a radiologic diagnosis. Gastrointest Radiol 1(2):157–161

Miettinen M, El-Rifai W et al (2002) Evaluation of malignancy and prognosis of gastrointestinal stromal tumors: a review. Hum Pathol 33(5):478–483

Ming SC (1976) II. Malignant potential of gastric polyps. Gastrointest Radiol 1(2):121–125

Nguyen BD (2002) CT and scintigraphy of aggressive lymphadenopathic mastocytosis. AJR Am J Roentgenol 178(3):769–770

Nix GA (1980) Early carcinoma of the ampulla and papilla of Vater. Clin Radiol 31(1):95–100

Park SH, Han JK et al (1999) Unusual gastric tumors: radiologic-pathologic correlation. Radiographics 19(6):1435–1446

Pattison CP, Combs MJ et al (1997) Helicobacter pylori and peptic ulcer disease: evolution to revolution to resolution. AJR Am J Roentgenol 168(6):1415–1420

Reese DF, Hodgson JR et al (1962) Giant hypertrophy of the gastric mucosa (Menetrier's disease):a correlation of the roentgenographic, pathologic, and clinical findings. Am J Roentgenol Radium Ther Nucl Med 88:619–626

Rutgeerts P, Onette E et al (1980) Crohn's disease of the stomach and duodenum: A clinical study with emphasis on the value of endoscopy and endoscopic biopsies. Endoscopy 12(6):288–294

Sherrick DW, Hodgson JR et al (1965) The Roentgenologic Diagnosis of Primary Gastric Lymphoma. Radiology 84:925–932

Sohn J, Levine MS et al (1995) Helicobacter pylori gastritis: radiographic findings. Radiology 195(3):763–767

Stolte M, Sticht T et al (1994) Frequency, location, and age and sex distribution of various types of gastric polyp. Endoscopy 26(8):659–665

Szemes GC and Amberg JR (1968) Gastric bezoars after partial gastrectomy. Radiology 90(4):765–768

Tada S, Iida M et al (1990) Barium meal study for amyloidosis of the small intestine: measurements on radiograph. Gastrointest Radiol 15(4):320–324

Taft DA and Hairston JT (1976) Duplication of the alimentary tract. Am Surg 42(7):455–462

Tishler JM (1979) Duodenal tuberculosis. Radiology 130(3):593–5.

Tomasulo J (1971) Gastric polyps. Histologic types and their relationship to gastric carcinoma. Cancer 27(6):1346–1355

Torigian DA, Levine MS et al (2001) Lymphoid hyperplasia of the stomach: radiographic findings in five adult patients. AJR Am J Roentgenol 177(1):71–75

Treitel H, Meyers MA et al (1970) Changes in the duodenal loop secondary to carcinoma of the hepatic flexure of the colon. Br J Radiol 43(507):209–213

Wehut WD, Olmsted WW et al (1976) Eosinophilic gastritis. Radiologic-pathologic correlation (RPC) from the Armed Forces Institute of Pathology (AFIP) Radiology 120(1):85–89

Wolfsen HC, Carpenter HA et al (1993) Menetrier's disease: a form of hypertrophic gastropathy or gastritis? Gastroenterology 104(5):1310–1319

Wu CS, Lin CJ et al (1997) Menetrier's disease: a new variant with duodenal involvement. Am J Gastroenterol 92(6):1041–1043

Yoo CC, Levine MS et al (1998) Gastric mucosa-associated lymphoid tissue lymphoma: radiographic findings in six patients. Radiology 208(1):239–243

CT of the Stomach

6.1

Teik C. See, Nicholas R. Carroll, and Alan H. Freeman

CONTENTS

T. C. See, MB, BS, MRCP, FRCR
Consultant Radiologist, Department of Radiology, Addenbrooke's Hospital, Box 219, Hills Road, Cambridge, CB2 2QQ, UK
N. R. Carroll, MB, BS, MRCP, FRCR
Consultant Radiologist, Department of Radiology, Addenbrooke's Hospital, Box 219, Hills Road, Cambridge, CB2 2QQ, UK
A. H. Freeman, MB, BS, FRCR
Consultant Radiologist, Department of Radiology, Addenbrooke's Hospital, Box 219, Hills Road, Cambridge, CB2 2QQ, UK

Traditional methods of examining the stomach, i.e., barium meal and endoscopy, confine themselves to demonstration of the mucosa, whilst giving indirect evidence of mural and extra gastric lesions. Computed tomography (CT) is of course excellent at demonstrating the latter, but an emerging role in the evaluation of mucosal lesions has become evident. This will accelerate with multi-slice CT and perhaps virtual gastroscopy (Lee 2000). To date the major role of CT has been in the diagnosis and staging of gastric carcinoma, but all tumours of the stomach; benign as well as malignant, are well demonstrated. In addition, various forms of gastritis may be identified as well as miscellaneous conditions such as Ménétrier's disease and varices (Fishman et al. 1996; Merino et al. 1999). CT also has a major role in the follow-up of post-gastrectomy patients, particularly after surgery for malignant conditions.

6.1.1 Preparation of the Patient

Good gastric distension is essential and various agents such as air, water, and corn oil have been tried. Ordinary tap water appears to be simplest and best, and the patient should drink as much as he comfortably can immediately before he arrives on the CT couch (Horton and Fishman 1998; Rossi et al. 1997). Ideally this should be a volume close to a litre. The small intestine will have been previously opacified by the ingestion of a 3% mixture of Gastrografin or alternative contrast agent. An antispasmolytic drug such as Buscopan or Glucagon is then administered to abolish gastric peristalsis. Finally an intravenous contrast medium such as Niopam 300 is injected at a rate of 2–3 ml per second using a total volume of 100–150 ml. Imaging is acquired at 35- and 70-second delays from the start of the injection to catch the arterial and portal phases, respectively. The region of the stomach that causes much difficulty is the gastro-oesophageal junction, because this is often collapsed, and it may therefore be necessary to image in a different position such as prone or decubitus.

Using this technique means that the whole of the gastric wall can be readily evaluated with the mucosal surface showing up as a hyperdense thin line, whereas the mural portion is of isodensity. The thickness of the well-distended wall should be no more than 2–3 mm.

Pathological changes in the stomach are demonstrated by thickening of either the mucosal or mural layers or both. This may be localised or generalised. Discrete masses both endo- and exogastric are well-demonstrated, as are of course the implications of malignancy such as involvement of the adjacent fat, lymphadenopathy, and liver metastases.

6.1.2 Pathology of the Stomach

6.1.2.1 Gastritis

This is a rather loosely used term that in a strict sense implies an increase in inflammatory cells in the gastric mucosa. However, it has become a generic term covering many entities that may be acute or chronic. Perhaps the most well known such entity is the relationship to *Helicobacter pylori* infection and peptic ulcer disease. This condition predominately affects the antrum and distal body, and indeed this is the most likely site for obtaining histological evidence of the organism. Often there may be little macroscopic evidence of change, and when present it is usually in the form of a non-erosive gastritis. However on occasion it may produce marked antral or greater curve wall thickening, thus simulating tumour (Urban et al. 1991). Ingestion of non steroidal antiinflammatory agents (NSAIDs) are a potent cause of acute gastritis, which is much more marked by erosive changes, resulting in a chemical gastropathy. Again this primarily affects the distal stomach. Alcohol abuse causes similar changes. A further group of conditions primarily affect the submucosal and mural layers of the stomach, typically including Crohn's disease and other granulomatous states such as TB and syphilis, as well as eosinophilic gastritis. The elderly patient may demonstrate changes of atrophic gastritis, which usually affects the whole stomach, but sometimes predominately affects the antrum, a condition referred to as the "rams horn sign" in barium meal literature. Gastric emphysema and emphysematous gastritis need to be distinguished. The former relates to a mechanical insult to the stomach, such as torsion, gastric outlet obstruction, or endoscopic injury and is usually associated with a good prognosis, whereas the latter is associated with the presence of a gas-forming organism, typically *Clostridium*, and is associated with an appalling prognosis. Finally, Ménétrier's disease is a form of hypertrophic gastritis characterised by underlying histological changes of inflammation and cystic glandular degeneration. This typically causes marked hypertrophy of the rugal pattern in the proximal stomach with relative sparing of the antrum. These patients are achlorhydric.

6.1.2.2 Gastric Ulcer

Although gastric ulcers may be found in any part of the stomach, the most common location is in the antrum, along the lesser curve aspect extending around the incisura angularis. Elderly patients may demonstrate a more random distribution, and often in these patients the ulcers are significantly larger with those over 3 cm being labelled as giant ulcers. Gastric ulcers may be benign or malignant, although statistically the great majority are benign. Differentiation on radiographic grounds may be suggested by several features. The sign of penetration is the most useful, that is to say that there is clear evidence of the ulcer burrowing cleanly through the gastric wall. Conversely, if the ulcer appears to have more of an intraluminal position and particularly if it is surrounded by a mass, then it clearly is more likely to be malignant. Position in the stomach is not very helpful, although any ulcer in the fundal region is almost certainly malignant.

6.1.2.3 Varices

Portal hypertension arises when there is an element of obstruction to the portal vein, most commonly as a consequence of cirrhosis of the liver. This results in enlargement of collateral veins between the intra-abdominal portal system and the superior vena cava (SVC). These most typically are demonstrated in the lower oesophagus (uphill varices) but may also be seen in the fundus of the stomach, where they may be so prominent as to give rise to a tumefactive mass. In this case there is usually an attendant portal gastropathy.

6.1.2.4 Intramural Pseudocyst

Pancreatic pseudocysts are well known for their ability to migrate within the abdominal cavity as well as in some cases entering the chest. On rare occasions they can migrate into the wall of the stomach, giving rise to an intramural mass. If the situation is in the antrum, there have been reports of associated gastric outlet obstruction (Vitello 1996).

6.1.2.5 Benign Tumours

The most common benign tumours are hyperplastic polyps, and these are not true neoplasms. These are usually small, though occasionally they may cause large masses which are difficult to distinguish from frank tumour. Adenomatous polyps are a true neoplasm and may undergo malignant change. They are usually solitary and most often are found in the antrum. Other benign tumours may be submucosal, such as a lipoma. Tumours that arise from the muscularis propria may have formally been regarded as benign leiomyomas, but are now referred to as gastrointestinal stromal tumours (GISTs) and should always be regarded as potentially malignant.

6.1.2.6 Malignant Tumours

These include carcinomas, lymphomas, GISTs, and secondary deposits. Adenocarcinoma accounts for approximately 75% of malignant tumours, lymphomas some 20%, and the rest the remaining 5%.

Primary carcinomas may arise anywhere in the stomach, but there has been a disturbing increase in recent years of the so-called junctional tumour. This tumour straddles the gastro-oesophageal junction and probably reflects the rising incidence of adenocarcinoma associated with Barrett's oesophagus. They are subdivided into three types. Type 1 junctional tumour is predominately oesophageal or arises within 5 cm of the gastro-oesophageal junction. A type 2 tumour straddles the gastro-oesophageal junction with equal involvement on either side. A type 3 tumour is predominately cardial in location. The stomach is the commonest GI tract organ to be involved in non-Hodgkin lymphoma (NHL) and is said to be involved in around 50% of cases (Lewin et al. 1978). Increased recognition is now being given to extranodal marginal zone B-cell lymphomas, otherwise known as MALT lymphoma (mucosa-associated lymphoid tissue). These used to be known as pseudolymphoma and comprise 7%–8% of all B-cell lymphomas. They appear to have an association with *Helicobacter pylori* infection and are therefore largely confined to the stomach (Wotherspoon et al. 1991). The gastric mucosa normally does not contain any lymphoid tissue, but lymphoid infiltration of this structure as a result of the infection is thought to be the origin of MALT lymphoma. They are divided into high or low grade, depending on their microscopic appearances (Chan et al. 1990). GISTs are commonest in the stomach but account for only approximately 1%–2% of malignant gastric tumours. Nodal metastases are rare, and they do have a more favourable prognosis than gastric adenocarcinoma, though haematogenous and intraperitoneal spread is well recognised. Many tumours can metastasise to the stomach, including breast, lung, and ovary, although the commonest is malignant melanoma.

6.1.3 Appearances at CT

6.1.3.1 Gastritis

As this is primarily a mucosal process, CT examination will most usually be normal. Sometimes the mucosa will appear hyperaemic, but this in itself is not a reliable sign. However if the submucosal layers are involved by reactive oedema, these will show up as a low-attenuation area resulting in a target sign if the stomach is viewed en face, an appearance similar to that seen in inflammatory bowel disease. This may be seen with the severer forms of antral gastritis, but is more to be expected in a chronic granulomatous condition such as Crohn's disease. Ménétrier's disease shows a uniform thickening of the gastric wall that may be as much as 1–2 cm. The appearance is most marked in the fundus and proximal body, and distinction from lymphoma can be difficult (Fig. 6.1.1)

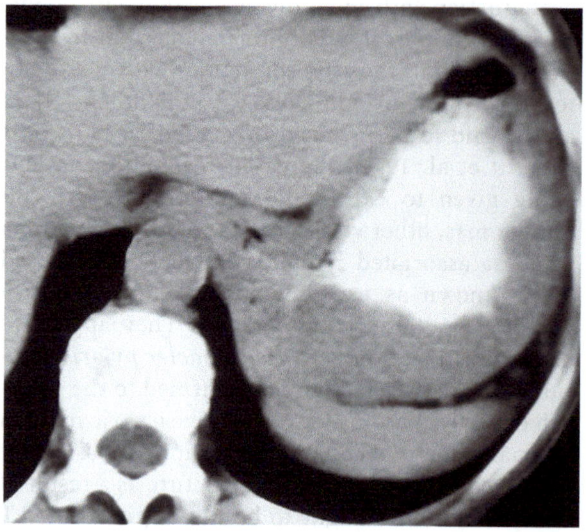

Fig. 6.1.1. Ménétrier's disease, demonstrated by marked thickening of the wall of the upper stomach

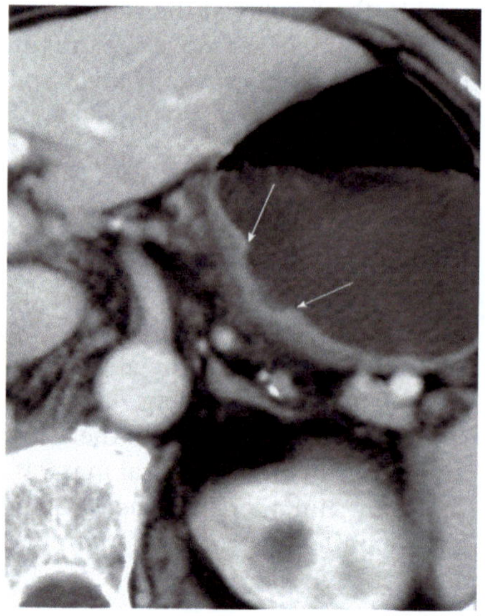

Fig. 6.1.2. A benign gastric ulcer on the posterior wall of the stomach. Note the sharp margins of the ulcer crater (*arrows*) and evidence of the ulcer burrowing into the gastric wall. Image courtesy of Prof. A.A. Stabile Ianora and the publishers of *La Radiologia Medica*, Turin

6.1.3.2 Gastric Ulcer

When seen in profile, the appearance of ulcers may vary from minor interruptions of the mucosa to major defects in the wall of the stomach. Typically a benign ulcer will demonstrate evidence of penetration through the mural layer of the stomach with a sharply marginated clean-cut edge (Jacobs et al. 1991; Stabile Ianora et al. 2001) (Fig. 6.1.2). Conversely a malignant ulcer is much more likely to demonstrate a heaped up and irregular margin, and the whole ulcer may assume more of an intraluminal configuration. (Fig. 6.1.3).

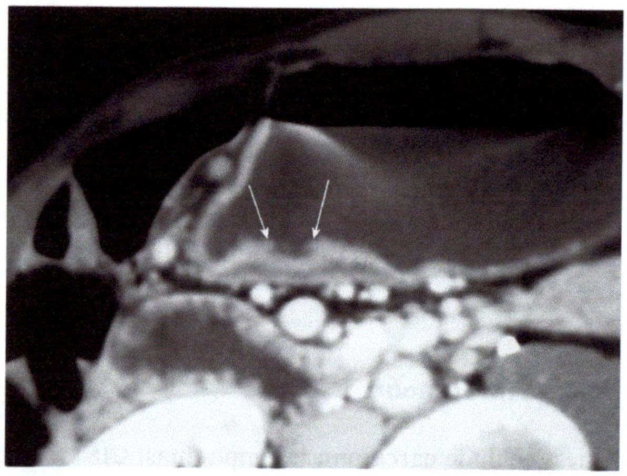

Fig. 6.1.3. A malignant gastric ulcer on the posterior wall of the stomach. Note the somewhat heaped up ulcer crater margins (*arrows*) and the more intraluminal position of the ulcer. Image courtesy of Prof A.A. Stabile Ianora and the publishers of *La Radiologia Medica* Turin

6.1.3.3 Gastric Varices

These are typically found in association with gastro-oesophageal varices as a consequence of portal hypertension secondary to cirrhosis. In this situation there is increased retrograde flow of blood through the coronary vein, which then reaches the systemic system via the short and left gastric veins, the azygos vein, and finally the SVC. In this situation the diagnosis of gastric varices is usually straightforward, but diagnostic confusion may occur if there are no associated oesophageal varices. This most commonly occurs if the splenic vein is obstructed distal to the coronary vein, and increased flow may then take place through the short gastric veins to retroperitoneal veins, typically the left renal. The usual cause for this occurrence is pancreatic cancer. Gastric varices are almost invariably found in the fundus but occasionally may be seen in the antrum. On the unenhanced images, varices will show as smooth lobulated filling defects, and there may well be a significant extraluminal component. Indeed the whole mass-like effect may well simulate a tumour with adjacent lymphadenopathy (Fig. 6.1.4a,b). Their true nature becomes apparent after administration of contrast medium, with the demonstration of avid enhancement of the varices (Fig. 6.1.4c). Of course there are likely to be other associated signs of cirrhosis such as a shrunken irregular liver, splenomegaly, ascites, and the opening of other collaterals such as via a recanalised umbilical vein (Balthazar et al. 1984).

6.1.3.4 Intramural Pseudocyst

The development of a pseudocyst is of course a well-recognised complication of pancreatitis. Most often these occur in the pancreatic bed, where they cause an extrinsic mass of low attenuation which displaces and distorts the stomach (Fig. 6.1.5) However, pseudocysts are well known for their ability to migrate, typically around the left pararenal area but sometimes much further afield such as to the mediastinum. Occasionally they can enter the wall of the stomach, and when they do this may present as an intramural mass. This is more likely to happen if there has been a transgastric drainage of a pseudocyst, but it may also be spontaneous (Wagholikar et al. 2003). At CT examination, pseudocysts are demonstrated as a smooth well-defined submucosal mass containing material of fluid attenuation. (Fig. 6.1.6a,b) They usually resolve spontaneously without ill effect, but as mentioned above they may cause obstructive symptoms if situated in the gastric antrum.

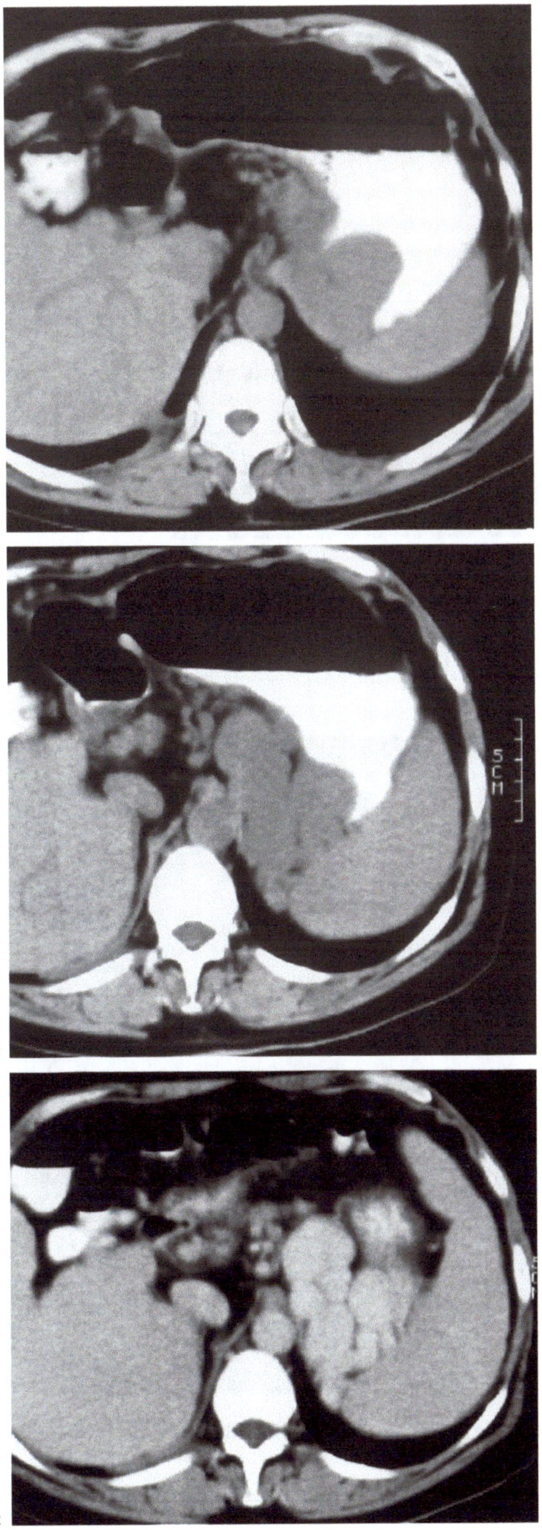

a b c

Fig. 6.1.4a–c. Gastric varices. The precontrast images (**a, b**) demonstrate masses indenting the fundus of the stomach which on (**a**) in particular could be confused with a fundal tumour. The nature of the abnormality becomes clear following contrast administration (**c**)

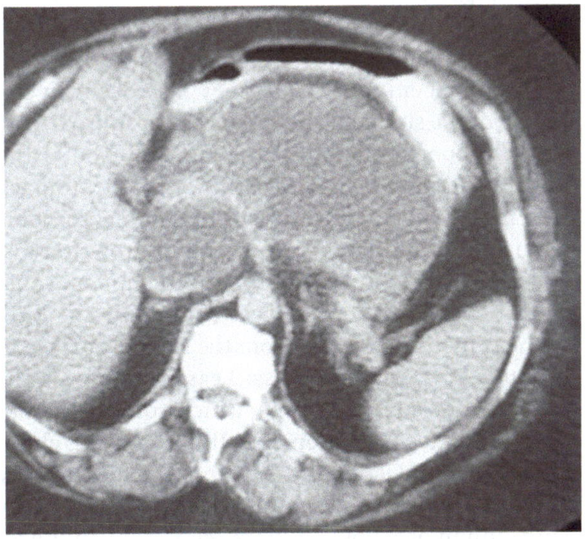

Fig. 6.1.5. A large pancreatic pseudocyst is displacing the stomach anteriorly and compressing it

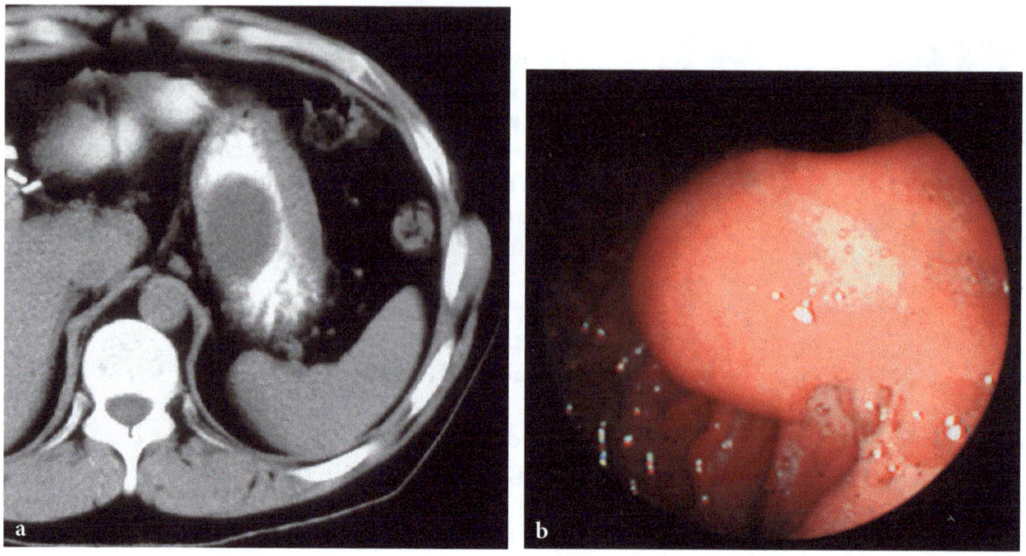

Fig. 6.1.6a,b. An intramural pseudocyst is demonstrated on CT as a well-defined, oval, low-attenuation mass related to the lesser curve of the stomach (**a**). The content was of fluid attenuation. Note the post-cholecystectomy clips. Endoscopy confirms the smooth submucosal mass (**b**), which disappeared spontaneously over the ensuing month

6.1.3.5 Benign Gastric Tumours

Small gastric polyps are rarely seen at CT, but an exception is the distinctive lipoma shown by its characteristic appearance of a well-defined mass of fat attenuation (Fig. 6.1.7).

GISTs are the most common mesenchymal neoplasm of the gastrointestinal tract, and the majority are found in the stomach, although a recent series reported a lower incidence of 50% (Ghanem et al. 2003). Although all are potentially malignant, smaller tumours (under 5 cm) are more likely to behave in a benign fashion. They may occur in any region of the stomach and are found in approximate equal proportion among the fundus, body, and antrum. Because they arise in the wall of the stomach they may exhibit a number of different macroscopic features depending on the pattern of growth. Most commonly they bulge into the gastric lumen, causing an endogastric mass. Less commonly the bulk of the tumour protrudes from the serosal surface to produce an exogastric mass. Least common is the dumbbell or hourglass type, which comprises both endo- and exogastric elements; this represents about 5% of cases. If GISTs protrude into the lumen, they are shown as rounded submucosal masses, typically with inhomogeneous hyperattenuation enhancement. They usually form a relatively acute angle with the adjacent mucosa (Fig. 6.1.8). If exophytic, they take the form of a mass growing away from the stomach which again demonstrates inhomogeneous enhancement. In this situation, the tumour usually forms an obtuse angle with the stomach due to its subserosal location (Fig 6.1.9).

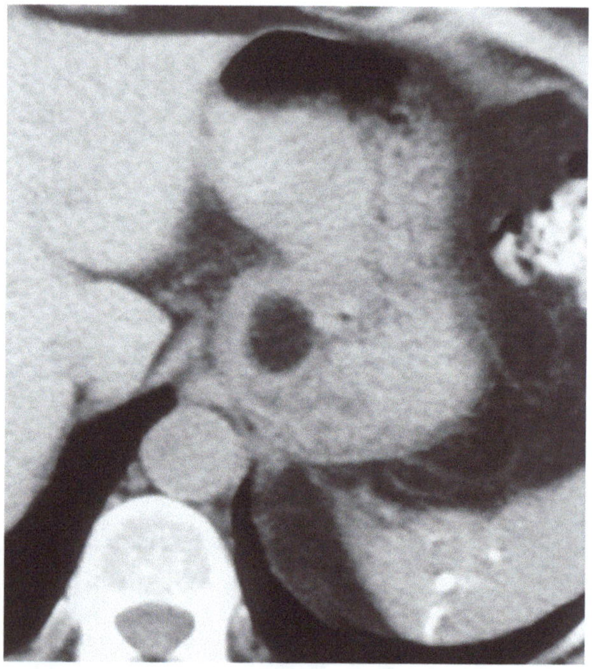

Fig. 6.1.7. A typical gastric lipoma identified by the attenuation of fat density

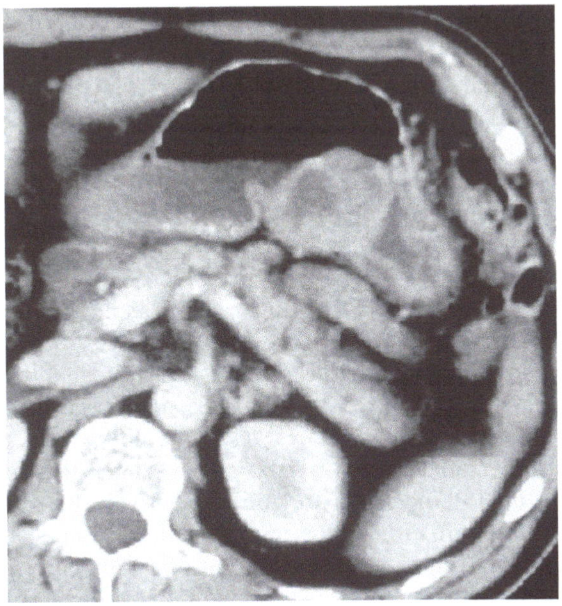

Fig. 6.1.8. An endogastric GIST arising from the posterior wall of the stomach. Note the intraluminal position with relatively acute angles to the adjacent gastric wall, as well as the heterogeneous attenuation

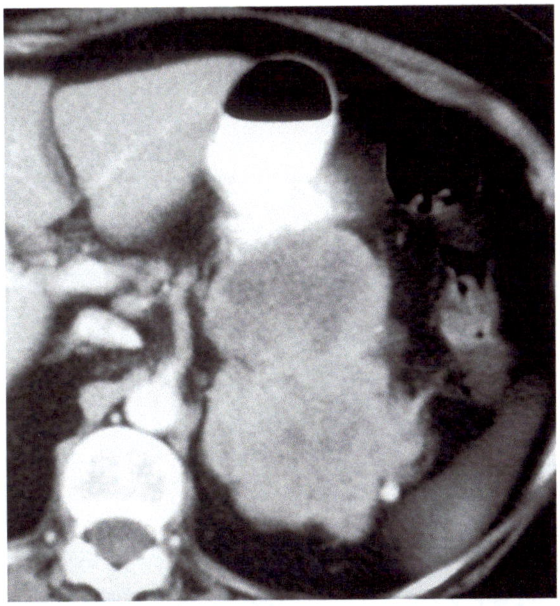

Fig. 6.1.9. An exogastric GIST arising from the posterior wall of the stomach. Note the more obtuse angle it forms with the body of the stomach and again a heterogeneous attenuation pattern. The size of this lesion together with the lack of definition of its margin suggest that this is frankly malignant. Image courtesy of Dr A. Padhani

6.1.3.6 Malignant Tumours: Carcinoma

Gastric carcinomas may demonstrate several forms at CT including (1) a thick walled ulcer, (Fig. 6.1.10a,b), (2) polypoid mass (Fig. 6.1.11), or (3) infiltration of the gastric wall with reduced distension and loss of mucosal detail (Fig. 6.1.12). Both ulcerated lesions and polypoid tumours are best

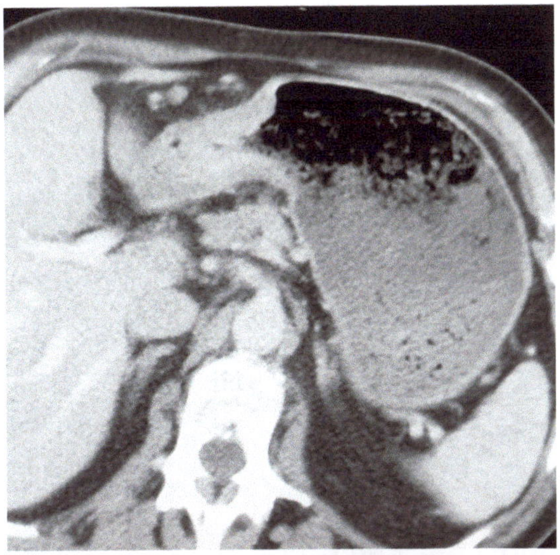

a

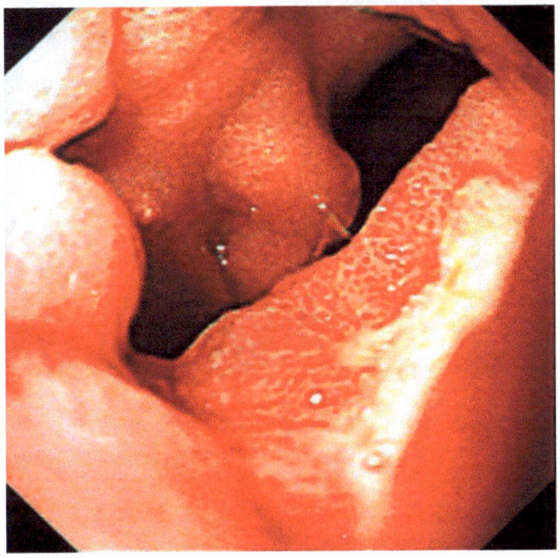

b

Fig. 6.1.10a,b. An infiltrating carcinoma of the gastric antrum demonstrated by marked local thickening of the antral wall (**a**). Note also the small lymph node in the perigastric fat just anterior to the tumour. The endoscopic view of the antrum confirms the thickened heaped up folds and also a shallow ulcer containing white slough (**b**). Despite this evidence that the tumour had impinged on the integrity of the mucosal surface, all initial biopsies were negative. Further deep biopsies were required to determine the nature of this largely submucosal tumour

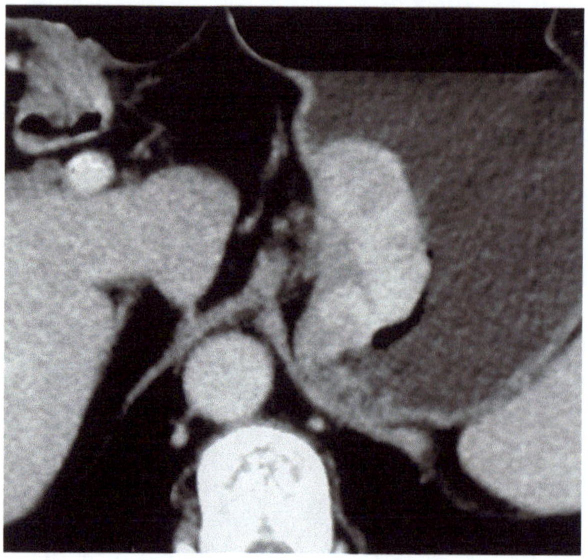

Fig. 6.1.11. A typical polypoid carcinoma arising from high on the lesser curve just below the cardia

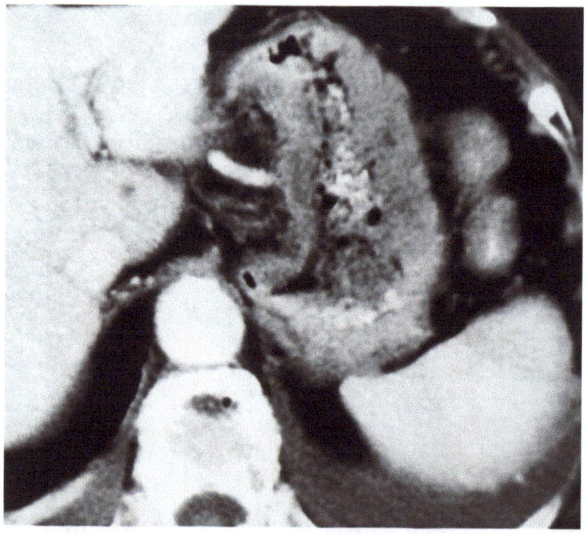

Fig. 6.1.12. A diffusely infiltrating carcinoma involving both walls of the stomach. This will eventually produce a linitis plastica appearance

demonstrated during intravenous contrast medium enhancement with the stomach fully distended with water. Infiltrating or scirrhous carcinomas are usually characterised by a degree of wall thickening, loss of mucosal detail, and variable intravenous contrast enhancement. There may be a substantial exophytic component.

CT examination is the mainstay of the staging of gastric carcinoma and other malignancies involving the stomach. Although laparoscopy for peritoneal disease and endoscopic ultrasound (EUS) for local and nodal staging are considered superior in their respective sphere, CT remains the main arbitrator as to whether or not patients are suitable for curative or palliative treatment. The use of multi-slice CT and subsequent three-dimensional (3D) reformatting has improved the ability of the technique to delineate the primary lesion, particularly when used with negative luminal contrast media as mentioned above (Horton and Fishman 2003).

Tumours of both the proximal and most distal parts of the stomach may be difficult to delineate using conventional helical CT, due to problems with partial volume effects in the gastric cardia (Fig. 6.1.13) and distal antrum, respectively. Placing the patient in either prone or lateral decubitus position may improve the resolution of proximal and distal gastric tumours. Further distension of the stomach with effervescent agents can also improve delineation of the tumour mass.

6.1.3.7 Staging

The primary role of CT is to assess for the presence of extra-gastric tumour spread, lymph node disease, intraperitoneal seeding, and haematogenous spread. See Appendix 1.

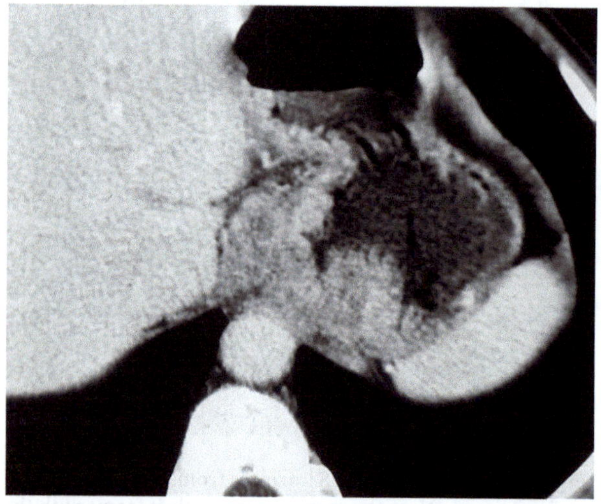

Fig. 6.1.13. A junctional tumour that involves the proximal body, cardia, and distal oesophagus (the latter not shown). Note the loss of the plane of cleavage between the tumour and the aorta

6.1.3.8 Direct Extension

Detection of early, in situ T1 and T2 disease is unreliable on CT. Tumour which however, has invaded through the muscular layer or subserosa into either the gastrocolic or gastrohepatic ligaments, or has invaded into the greater or lesser omentum without perforation of the visceral peritoneum, is still classified as T2 disease. If however, there is perforation of the visceral peritoneum without invasion of adjacent structures, the classification will be T3.

Continued spread of tumour results in invasion of adjacent organs via the ligaments and peritoneal reflections. The liver may be directly invaded via the gastrohepatic ligament, the transverse colon via the gastrocolic ligament, and the pancreas via the posterior wall and lesser sac. Tumour thrombosis may also occur in the portal vein (Fig. 6.1.14a,b). Many of these features are better appreciated following 3D reformatting of multi-slice imaging, which in itself has markedly improved the ability of CT to perform accurate T staging.

6.1.3.9 Lymphatic Spread

CT is only able to reliably detect relatively enlarged nodes in the perigastric tissue, e.g. in the gastrohepatic ligament (Fig. 6.1.15a). Although adenopathy in local nodes has a prognostic effect (Karpeh et al. 2000), the presence of such nodes does not

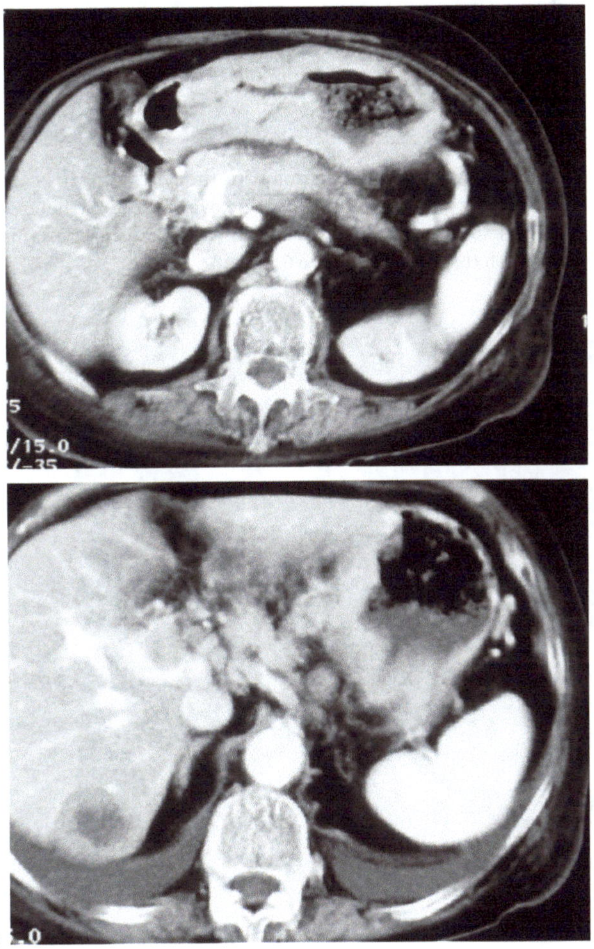

a b

Fig. 6.1.14a,b. Haematogenous spread from a gastric carcinoma. The extensive tumour together with thrombus in the splenic vein is shown on (**a**), whereas (**b**) demonstrates tumour thrombus in the portal vein as well as a liver metastasis. Note bilateral pleural effusions

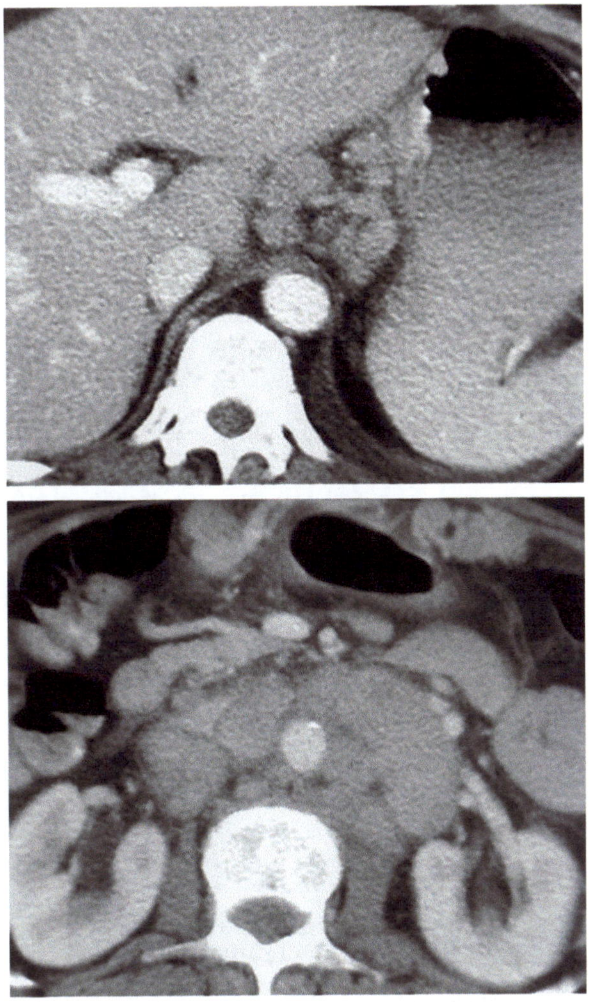

a b

Fig. 6.1.15a,b. Lymph node metastases from gastric carcinoma demonstrated in the left gastric and celiac axis territory (**a**) and para-aortic (**b**) alter the surgical management. More distant lymphatic drainage occurs at the porta, peripancreatic area, and finally other sites such as the para-aortic nodes (Fig. 6.1.15b). Nodal staging is determined by the number of nodes involved in the various sites, demonstrated in Table 6.1.1. Although CT is able to detect a substantial number of nodes over 1 cm in size, tumour is often found in nodes of less than 5 mm, which is below the resolution of the images obtained. Despite use of multi-slice dynamic CT with optimal contrast, sensitivity for the detection of nodal metastases remains disappointingly low (Mani et al. 2001). It is likely that PET/CT will play an increasing role here.

6.1.3.10 Intraperitoneal Seeding

Seeding with tumour within the peritoneal cavity is characterised by nodules or fluid collections around peritoneal reflections and within the mesentery or generalised ascites (Fig. 6.1.16a,b). Full CT examination should include the pelvis to exclude the presence of metastases to the ovaries (Krukenberg tumours). Typically these are bilateral and are usually associated with signet ring tumours of the stomach. Unlike the cystic lesions of primary ovarian carcinoma, these more commonly demonstrate a solid heterogeneous pattern (Fig. 6.1.17).

Laparoscopy and laparoscopic ultrasound are more sensitive for the presence of peritoneal disease than CT, but it is clear that a combination of staging modalities is most effective in the management of these tumours (Wakelin et al. 2002).

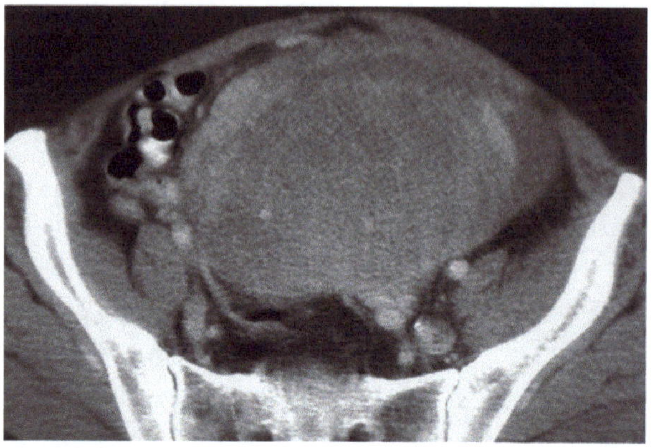

Fig. 6.1.17. A Krukenberg tumour in the pelvis. In this case it is a solitary tumour involving one ovary. Note the heterogeneous solid nature of the tumour mass. This is the same case as that shown in Figure 6.1.15a,b

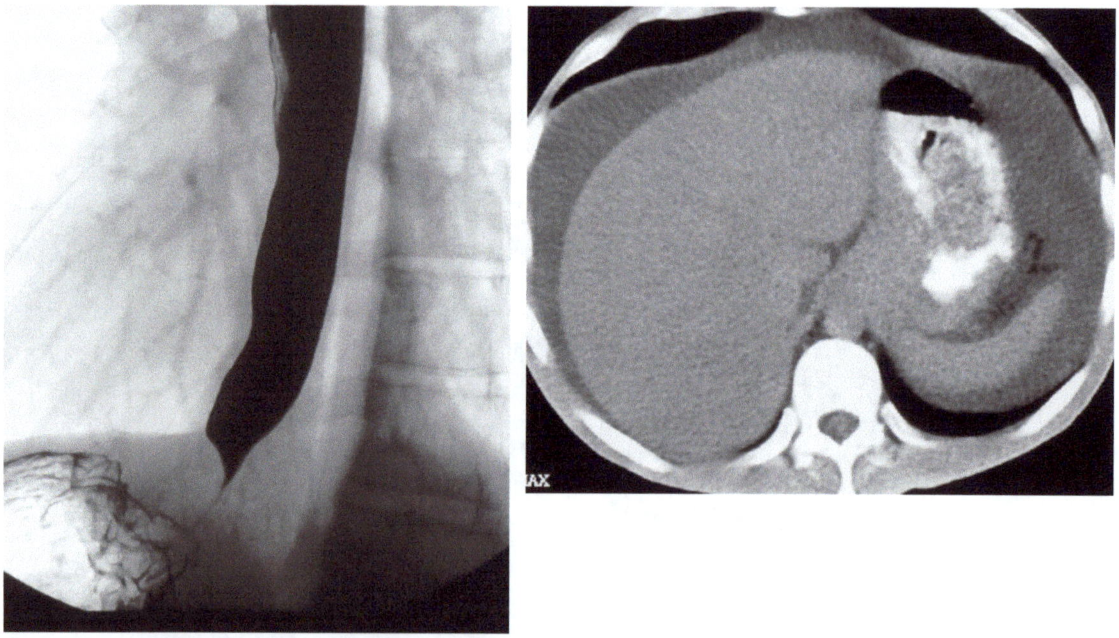

a b

Fig. 6.1.16a,b. Barium swallow in this twenty-six-year-old male reveals an appearance reminiscent of achalasia. The true nature of the problem can be discerned from the irregular impression on the gastric fundus caused by a carcinoma (**a**). Follow-up CT demonstrates evidence of generalised abdominal involvement with widespread ascites. Note the tumour mass at the cardia together with obliteration of the left crus and anterior margin of the aorta

A CT examination should also include the chest to exclude lung metastases, second only to the liver as a location of haematogenous spread. The examination should also include careful assessment of the adrenals. Sensitivity for the detection of metastases by contrast-enhanced CT (CECT) remains at approximately 80%, compared to 90% for FDG PET in a comparative study (Kinkel et al. 2002).

6.1.3.11 Lymphoma

The stomach is the most common site of gastro-intestinal involvement by non-Hodgkin lymphoma (Megibow et al. 1983). Approximately 50% of all gastro-intestinal lymphomas involve the stomach, and overall these tumours account for approximately 3%–5% of gastric malignancy.

As with gastric adenocarcinoma, CT is the primary imaging in the assessment of both the local and nodal disease. Lymphoma of the gastric wall may result in marked increase in thickness with a bland homogeneous appearance to the mucosa (Sato et al. 1986; Buy and Moss 1982). This thickening may be segmental or diffuse, and more than one region of the stomach may be involved. Lymphoma of the gastric wall may also present as polypoid intraluminal masses or sometimes as an ulcerated lesion. Spread of tumour through the hiatus into the distal oesophagus and beyond the pylorus into the duodenum is not uncommon (Cho et al. 1996). Full examination of the chest, abdomen, and pelvis is essential for the detection of associated lymph node involvement and other organ disease. This should always be contrast medium-enhanced for initial staging, though this is not so important for follow-up studies.

MALT lymphomas associated with Helicobacter pylori infection are usually low-grade and produce similar CT findings to NHL, but with some variation. Most typical is diffuse thickening, which mainly affects the body of the stomach but can affect all parts of the stomach from fundus to antrum (Fig. 6.1.18a–c). Polypoid masses are less commonly seen (Brown et al. 2000; Kessar et al. 1999). Abdominal lymphadenopathy is seen in about half the cases (Fig. 6.1.19a,b), and it has been postulated that the presence of extensive extra gastric disease together with marked thickening of the wall of the stomach may indicate a subgroup of low-grade MALTs which have a more aggressive outcome and border on high-grade (Park et al. 2002).

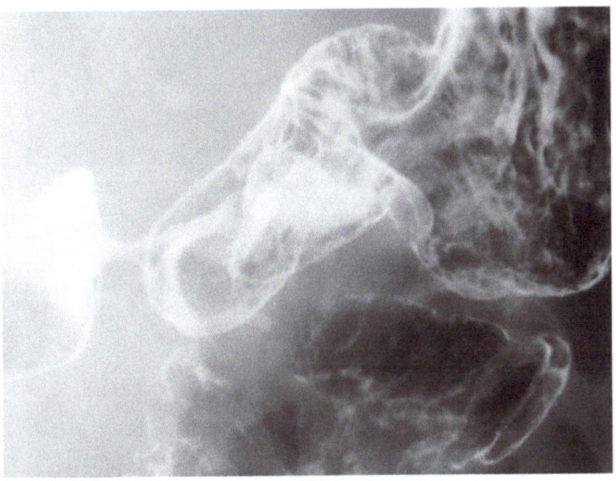
a

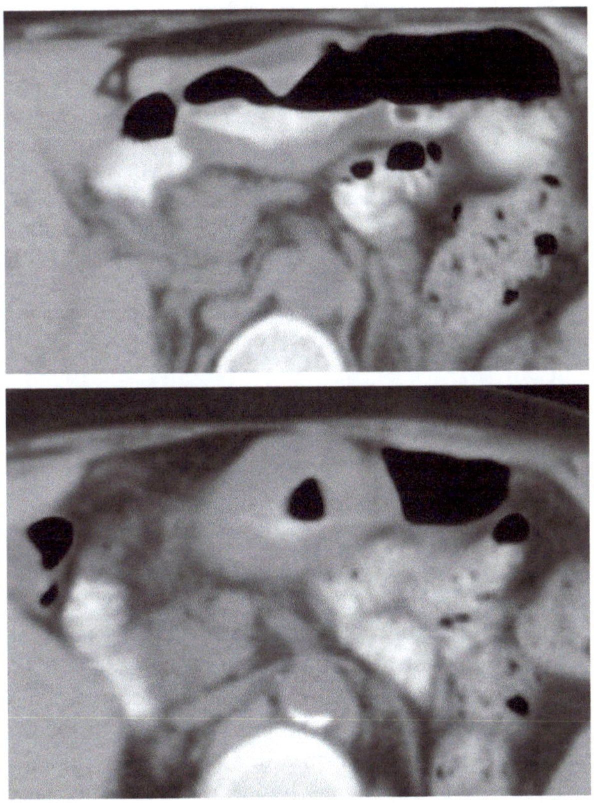
b
c

Fig. 6.1.18a–c. Gastric MALT lymphoma with the barium meal showing lobulated thickening of the wall of the gastric antrum resulting in an intraluminal mass (**a**). CT of this patient confirms the irregular thickening of the antral wall (**b**), whilst the degree of thickening is best appreciated on (**c**)

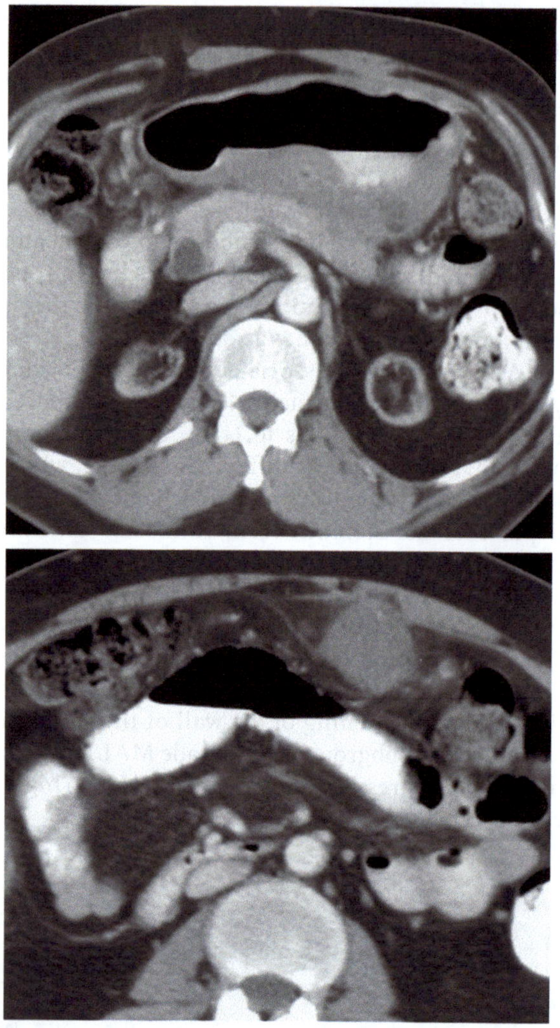

Fig. 6.1.19a,b. A second case of gastric MALT lymphoma showing marked thickening of the posterior wall of the stomach (**a**). Note the bilateral shrunken kidneys in this renal transplant patient (as was the case from Figure 6.1.18). There is also marked extranodal lymphadenopathy in the region of the omentum, suggesting that the underlying condition is more likely to be high-grade (**b**)

6.1.3.12
Gastro-intestinal Stromal Tumour

Larger, more malignant-behaving GISTs may have either luminal or exogastric patterns of growth (Davis et al. 2000; Pannu et al. 1999) CT is excellent at demonstrating the extent of exogastric mass and possible invasion of adjacent structures. They have varying patterns of enhancement following contrast administration. Small tumours usually display a heterogeneous hyperattenuation pattern, but as they grow, large areas of hypoattenuation may occur due to ulceration and advanced necrosis within the tumour (Fig. 6.1.20a). Occasionally a large predominantly exogastric necrotic GIST may resemble a water filled stomach and care must be taken to identify the gastric lumen (Fig. 6.1.20b). CT may also detect both peritoneal and haematogenous spread. Lymph node involvement is rare.

New forms of chemotherapeutic treatment may result in dramatic reduction and advanced necrosis of the lesions on subsequent follow-up CT. Tumour size, as judged by Response Evaluation Criteria of Solid Tumors (RECIST) criteria, may not adequately define response to therapy when the predominant

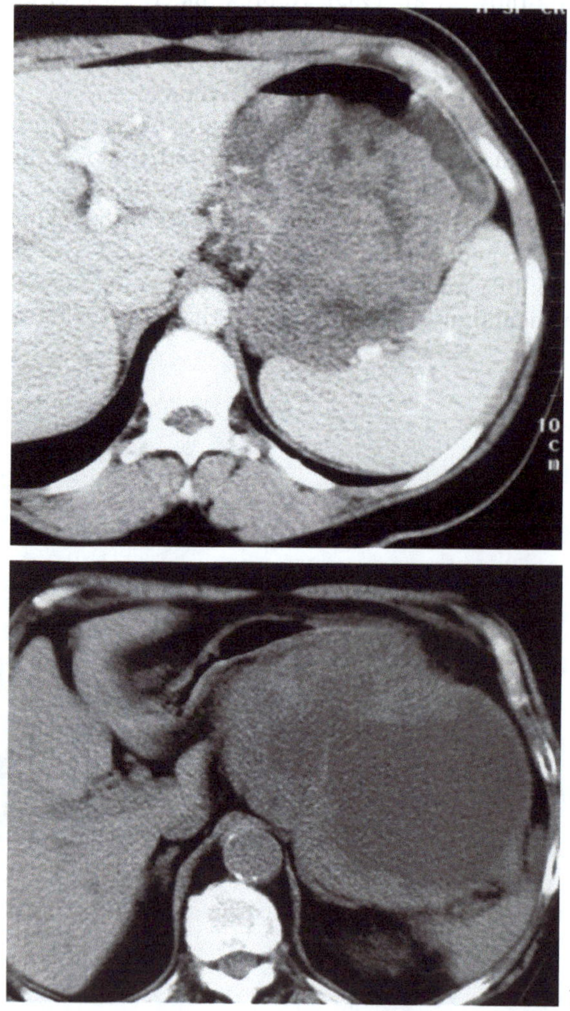

Fig. 6.1.20a,b. The whole of the lumen of the stomach is filled with a huge frankly malignant GIST, displaying a heterogeneous pattern with areas of low attenuation due to necrosis (**a**). A large low-attenuation exophytic GIST has a superficial resemblance to a fluid-filled stomach, but of course the main organ is grossly compressed and displaced to the right

changes are of attenuation rather than tumour dimension (Fig. 6.1.21a,b). PET/CT is probably a more accurate judge in this situation.

6.1.3.13 Metastases

Although gastric metastases are rare (less than 2% of autopsy patients who die of carcinoma), CT is highly effective for their demonstration. They may result from direct spread such as from a carcinoma of the pancreas or kidney (Fig. 6.1.22) or from a haematogenous route. The latter are exemplified by melanomas that produce submucosal masses and may have a substantial exophytic component (Fig. 6.1.23), or breast carcinoma, which typically produces a scirrhous reaction in the antrum (Fig. 6.1.24).

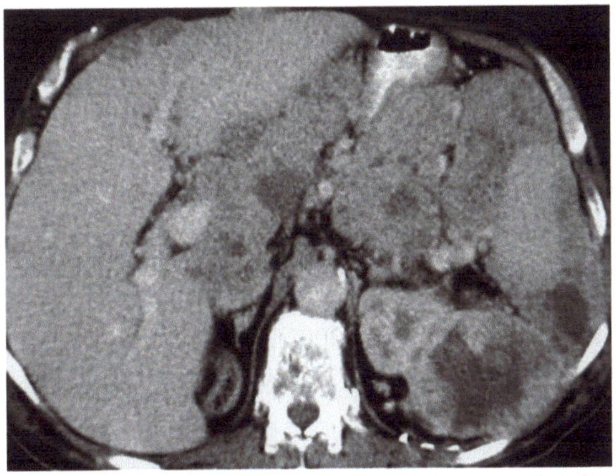

Fig. 6.1.22. Secondary involvement of the stomach by a renal carcinoma. The primary tumour arises from the left kidney and spreads around the spleen, stomach, and portal areas, resulting in obliteration of the gastric lumen

a

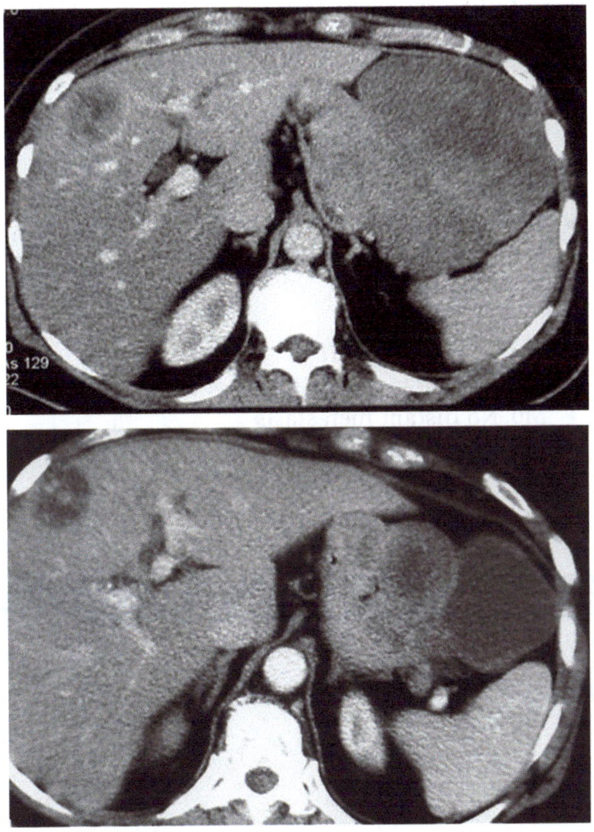

b

Fig. 6.1.21a,b. GIST response to Glivec therapy. The initial CT demonstrates a huge predominately exophytic GIST arising from the greater curve of the stomach (**a**). Note the metastasis in the liver. Following three months of Glivec therapy, there has been dramatic reduction in the size of the main tumour and it is of lower attenuation (**b**). However, there has been relatively little change in the appearance of the metastasis

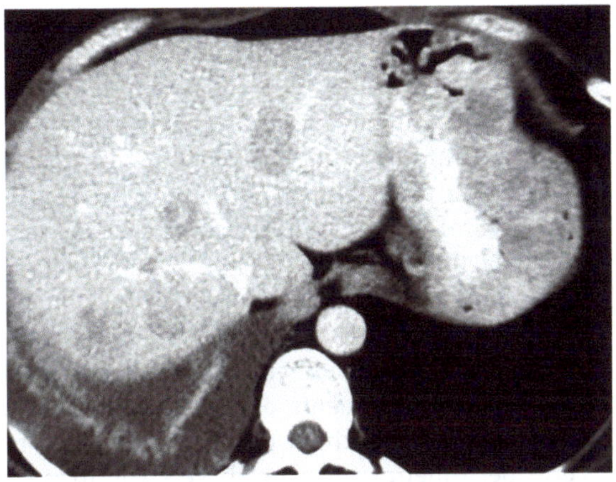

Fig. 6.1.23. Secondary involvement of the stomach from malignant melanoma. Note the exophytic mass primarily affecting the greater curve, together with liver metastases, ascites, and a pleural effusion

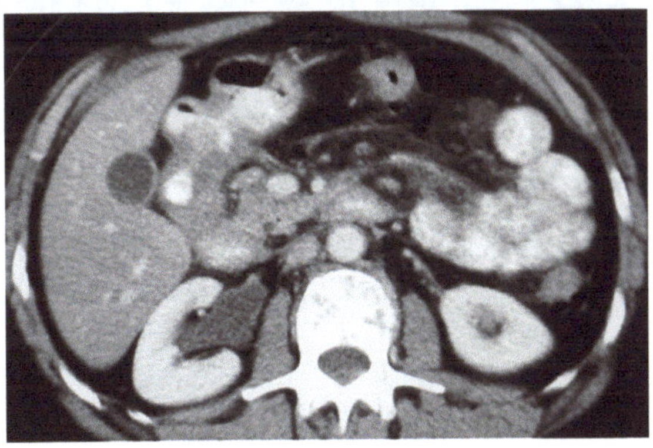

Fig. 6.1.24. Secondary involvement of the stomach from breast carcinoma. The antrum, pyloric region and proximal duodenum are most affected, with irregular thickening of the wall

6.1.4 Gastric Cancer Appendix 1

6.1.4.1 TNM Staging System

The American Joint Committee on Cancer (AJCC) designated staging incorporating the TNM classification (Greene et al. 2002), with previous refinements (Roder et al. 1998; Ichikura et al. 1999). TNM definitions:

Primary tumour (T)

- TX Primary tumour cannot be assessed
- T0 No evidence of primary tumour
- Tis Carcinoma in situ: Intraepithelial tumour without invasion of the lamina propria
- T1 Tumour invades lamina propria or submucosa
- T2 Tumour invades the muscularis propria or the subserosa*
  T2a Tumour invades muscularis propria.
  T2b Tumour invades subserosa
- T3 Tumour penetrates the serosa (visceral peritoneum) without invading adjacent structures ** ***
- T4 Tumour invades adjacent structures ***

* Note: A tumour may penetrate the muscularis propria with extension into the gastrocolic or gastrohepatic ligaments or into the greater or lesser omentum without perforation of the visceral peritoneum covering these structures. In this case, the tumour is classified T2. If there is perforation of the visceral peritoneum covering the gastric ligaments or omentum, the tumour should be classified T3.

** Note: the adjacent structures of the stomach include the spleen, transverse colon, liver, diaphragm, pancreas, abdominal wall, adrenal gland, kidney, small intestine, and retroperitoneum.

*** Note: Intramural extension to the duodenum or oesophagus is classified by the depth of greatest invasion in any of these sites, including stomach.

Regional lymph nodes (N). The regional lymph nodes are the perigastric nodes, found along the lesser and greater curvatures, and the nodes located along the left gastric, common hepatic, splenic, and celiac arteries. For pN, a regional lymphadenectomy specimen will ordinarily contain at least 15 lymph nodes. Involvement of other intra-abdominal lymph nodes, such as the hepatoduodenal, retropancreatic, mesenteric, and para-aortic is classified as distant metastasis.

- NX Regional lymph node(s) cannot be assessed
- N0 No regional lymph node metastasis
- N1 Metastasis in 1 to 6 regional lymph nodes
- N2 Metastasis in 7 to 15 regional lymph nodes
- N3 Metastasis in more than 15 regional lymph nodes

Distant metastasis (M)

- MX Distant metastasis cannot be assessed
- M0 No distant metastasis
- M1 Distant metastasis

Table 6.1.1. AJCC stage groupings

Stage 0	Stage 1A	Stage 1B	Stage 11	Stage IIIA	Stage IIIB	Stage IV
Tis, NO, MO	T1, NO, MO	T1, N1, MO T2, NO, MO	T1, N2, MO T2, N1, MO T3, NO, MO	T2, N2, MO T3, N1, MO T4, NO, MO	T3, N2, MO	T4, N1, MO T1, N3, MO T2, N3, MO T3, N3, MO T4, N2, MO T4, N3, MO Any T, Any N M1

References

Balthazar EJ, Megibow A, Naidich D, Le Fleur RS (1984) Computed tomographic recognition of gastric varices. AJR Am J Roentgenol 142:1121–1125

Brown JA, Carson BW, Gascoyne RD, Cooperberg PL, Connors JM, Mason AC (2000) Low grade gastric MALT lymphoma: radiographic findings. Clin Radiol 55:384–389

Buy JN, Moss AA (1982 Computed tomography of gastric lymphoma. AJR Am J Roentgenol 138:859–865

Chan JK, Ng CS, Isaacson PG (1990) Relationship between high-grade lymphoma and low-grade B-cell mucosa-associated lymphoid tissue lymphoma (MALToma) of the stomach. Am J Pathol 136:1153–1164

Cho KC, Baker SR, Alterman DD, Fusco JM, Cho S (1996) Transpyloric spread of gastric tumors: comparison of adenocarcinoma and lymphoma. AJR Am J Roentgenol 167:467–469

Davis GB, Blanchard DK, Hatch GF et al (2000) Tumors of the stomach. World J Surg 24:412–420

Fishman EK, Urban BA, Hruban RH (1996) CT of the stomach: spectrum of disease. Radiographics 16 :1035–1054

Ghanem N, Altehoefer C, Furtwangler A, Winterer J, Schafer O, Springer O, Kotter E, Langer M (2003) Computed tomography in gastrointestinal stromal tumors. Eur Radiol 13:1669–1678

Greene FL, Fritz AG, Balch CM, Haller DG, Page DL, Fleming ID, Morrow M (eds) (2002) American Joint Committee on Cancer. AJCC Cancer Staging Handbook, 6th edition, Springer, New York

Horton KM, Fishman EK (1998) Helical CT of the stomach: evaluation with water as an oral contrast agent. AJR Am J Roentgenol 171:1373–1376

Horton KM, Fishman EK (2003) Current role of CT in imaging of the stomach. Radiographics 23:75–87

Ichikura T, Tomimatsu S, Uefuji K et al (1999) Evaluation of the New American Joint Committee on Cancer/International Union against cancer classification of lymph node metastasis from gastric carcinoma in comparison with the Japanese classification. Cancer 86:553–558

Jacobs JM, Hill MC, Steinberg WM (1991) Peptic ulcer disease: CT evaluation. Radiology 178:745–748

Karpeh MS, Leon L, Klimstra D, Brennan MF (2000) Lymph node staging in gastric cancer: is location more important than number? An analysis of 1,038 patients. Ann Surg 232:362–371

Kessar P, Norton A, Rohatiner AZ, Lister TA, Reznek RH (1999) CT appearances of mucosa-associated lymphoid tissue (MALT) lymphoma. Eur Radiol 9:693–696

Kinkel K, Lu Y, Both M, Warren RS, Thoeni RF (2002) Detection of hepatic metastases from cancers of the gastrointestinal tract by using non-invasive imaging methods (US, CT, MR imaging, PET): a meta-analysis. Radiology 224:748–756

Lee DH (2000) Two-dimensional and three-dimensional imaging of gastric tumours using spiral CT. Abdom Imaging 25:1–6

Lewin KJ, Ranchod M, Dorfman RF (1978) Lymphomas of the gastrointestinal tract: a study of 117 cases presenting with gastrointestinal disease. Cancer 42:693–707

Mani NB, Suri S, Gupta S, Wig JD (2001) Two-phase dynamic contrast-enhanced computed tomography with water-filling method for staging of gastric carcinoma. Clin Imaging 25:38–43

Megibow AJ, Balthazar EJ, Naidich DP, Bosniak MA (1983) Computed tomography of gastrointestinal lymphoma. AJR Am J Roentgenol 141:541–547

Merino S, Saiz A, Moreno MJ et al (1999) CT evaluation of gastric wall pathology. Br J Radiol 72:1124–1131

Pannu HK, Hruban RH, Fishman EK (1999) CT of gastric leiomyosarcoma: patterns of involvement. AJR Am J Roentgenol 173:369–373

Park MS, Kim KW, Yu JS, Park C, Kim JK, Yoon SW, Lee KH, Ryu YH, Kim H, Kim MJ, Lee JT, Yoo HS (2002) Radiographic findings of primary B-cell lymphoma of the stomach: low-grade versus high-grade malignancy in relation to the mucosa-associated lymphoid tissue concept. AJR 179:1297–1304

Roder JD, Bottcher K, Busch R et al (1998) Classification of regional lymph node metastasis from gastric carcinoma. German Gastric Cancer Study Group. Cancer 82:621–631

Rossi M, Broglia L, Maccioni F et al (1997) Hydro-CT in patients with gastric cancer: preoperative radiologic staging. Eur Radiol 7:659–664

Sato T, Sakai Y, Ishiguro S, Furukawa H (1986) Radiologic manifestations of early gastric lymphoma. AJR Am J Roentgenol 146:513–517

Stabile Ianora AA, Wolowiec A, Francioso G, Scardapane A, Rotondo A, Angelelli G (2001) Aspetti delle ulcere benigne e maligne dello stomaco in Tomografia Computerizzata. Radiol Med 102:32–36

Urban BA, Fishman EK, Hruban RH (1991) Helicobacter pylori gastritis mimicking gastric carcinoma at CT evaluation. Radiology 179:689–691

Vitello JM (1996) Gastric intramural pseudocyst with associated gastric outlet obstruction: recognition and management. South Med J 89:534–537

Wagholikar GD, Ibrarullah M, Venkataramanapa M (2003) Gastric intramural pseudocyst-a complication of percutaneous drainage of an acute pancreatic pseudocyst. Am J Gastroenterol 98:229–231

Wakelin SJ, Deans C, Crofts TJ, Allan PL, Plevris JN, Paterson-Brown (2002) A comparison of computerised tomography, laparoscopic ultrasound and endoscopic ultrasound in the preoperative staging of oesophago-gastric carcinoma. Eur J Radiol 41:161–167

Wotherspoon AC, Ortiz-Hidalgo C, Falzon MR, Isaacson PG (1991) Helicobacter pylori-associated gastritis and primary B-cell gastric lymphoma. Lancet 338:1175–1176

Multislice CT of the Stomach

6.2

Ahmed Ba-Ssalamah, Martin Uffmann, Peter Pokieser, and Mathias Prokop

CONTENTS

A. Ba-Ssalamah, MD
M. Uffmann, MD
P. Pokieser, MD
M. Prokop, MD
Department of Radiology, University of Vienna, Währinger Gürtel 18–20, 1090 Vienna, Austria

6.2.1 Introduction

Multislice CT offers new opportunities for the imaging of gastrointestinal organs. With thin collimation, excellent imaging of the stomach becomes possible and allows for high-quality multiplanar reformations and 3D visualization. Adequate distension of the stomach using water as a negative contrast agent (hydro-CT) is a prerequisite for assessing the stomach wall. While such techniques have already been used with single-slice spiral CT to improve staging of gastric malignancies, single slice suffers substantially from relatively large slice thickness (Fishman et al. 1996; Baert et al. 1989; Merino et al. 1999). The much faster speed of multislice CT means that optimal contrast material injection techniques are essential (Fleischmann et al. 2000) in order to improve delineation of tumour from normal tissue. Indeed, the combination of hydro-CT with near isotropic multislice imaging offers improved diagnosis to a large variety of gastric diseases. Compared with endosonography, multislice CT is able not only to visualize the immediate vicinity of the stomach, but also more distant regions, such as para-aortic lymph nodes or abdominal organs. It is expected that multislice CT will be able to help in the decision between conservative and surgical therapy in selected patients.

This chapter reviews the applications of multislice CT for a variety of diseases of the stomach.

6.2.2 CT Technique

Optimum CT technique requires high spatial resolution, good gastric distension and an appropriate timing of contrast media injection in order to detect subtle changes in the gastric wall and to accurately stage tumours. Table 6.2.1 provides an overview of techniques for various multislice CT machine types.

The CT examinations in our department are performed on a four-detector-row CT machine with a 0.5-s tube rotation (Somatom Volume Zoom, Siemens, Forchheim, Germany). To acquire a near isotropic data set, the use of 4×1-mm collimation and reconstructed 1.25-mm-thick sections every 0.7 mm appears optimal. For diagnostic viewing, 3- to 4-mm-thick axial sections are reconstructed, either directly from the scan data or from the thin-section volumetric data set ("secondary raw data set") using the multiplanar reformatting (MPR) functionality of the scanner console. In addition, coronal and sagittal reformations in the region of the stomach are routinely performed. Because of high image noise on the original 1.25-mm-thick sections, the width of these reformations was increased to 3–5 mm, depending on the size of the patient. Interactive reformations are helpful whenever diagnostic questions remain unresolved on standard MPR, using a dedicated CT workstation (MagicView 1000, Siemens, Forchheim, Germany).

Contrast material injection for the stomach is timed in a manner that assures portal phase imaging. If tumour staging is required, an additional arterial phase examination of the liver is added to the protocol. In such cases, the scan range includes only the liver and the stomach in the arterial phase, and then the entire abdomen down to the level of the iliac crest for the portal venous phase (see Table 6.2.1). The use of 125 kVp and 150 mAs_{eff} as the exposure settings appears optimal. The resulting volume CT dose index ($CTDI_{vol}$), as an indicator of average local dose, was 17.1 mGy for each multislice acquisition. This number may be varied with patient size: 125 kVp and 10 mGy appears sufficient for slim patients, but for very obese patients, 140 kVp and up to 30 mGy should be used for optimal image quality.

6.2.3 Gastric Cancer

Gastric cancer remains a deadly disease, with overall 5-year survival rates of <20%. Early gastric cancers, however, are curable lesions with 5-year survival rates of more than 90%. The peak incidence is between 50 and 70 years of age (Moore

Table 6.2.1. Suggested CT technique for examination of the stomach

Patient preparation and positioning
• Fasting: no solid food for at least 6 h
• Oral contrast: 1000–1500 ml water or flavoured methylcellulose preparation
• Hypotonia: 20 mg scopolamine intravenously
• Patient position: prone position if known lesion in the antrum or pyloric wall
• Supine position in all other lesions
Scanning technique
• Slice collimation: 0.75–1.25 mm (4-, 8- ,16-row scanners)
• Pitch: >1.0 (e.g., 6:4 on most 4-row scanners)
• CT dose index ($CTDI_{vol}$): 15 mGy (10–30 mGy depending on patient size)
• Reconstruction slice thickness: 1.0–1.5 mm secondary raw data set for volumetric reconstruction
• Reconstruction increment: 0.7 mm
Imaging
• Axial, coronal, sagittal reformations: 4-mm thickness (3–6 mm, depending on image noise)
• Interactive multiplanar reformations: optional for equivocal and difficult cases
Contrast material (CM) injection
• Contrast volume + saline flush: 120 ml (or 1.5 ml/kg body weight) CM + 60 ml saline
• Flow rate: 4 ml/s (or 30-s injection duration)
• Start delay
– Arterial phase: 30 s (or bolus tracking: 10 s after aortic arrival) for tumour staging
– Portal venous phase: 60 s (or bolus tracking: 40 s after aortic arrival) for stomach

1986). Gastric carcinoma has striking geographic variations, with the highest incidences reported in Japan. Conditions that predispose patients to the development of gastric carcinoma include atrophic gastritis, pernicious anaemia, gastric polyps, partial gastrectomy, and Ménétrier's disease (Oiso 1975). About 30% of cancers are located in the antrum, 30% in the body, and 30% in the fundus or cardia region. The remaining 10% are diffusely infiltrating lesions involving the entire stomach. Most gastric cancers are adenocarcinomas of mucous cell origin (Parker et al. 1996). Signet-ring cell carcinomas account for 5–15% of all gastric cancers and typically cause scirrhous infiltration of the gastric wall (Balthazar et al. 1980). Scirrhous carcinomas frequently involve the distal half of the stomach, arise near the pylorus, and gradually extend upward from the antrum into the body and fundus. In advanced cases, the entire stomach is infiltrated by tumour.

6.2.3.1 Tumour Detection and Classification

Gastric carcinomas may present as a focal area of mural thickening with or without ulceration, or as a generalized mural thickening. Sometimes they present as a polypoid lesion.

In early gastric cancers, malignant invasion is limited to the mucosa or submucosa, regardless of the presence of lymph node metastases (Maruyama and Baba 1994). Early cancers are classified into three types (Davis 1993; Fig. 6.2.1), and type I lesions can be better detected than type-II and type-III lesions (Fig. 6.2.2).

Advanced gastric cancer invades the muscularis propria (Maruyama and Baba 1994). Advanced cancer may present as large, segmental lesions (Fig. 6.2.3a), or diffuse wall thickening with irregular lobulation and, often, ulceration (Fig. 6.2.3b). Signet-ring cell cancer usually presents as a scirrhous tumour of the stomach that leads to obliteration of gastric folds and diffuse thickening of the gastric wall (linitis plastica; Fig. 6.2.3c). Gastric carcinoma can present as large polypoid, fungating lesions (Fig. 6.2.4a).

Carcinoma of the gastric cardia may be difficult to visualize on CT because of the normal soft tissue thickening that occurs at the gastroesophageal junction. This is due to the reflections of the phrenoesophageal ligament and the attachments of the gastrohepatic ligament onto the adjacent lesser curvature. Full distension of the stomach helps to distinguish a focal tumour from the normal gastroesophageal junction.

6.2.3.2 T Staging

CT criteria for differentiating the various T stages are given in Table 6.2.2 (D'Elia et al. 2000). In early advanced gastric cancers, (T2) malignant invasion is limited to the muscularis propria. The outer border may be smooth (Fig. 6.2.3a) or show a few small linear strands of soft tissue extending into the fat plane in cases with a desmoplastic or inflammatory reaction (Fig. 6.2.3b). The probability of transmural extension of tumour (T3) is directly correlated with mural thickness. In transmural extension, the serosal contour becomes blurred, and strand-like densities may be seen extending into the perigastric

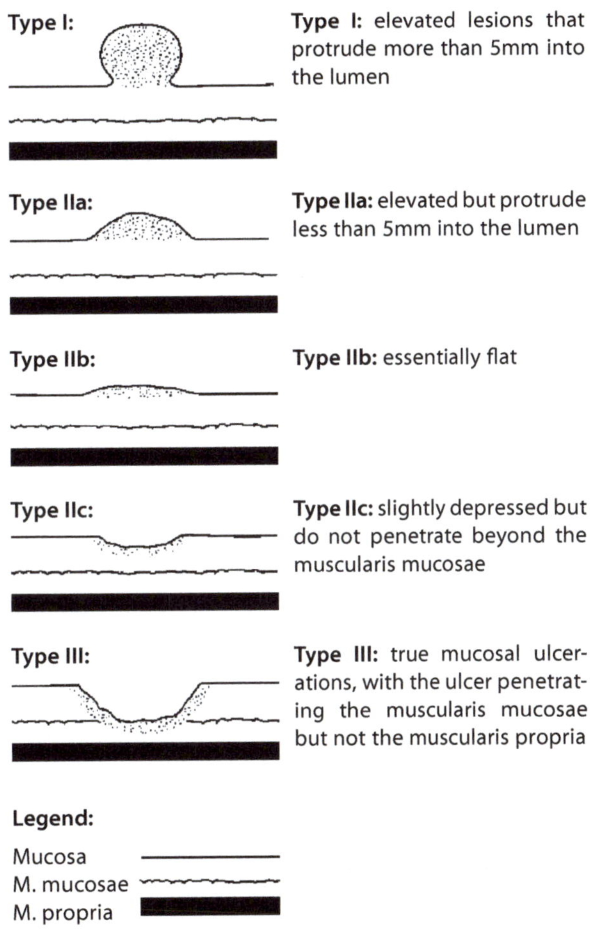

Fig. 6.2.1. Types of early gastric cancer. (Modified from Davis 1993)

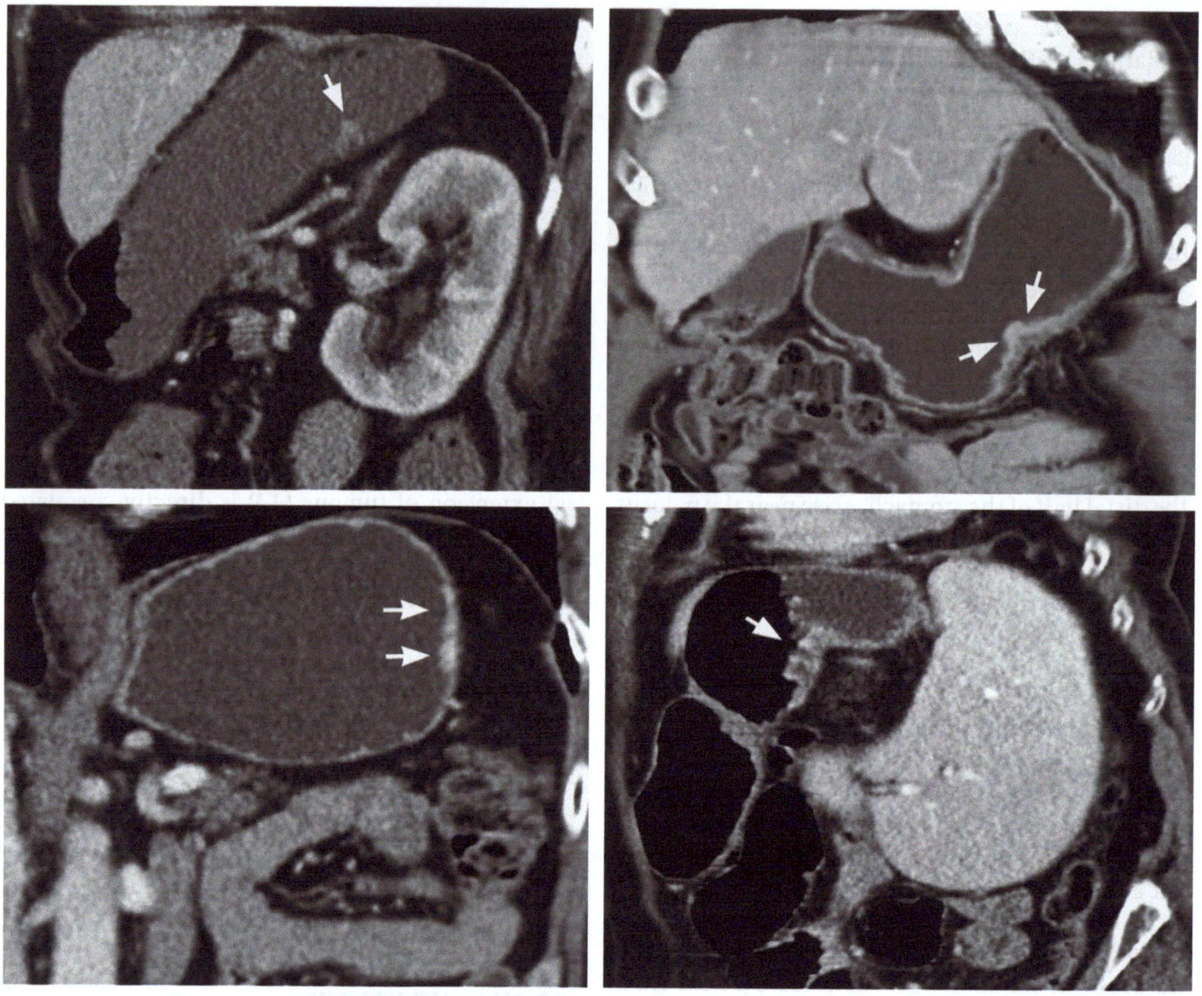

Fig. 6.2.2a–d. Early gastric cancer (pT1). **a** Type I: The sagittal reformation shows an enhancing polypoid lesion that protrudes more than 5 mm into the lumen (*arrow*). **b** Type IIa: The coronal reformation shows an elevated lesion in the greater curvature that protrudes less than 5 mm into the lumen. There is a strong focal enhancement of the inner layer (*arrows*) of the gastric wall. **c** Type IIb: Coronal reformation shows focal thickening of gastric wall with strong enhancement but an essentially flat surface. The other nodular protrusions of the gastric wall correspond to normal folds that are stretched out because of gastric dilatation (*arrows*). **d** Type III: Oblique sagittal reformation demonstrates focal thickening of the gastric wall with central ulceration (*arrow*)

fat (Fig. 6.2.4). Tumour spread frequently occurs via ligamentous and peritoneal reflections to adjacent organs (T4; Fig. 6.2.5). The liver may be invaded via the gastrohepatic ligament, the pancreas via the lesser sac (Fig. 6.2.5a) and the transverse colon via the gastrocolic ligament (Fig. 6.2.5b). The distal oesophagus is directly involved by carcinoma of the cardia in about 60% of patients (Fig. 6.2.5c), whereas the duodenum is involved by carcinoma of the antrum in 13–18% of patients. Infiltration into the transverse mesocolon (T4) is often hard to distinguish from infiltration of the mesenteric fat. Coronal or sagittal reformations are best suited for this purpose (Fig. 6.2.5b).

6.2.3.3 N Staging

Because of the abundant lymphatics in the stomach, lymphatic spread is found in 74–88% of patients with gastric carcinoma (Fukuya et al. 1995). The frequency of lymphatic metastases is related to the size and depth of penetration of the tumour. According to the American Joint Committee of Cancer (AJCC; Kapeh et al. 2000), N staging depends on the number of positive perigastric lymph nodes (N1=1–5, N2=6–15 and N3=more than 15 affected lymph nodes; Figs. 6.2.6, 6.2.7). Lymph node assessment for metastatic spread remains a challenge

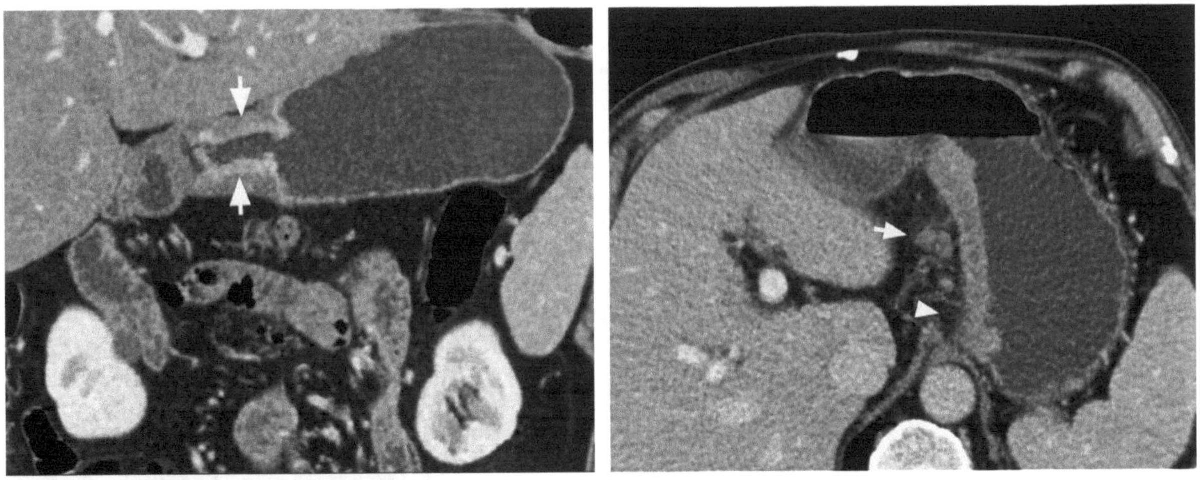
a b

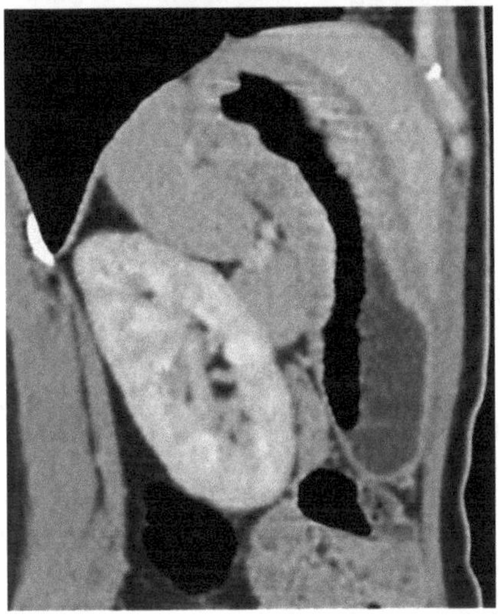
c

Fig. 6.2.3a–c. Advanced gastric cancer (pT2). **a** Coronal reformation shows focal wall thickening of the antrum with marked enhancement of the mucosal layer (*arrows*). At histology, the outer layers of the muscularis propria were intact, whereas the inner layers were infiltrated. The subtle irregularities of the mucosal surface correspond to ulceration at histology. Note the clear fat plane around the tumour. **b** Large carcinoma at the lesser curvature. Note that there is an area with irregular delineation of the tumour from the surrounding fat (*arrowhead*), which corresponds to a desmoplastic reaction at histology. There are two slightly hyperenhancing lymph nodes adjacent to each other (*arrow*); both proved to be metastases positive at histology. **c** Sagittal reformation shows diffuse thickening of the gastric wall in the fundus and corpus region due to linitis plastica. Note the lack of the gastric folds and the decreased distension in the affected region.

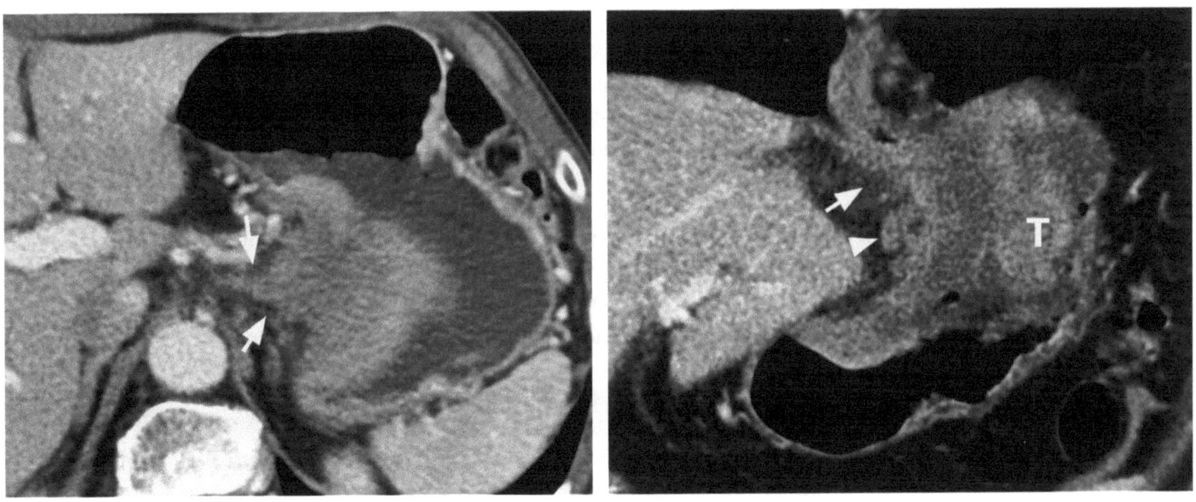

a b

Fig. 6.2.4a,b. Advanced gastric cancer (pT3). **a** A large polypoid carcinoma with gross infiltration of the perigastric fatty tissue (*arrows*). **b** Oblique coronal reformation tilted posteriorly to display the corpus and fundus of the stomach and distal oesophagus. There is a large tumour (*T*) that protrudes from the posterior wall into the lumen and appears as a filling defect within the water-filled stomach. Note the increased density stranding in the perigastric fat (*arrow*) and the oval lymph node that proved to be hyperplastic at histology (*arrowhead*)

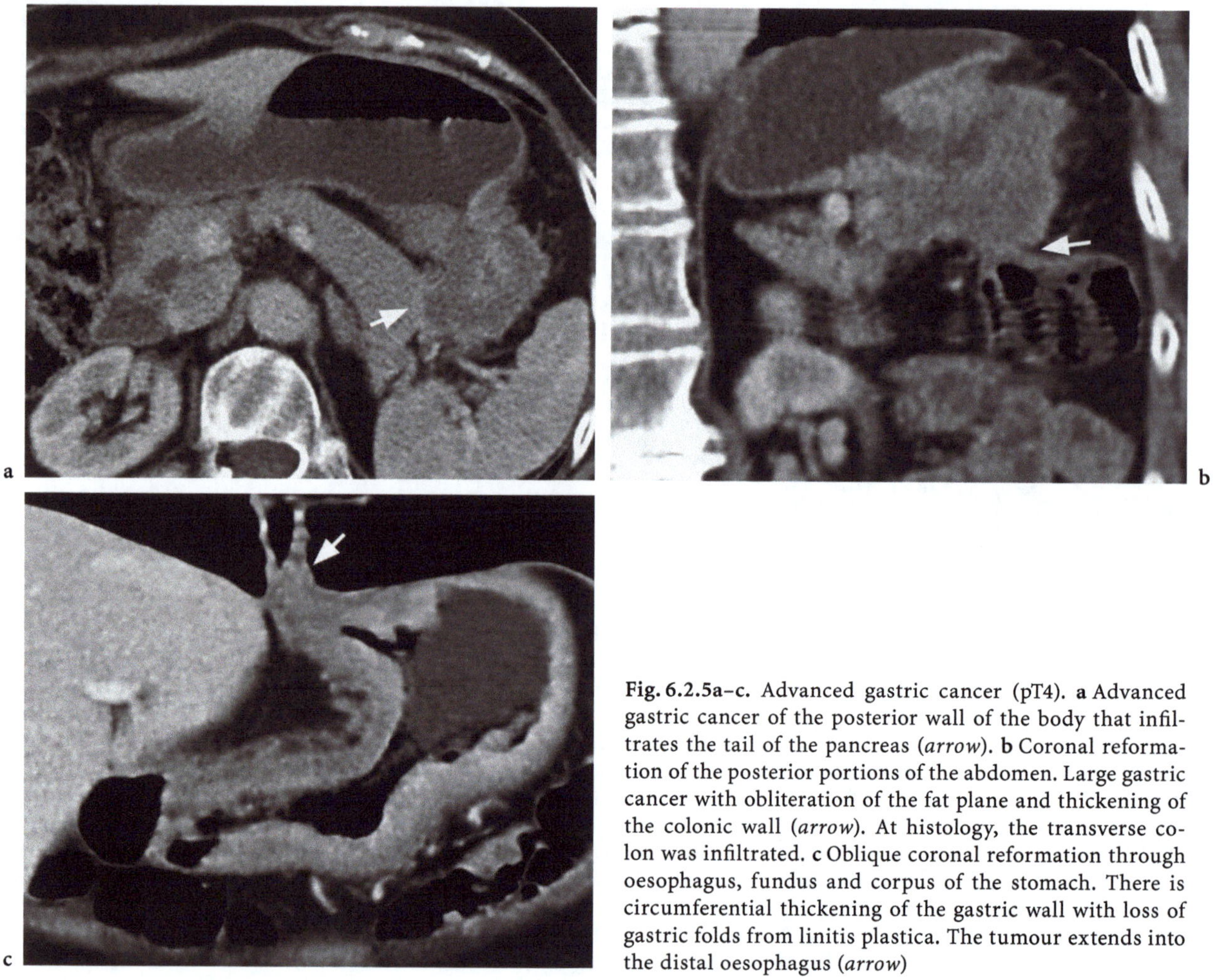

Fig. 6.2.5a–c. Advanced gastric cancer (pT4). **a** Advanced gastric cancer of the posterior wall of the body that infiltrates the tail of the pancreas (*arrow*). **b** Coronal reformation of the posterior portions of the abdomen. Large gastric cancer with obliteration of the fat plane and thickening of the colonic wall (*arrow*). At histology, the transverse colon was infiltrated. **c** Oblique coronal reformation through oesophagus, fundus and corpus of the stomach. There is circumferential thickening of the gastric wall with loss of gastric folds from linitis plastica. The tumour extends into the distal oesophagus (*arrow*)

Table 6.2.2. The CT criteria for T- and N-staging. (Modified from D'Elia et al. 2000)

T staging
• TO: no evidence of alteration of the gastric wall with normal fat plane
• T1: Non-transmural strong enhancement with focal wall thickening or strong enhancement only without wall thickening in a single layer pattern, or thickening and strong enhancement without abrupt obliteration of middle and outer layers in multilayered pattern
• T2: transmural enhancement with focal wall thickening in a single layer pattern, or both abnormal enhancement and abrupt obliteration of middle in three-layered pattern, or outer layers in two-layered pattern. Smooth outer border of thickened gastric wall or few small linear strands of soft tissue extending into fat plane
• T3: Reticular or irregular outer border of thickened gastric wall, or blurred fat plane around the lesion
• T3/T4: Obliteration of the fat plane between the gastric tumour and adjacent organs (indeterminant)
• T4: gross infiltration of adjacent organs
N staging
• Regional lymph nodes are considered involved when the short-axis diameter is >6 mm for the perigastric lymph nodes and >8 mm for the extraperigastric lymph nodes
Other criteria for malignant involvement include:
• Nearly round shape (L/T ratio <1.5)
• Fatty hilum eccentric or missing
• Strong or heterogeneous enhancement

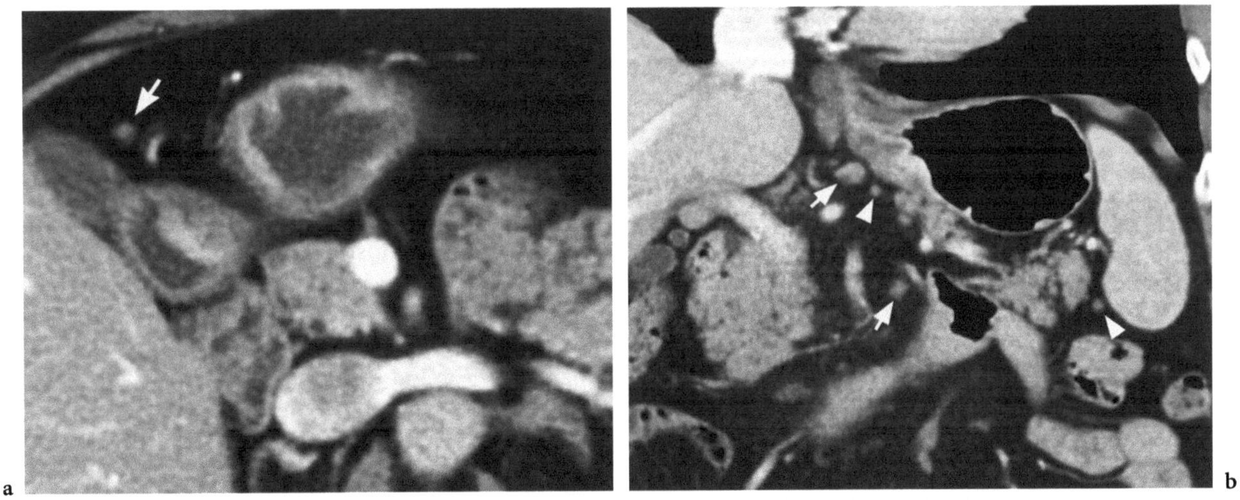

Fig. 6.2.6a,b. Normal lymph nodes in gastric cancer. **a** Small slightly oval lymph node 4 mm in diameter without significant contrast enhancement (*arrow*). **b** Coronal reformation through the gastric fundus. Large gastric cancer of the cardia (pT2), with multiple lymph nodes. Note the two inhomogeneous contrast-enhancing nodes ≥8 mm (*arrows*) as well as multiple lymph nodes of <6 mm in diameter (*arrowheads*). At histology all lymph nodes were negative for metastatic disease

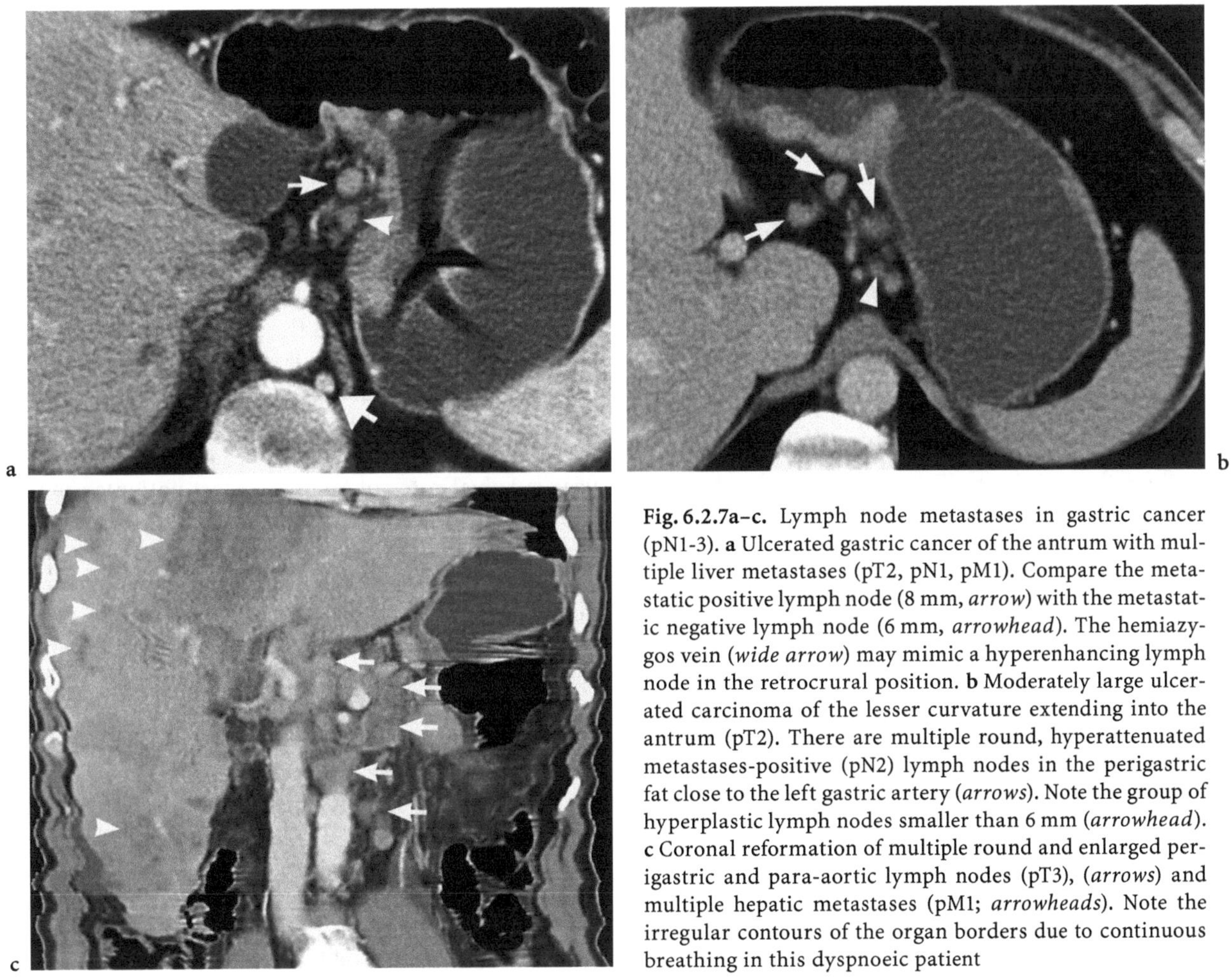

Fig. 6.2.7a–c. Lymph node metastases in gastric cancer (pN1-3). **a** Ulcerated gastric cancer of the antrum with multiple liver metastases (pT2, pN1, pM1). Compare the metastatic positive lymph node (8 mm, *arrow*) with the metastatic negative lymph node (6 mm, *arrowhead*). The hemiazygos vein (*wide arrow*) may mimic a hyperenhancing lymph node in the retrocrural position. **b** Moderately large ulcerated carcinoma of the lesser curvature extending into the antrum (pT2). There are multiple round, hyperattenuated metastases-positive (pN2) lymph nodes in the perigastric fat close to the left gastric artery (*arrows*). Note the group of hyperplastic lymph nodes smaller than 6 mm (*arrowhead*). **c** Coronal reformation of multiple round and enlarged perigastric and para-aortic lymph nodes (pT3), (*arrows*) and multiple hepatic metastases (pM1; *arrowheads*). Note the irregular contours of the organ borders due to continuous breathing in this dyspnoeic patient

even with multislice CT; however, improved evaluation appears possible if both morphological and enhancement criteria are used (Table 6.2.2).

6.2.3.4 M Staging

Haematogenous metastases from gastric carcinoma most commonly involve the liver, because venous drainage of the stomach is via the portal vein (Fig. 6.2.7c). Other less common sites of haematogenous spread include the lungs, adrenals, kidneys, bones and brain. Lymph node involvement outside the perigastric location is considered M1 disease. Advanced cancers can develop peritoneal metastases (Fig. 6.2.8). Some patients with signet-ring cell gastric carcinomas may have transperitoneal seeded metastases to the ovaries, which are known as Krukenberg tumours.

6.2.3.5 Follow-Up After Partial Gastrectomy

A gastric "stump" cancer is defined as a primary carcinoma that occurs in the gastric remnant which follows partial gastrectomy for gastric ulcers or other benign disease. They may appear after latent periods of 15–25 years from the time of gastrectomy (Fig. 6.2.9a). Affected individuals usually have undergone a Billroth II, rather than a Billroth I, procedure. These tumours tend to be located in the distal portion of the gastric remnant near the gastrojejunal anastomosis. It has been postulated that recurrent bile reflux above the anastomosis causes chronic gastritis, intestinal metaplasia and, eventually, gastric carcinoma. Not all thickening of the anastomotic region is due to tumour involvement (Fig. 6.2.9b). Other postoperative changes, such as following a Nissen procedure for gastric reflux, can sometimes lead to marked fold thickening (Fig. 6.2.9c), and postoperative complications, such as seroma, may cause confusion (Fig. 6.2.9d).

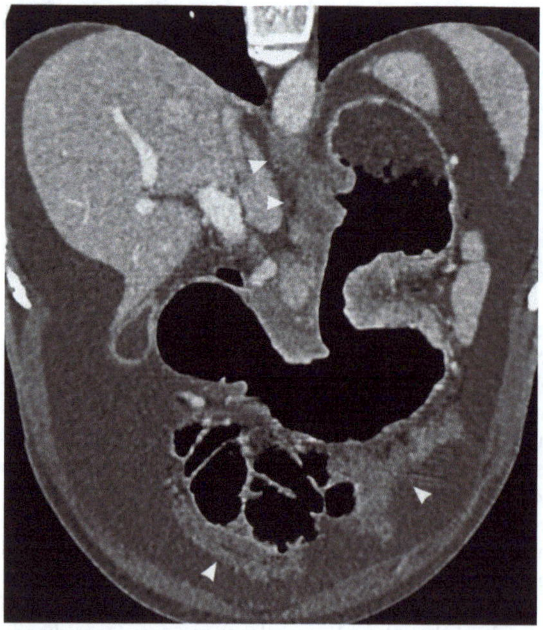

Fig. 6.2.8. Extension of gastric cancer. Oblique coronal reformation performed to display fundus, corpus and antrum of the stomach. Surgical proven advanced cancer in the gastric body with ascites and peritoneal carcinomatosis (*arrowheads*)

6.2.4 Other Gastric Malignancies

6.2.4.1 Gastric Lymphoma

Lymphoma involves the stomach more frequently than any other portion of the gastrointestinal tract. Gastric lymphoma accounts for 50% of all gastrointestinal lymphomas, 25% of all extranodal lymphomas and 3–5% of all malignant neoplasms in the stomach (Lewin et al. 1978). Primary gastric lymphoma is confined to the stomach and regional lymph nodes. Secondary gastric lymphoma is generalized lymphoma associated with gastric involvement. Primary gastric lymphoma has a much better prognosis than gastric carcinoma, with overall 5-year survival rates of 50–60%. Most patients are in the sixth or seventh decade of life.

Lymphoma may involve any portion of the stomach. Transpyloric spread of tumour into the duodenum occurs in about 30% of patients (Cho et al. 1996). Despite extensive lymphomatous infiltration, the stomach usually remains pliable and distensible without significant luminal narrowing.

Early gastric lymphoma is a lesion that is confined to the mucosa and submucosa (Fig. 6.2.10a), with an average size of only 3.5 cm at the time of diagnosis (Sato et al. 1986); however, gastric lymphomas are usually advanced lesions with a mean diameter of 10 cm (Fig. 6.2.10b). Most cases involve the antrum and body, although the entire stomach can be involved.

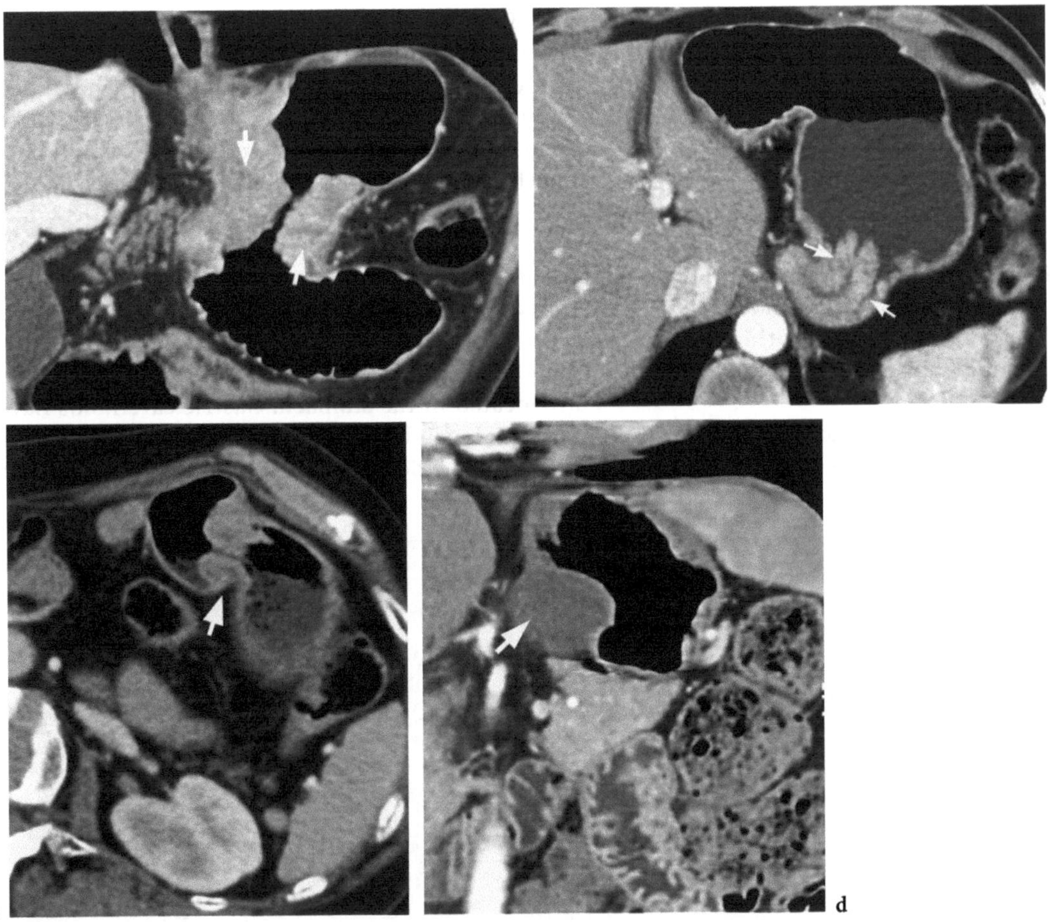

Fig. 6.2.9a–d. Postoperative findings. **a** Oblique coronal reformation to display the gastroesophageal junction as well as the gastroenterostomy after partial gastrectomy for adenocarcinoma of the stomach. There is a histologically proven large recurrent tumour in the region of the anastomosis that infiltrates the remaining portions of lesser curvature up to the gastroesophageal junction (*arrows*). **b** Oblique axial section tilted laterally to display the gastrojejunostomy after the BII resection. Despite substantial thickening (*arrow*) of the anastomotic region, there was no evidence of malignancy on multiple biopsies. **c** Marked fold thickening of the gastroesophageal junction line after fundoplication (*arrows*). **d** Coronal reformation through the gastric fundus. Round homogenous biopsy-proven seroma adjacent to the lesser curvature after BII resection of the stomach (*arrow*)

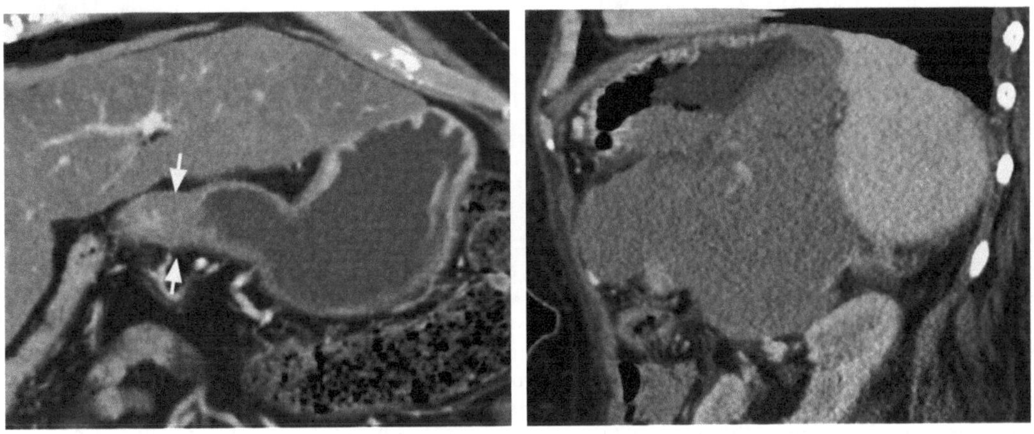

Fig. 6.2.10a,b. Gastric lymphoma. **a** Coronal reformation demonstrates biopsy-proved early gastric lymphoma with focal thickening of the antral wall (*arrows*). **b** Sagittal reformation shows bulky disease from a biopsy-proven advanced B-cell lymphoma

There are four gross pathological types of gastric lymphoma (Fischback et al. 1992): infiltrative gastric lymphomas manifest as a focal or diffuse enlargement of rugal folds due to submucosal spread of tumour (Fig. 6.2.11a). One or more ulcerated lesions characterize ulcerative gastric lymphoma (Fig. 6.2.11b). Polypoid gastric lymphomas are characterized by intraluminal masses that may simulate polypoid carcinomas (Fig. 6.2.11c). Multiple submucosal nodules ranging in size between several millimetres and several centimetres characterize the nodular form of gastric lymphoma (Fig. 6.2.11d).

Computed tomography is the primary imaging modality for the pretreatment evaluation of abdominal lymphoma. In patients with suspected gastric lymphoma, multislice CT may provide both detection of a stomach lesion and staging of generalized lymphoma in the abdomen and chest; however, the appearance of lymphoma and gastric carcinoma may be very similar (Table 6.2.3).

6.2.4.2 Carcinoid Tumours

Only about 2–3% of all gastrointestinal carcinoids are located in the stomach. Gastric carcinoids have an equal gender distribution and usually occur in patients older than the age of 40 years. Gastric

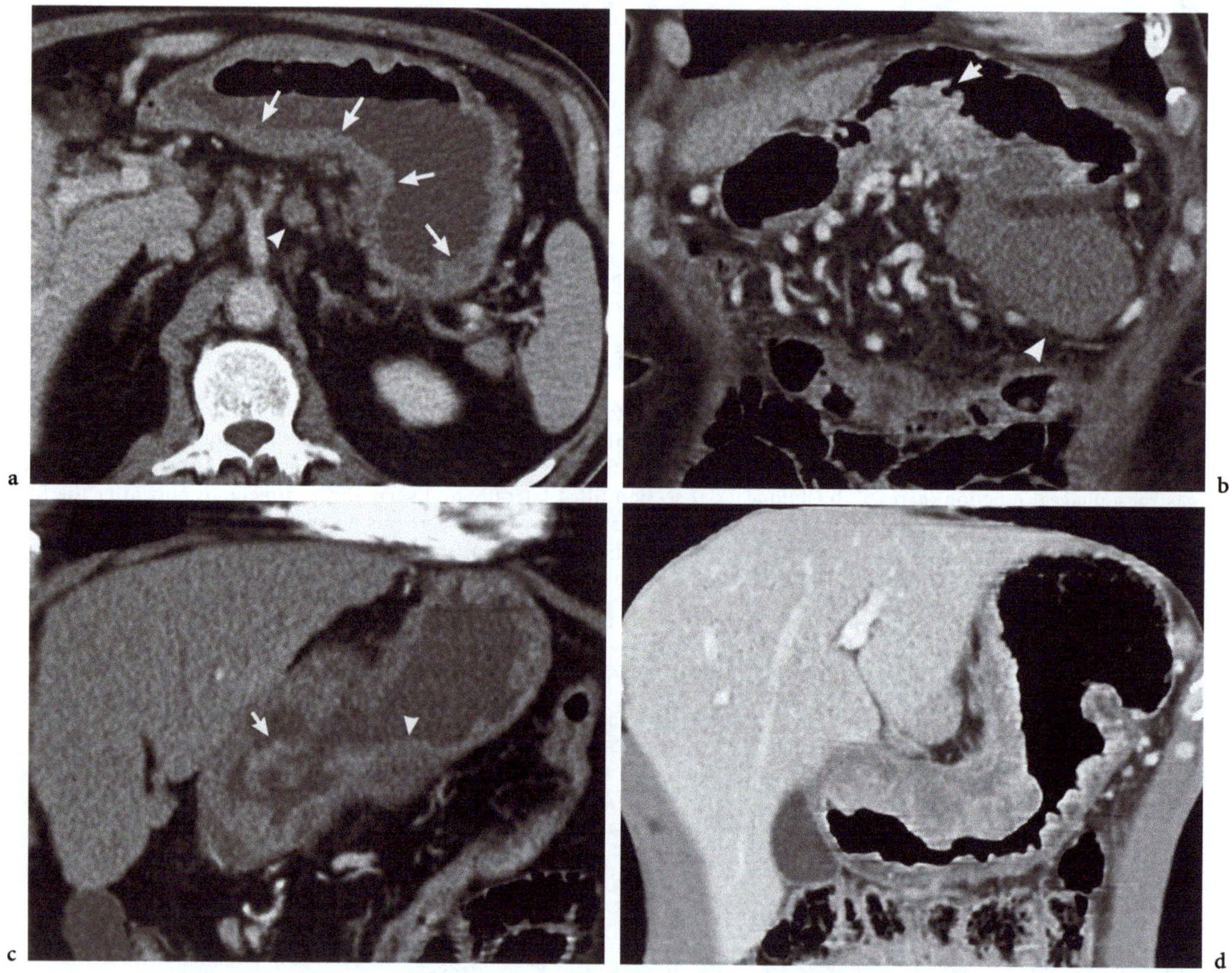

Fig. 6.2.11a–d. Morphological types of gastric lymphoma. **a** Biopsy-proven infiltrative type with large areas of gastric wall thickening (*arrows*) and enlarged lymph nodes (*arrowhead*). **b** Coronal reformation shows biopsy-proven polypoid type advanced gastric lymphoma with ulceration (*arrow*) and large extension into the mesenteric root (*arrowhead*). **c** Coronal reformation of biopsy-proven polypoid type with segmental thickening (*arrowhead*) and a large polypoid filling defect arising from the posterior wall of the stomach (*arrow*) in advanced gastric lymphoma. **d** Coronal reformation of biopsy-proven nodular type with nodular thickening of the gastric wall

Table 6.2.3. The CT features of gastric malignancies

Adenocarcinoma of the stomach	Gastric lymphoma	Gastric leiomyosarcoma[a]
Focal area of increased wall thickening Diffuse infiltration (linitis plastica) Presence of a bulky or ulcerated mass Intraluminal, exophytic or mixed Abnormal perigastric fat Local lymphadenopathy Seeding along peritoneal ligaments Metastases	Thickening of the stomach wall >1 cm Diffuse infiltration that involves >50% of the stomach wall Circumferential involvement of most of the stomach Segmental infiltration of the stomach Homogeneous wall thickening with preservation of the overlying rugal folds Localized polypoid formation with ulcer/perforation Presence of nodes on either side of the mesenteric vessels ("sandwich sign")	Large, heterogeneous masses extending outside the gastric wall Central necrosis and liquefaction Large ulceration Calcification

[a]Gastrointestinal stromal tumours

lesions often bleed regardless of size and rarely produce the carcinoid syndrome (Godwin 1975). Metastases are found in 20–30% of patients with gastric carcinoids at the time of diagnosis, but long-term survival has been reported even when regional or hepatic metastases are present.

The majority of patients with gastric carcinoids have one or more submucosal-appearing masses ranging from 1 to 4 cm in size. Gastric carcinoids may also present as sessile or pedunculated polyps that are indistinguishable from hyperplastic or adenomatous polyps. Advanced gastric carcinoid tumours may appear as polypoid or ulcerated intraluminal masses that simulate gastric carcinoma (Fig. 6.2.12). Characteristically, they are hypervascular and hyperattenuating in arterial phase scans.

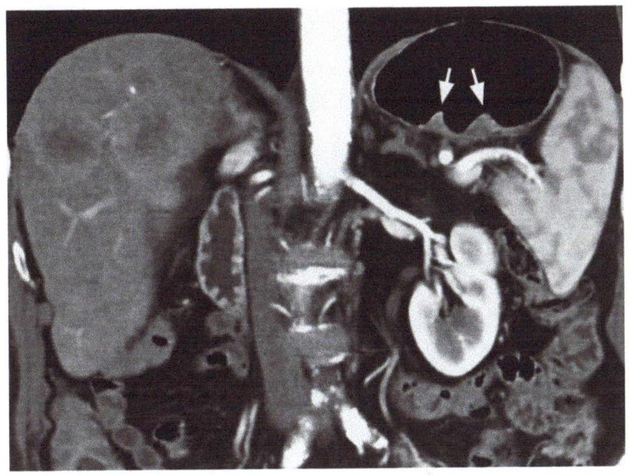

Fig. 6.2.12. Coronal reformation shows biopsy-proven carcinoid tumour presenting as an ulcerated mass. Note the thickened rim of the ulcer (*arrows*) on the coronal reformation. Note the presence of two liver metastases

6.2.4.3 Metastases

Gastric metastases are found at autopsy in <2% of patients who die of carcinoma. The majority of lesions are haematogenous metastases from malignant melanoma, or carcinoma of the breast and lung. Less commonly metastases from tumours of the cervix- (Fig. 6.2.13a), oesophagus- (Fig. 6.2.13b) and liver- (Fig. 6.2.13c), may be observed.

Continuous tumour invasion into the stomach may occur from tumours arising in neighbouring structures such as the pancreas (Fig. 6.2.14a), oesophagus (Fig. 6.2.14b), gall bladder, liver, colon and kidney.

6.2.5 Miscellaneous Tumours

6.2.5.1 Gastrointestinal Stromal Tumours

Gastrointestinal stromal tumours (GISTs) are part of the group of mesenchymal tumours. Many, but not all, mesenchymal tumours previously diagnosed as leiomyomas, leiomyoblastomas, leiomyosarcomas, etc., are now considered GISTs based on specific immunohistochemical criteria (Miettinen and Lasota 2001). The malignant variety of GISTs represents only

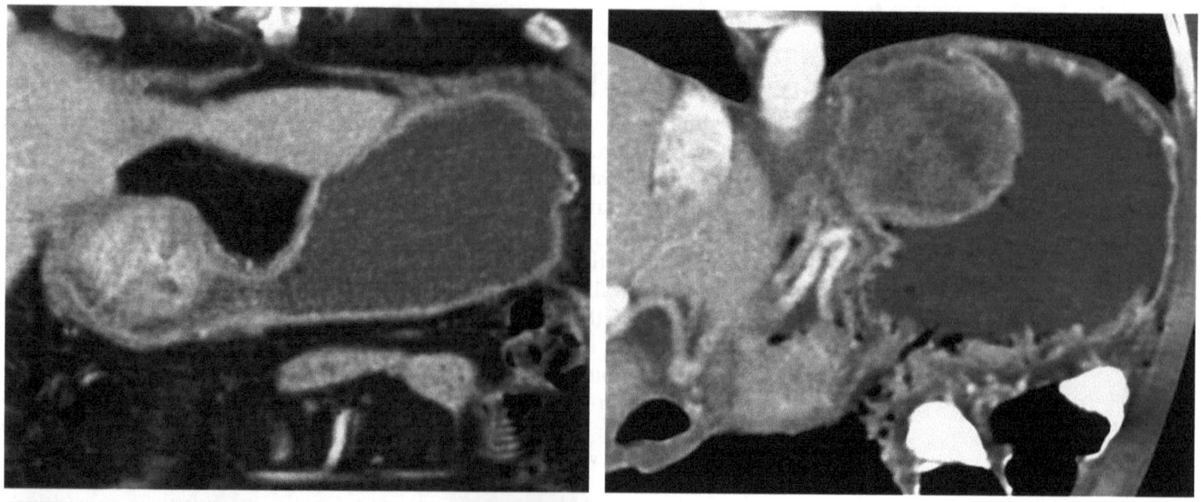

a b

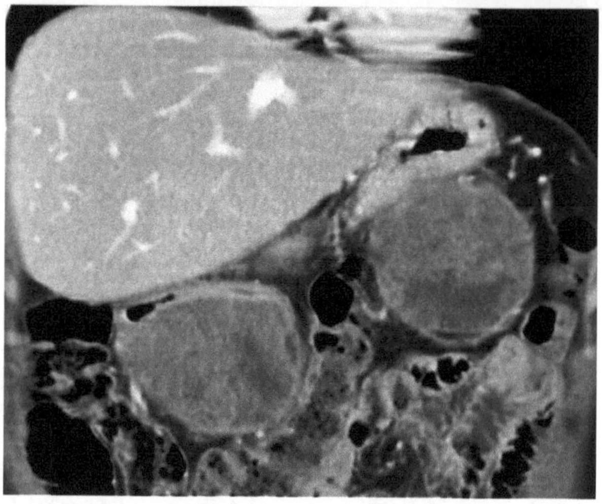

c

Fig. 6.2.13a–c. Metastases to the stomach. **a** Coronal reformation of the gastric antrum and corpus. Calcified rounded metastases in the antrum due to ovarian cancer. At histology, all gastric wall layers were infiltrated and psammoma bodies were found. **b** Coronal reformation of biopsy-proven gastric metastases from oesophageal carcinoma. Note the submucosal location. **c** Coronal reformation in a patient with cholangiocarcinoma. Histology revealed two subserosal metastases to the stomach

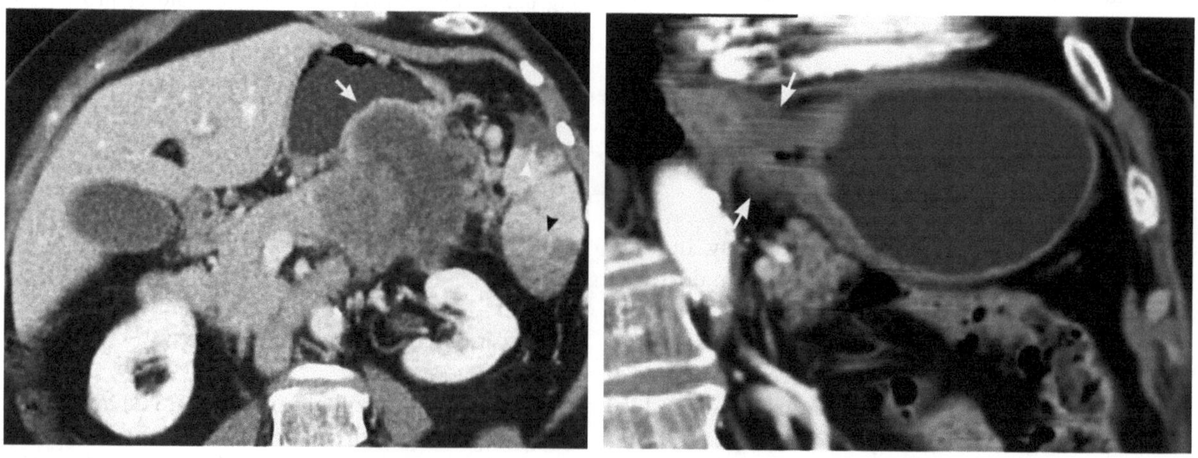

a b

Fig. 6.2.14a,b. Direct invasion of the stomach by neighbouring tumour. **a** Oblique coronal reformation through the pancreas demonstrates the direct invasion of the stomach by an adenocarcinoma of the pancreatic tail (*arrow*). There is a splenic infarct (*white arrowhead*) and splenic hypoperfusion (*black arrowhead*) due to tumour obstruction of the splenic artery and vein. **b** Parasagittal reformation through the gastroesophageal junction demonstrates surgical proved direct infiltration of the stomach by oesophageal carcinoma (*arrows*) about 3% of all malignant gastrointestinal tumours (Davis et al. 2000). Approximately 60–70% are found in the stomach (Miettinen and Lasota 2001). It is known that 10–30% of GISTs are malignant and the risk for malignancy increases with extragastric location, size greater than 5 cm and extension into adjacent organs (DeMatteo et al. 2000; Miettinen et al. 1999). Preoperatively and intraoperatively it is difficult to distinguish benign and malignant lesions; all may demonstrate a mixture of intramural, endogastric and exogastric appearances (Fig. 6.2.15).

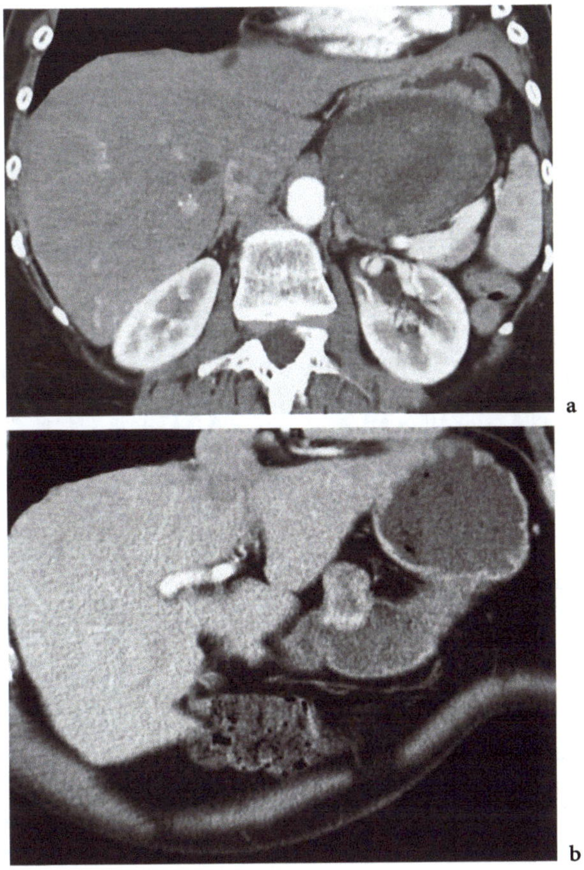

Fig. 6.2.15a,b. Gastrointestinal stromal tumours (GIST). **a** Oblique coronal reformation demonstrates a large inhomogeneous rounded mass that compresses the fundus of the stomach. Note the obtuse angle on the medial side and the rounded angle on the lateral side that were compatible with the subserosal location of this GIST. **b** Coronal reformation shows a biopsy-proven GIST arising from the lesser curvature with endo- and exogastric extension

6.2.5.2 Leiomyosarcoma

Gastric leiomyosarcomas occur more frequently in men than in women by a ratio of approximately 2:1 (Megibow et al. 1985). Affected individuals are usually middle-aged or elderly. Gastric leiomyosarcomas generally have a better prognosis than gastric carcinomas, with reported 5-year survival rates ranging from 20 to 55%. Tumours smaller than 5 cm have the best chance of cure. By contrast, tumours >8 cm at the time of diagnosis are often found to be advanced and unresectable. In patients with advanced leiomyosarcomas, CT may reveal metastases in the liver or peritoneal cavity. Unlike adenocarcinomas, however, leiomyosarcomas rarely metastasize to regional lymph nodes. The majority of leiomyosarcomas (90%) involve the fundus and body, and the remaining 10% involve the antrum.

Intramural leiomyosarcomas (50% of lesions) typically appear as large, lobulated submucosal masses in the gastric fundus or body. Endogastric leiomyosarcomas (15%) may appear as polypoid intraluminal masses indistinguishable from primary gastric carcinomas. Exogastric lesions (35%) may be manifested as giant soft tissue masses that cause extrinsic compression of the adjacent gastric wall.

6.2.5.3 Leiomyoma

Leiomyomas are pure submucosal lesions. About 80% are endogastric lesions that remain intramural but grow toward the lumen; another 15% are exogastric lesions that remain subserosal but grow outward from the stomach toward the peritoneal cavity. The remaining 5% of tumours have both endogastric and exogastric components (Kavlie and White 1972; Goodman et al. 1990).

The vast majority of leiomyomas in the stomach occur as solitary lesions, but multiple tumours are present in 1–2% of patients. Leiomyomas may be found in the antrum, body, or fundus of the stomach. Gastric leiomyomas may vary in size from tiny lesions of a few millimetres to enormous masses that significantly encroach on the lumen.

On multislice CT, gastric leiomyomas present as smooth masses of uniform soft tissue attenuation with a density similar to that of skeletal muscle. Leiomyomas may contain irregular streaks or clumps of mottled calcification and are the most common calcified benign gastric tumours. Their margins are smooth, although surface ulceration may be present in 50–70% of leiomyomas >2 cm in size (Fig. 6.2.16).

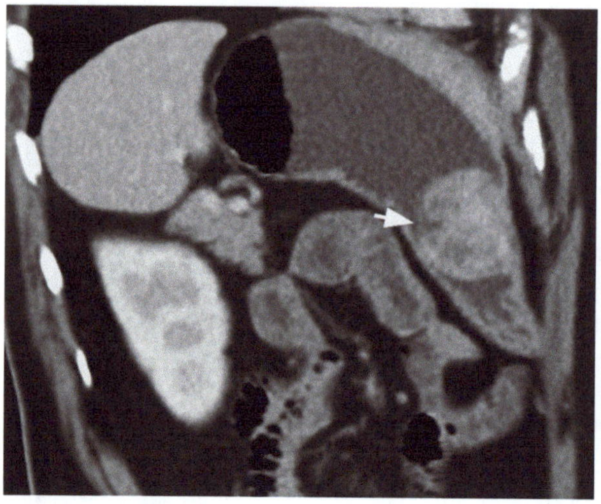
a
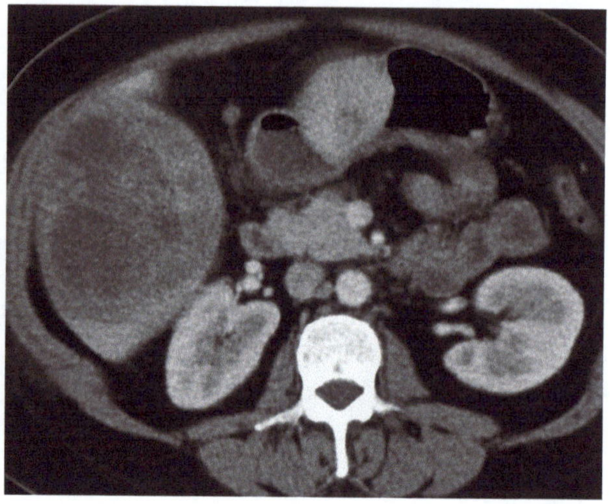
b

Fig. 6.2.16a,b. Leiomyoma of the stomach. **a** Sagittal reformation from a prone scan. Round submucosal hyperenhancing soft tissue mass with a small central ulcer (*arrow*). At histology, a benign GIST was found. **b** Hypervascular mass in the gastric antrum with an eccentric inhomogeneity. Histology proved benign leiomyoma. The large liver lesion was due to a hepatic abscess

Other unusual malignancies that have been reported in the stomach include liposarcoma, fibrosarcoma, neurofibrosarcoma, haemangioendothelioma, haemangiopericytoma, plasmacytoma, chorion carcinoma and Kaposi's sarcoma. Rarely, the stomach may be involved by leukaemia or multiple myeloma.

6.2.6 Benign Gastric Tumours

Between 85 and 90% of all neoplasms in the stomach are benign, equally distributed between mucosal and submucosal lesions.

6.2.6.1 Neural Tumours

Neural tumours constitute about 5–10% of benign gastric tumours (Hoare and Elkington 1976). The majority are nerve sheath tumours (neurinomas, schwannomas or neuromas). Most nerve sheath tumours are benign, but sarcomatous changes in these lesions have occasionally been reported. Neural tumours in the stomach usually appear on CT as submucosal masses (with or without ulceration) that are indistinguishable from other mesenchymal tumours (Fig. 6.2.17).

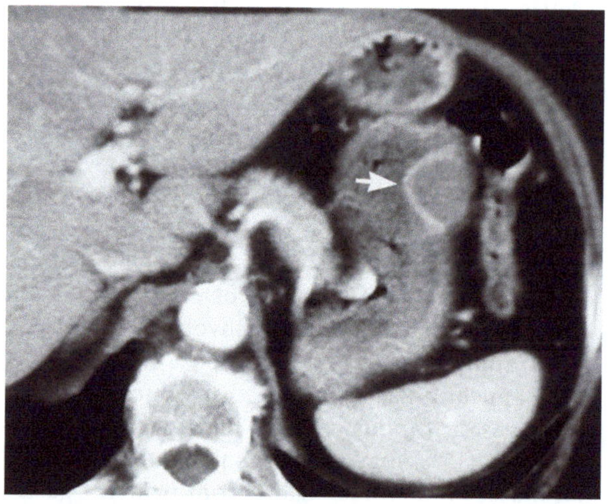

Fig. 6.2.17. Biopsy-proven schwannoma. There is a submucosal soft tissue mass that shows only minor enhancement but a preserved and strongly enhancing mucosa (*arrow*). Note that the perigastric fat plane around the tumour is clear

6.2.6.2 Gastric Polyps

6.2.6.2.1 Hyperplastic Polyps

Hyperplastic polyps account for 75–90% of all gastric polyps (Feczko et al. 1985). Hyperplastic polyps are often seen in the setting of chronic gastritis, atrophic gastritis or bile reflux gastritis. Although these polyps have no malignant potential, patients with hyperplastic polyps are at increased risk for harbouring separate, coexisting gastric carcinomas.

On multislice CT, most hyperplastic gastric polyps are smooth, sessile, round, or oval lesions, ranging from 5 to 10 mm in size. They occur usually as multiple lesions of similar size, clustered in the gastric body or fundus on the posterior gastric wall (Fig. 6.2.18a).

6.2.6.2.2 Adenomatous Polyps

Adenomatous polyps are rare in the stomach of the general population (Feczko et al. 1985). They are larger (about 2 cm in diameter) than hyperplastic polyps and more commonly pedunculated. Adenomatous polyps are solitary, and usually sited in the antrum; However, those that are larger harbour carcinomatous foci in approximately 40% of cases (Ginsberg et al. 1996) or will develop carcinomatous foci within 4 years. They may appear sessile or pedunculated and tend to have a more lobulated appearance (Fig. 6.2.18b).

a

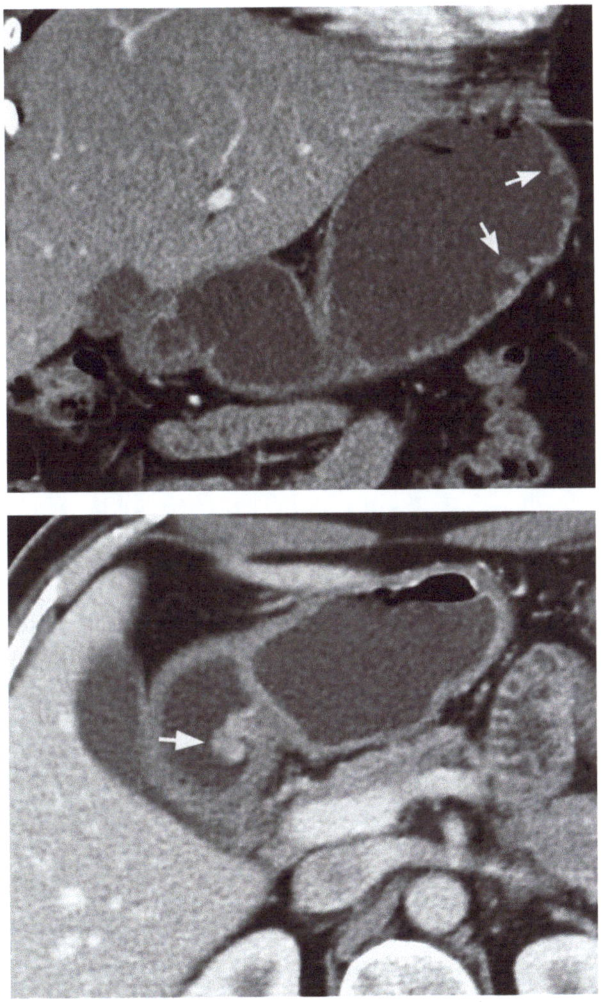

b

Fig. 6.2.18a,b. Polypoid lesions. **a** Coronal reformation. Biopsy-proven multiple hyperplastic polyps of the gastric wall (*arrows*). **b** Biopsy-proven adenomatous polyp in the gastric antrum (*arrow*)

6.2.7 Gastric Inflammation

6.2.7.1 Gastritis

Gastritis is a very common disease. Predisposing factors include alcohol, aspirin, NSAIDs, stress, viral or fungal infection and *Helicobacter pylori* infection. *Helicobacter* gastritis is identified in nearly 80% of patients with gastric ulcers and in nearly 100% of chronic gastritis cases. In many cases, gastric carcinoma and lymphoma are related to *Helicobacter* gastritis (Levine et al. 1996). The gastric antrum is the most common site of involvement; however, this disease often involves the proximal half of the stomach or the entire stomach. Thickened folds of the gastric wall are the best CT sign of conventional (Fig. 6.2.19a) or *Helicobacter pylori*-related gastritis (Fig. 6.2.19b); however, polypoid and lobulated folds are difficult to distinguish from gastric cancer and lymphoma. Biopsy is required in questionable cases.

6.2.7.2 Gastric Ulcer Disease

Gastric ulcer is a mucosal defect that reaches the muscularis mucosa and beyond. Ulcers occur usually in a solitary fashion. Gastric ulcer disease with or without perforation is one of the most important causes of acute abdomen (Fig. 6.2.20; Jacobs et al. 1991).

The vast majority (90%) of gastric ulcers develop along the lesser curvature or posterior wall of the gastric antrum or body of the stomach. Less than 5% of gastric ulcers occur on the anterior wall. Aspirin, NSAIDs, alcohol, coffee, corticosteroids and stress have been associated with gastric ulcer disease.

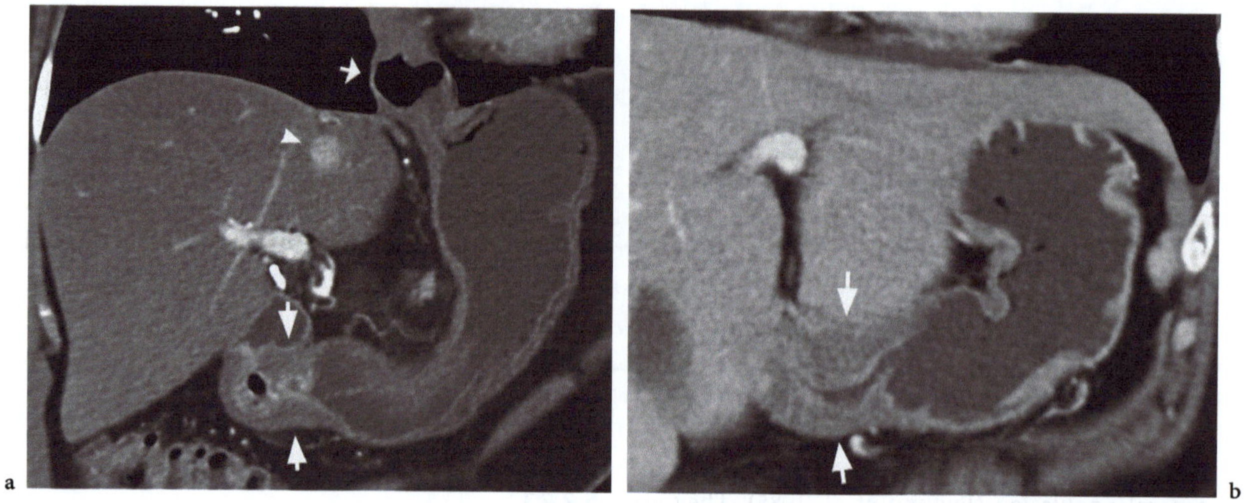

Fig. 6.2.19a,b. Gastritis. **a** Oblique coronal reformation. Marked thickening of the antrum in a pattern that is hard to distinguish from carcinoma. Note the contrast-enhancing mucosal lining and irregular folds (*arrows*). There was no ulcer at endoscopy and multiple biopsies showed acute gastritis only. Note the small axial hernia (*wide arrow*). Due to the oblique orientation of the cut plane through the oesophagus and stomach, the inferior vena cava appears as a round hypervascular lesion in the liver (*arrowhead*). **b** Biopsy-proved *Helicobacter pylori*-induced gastritis of the antrum with focal thickening and enhancement of the gastric wall. Note the preserved mucosal lining

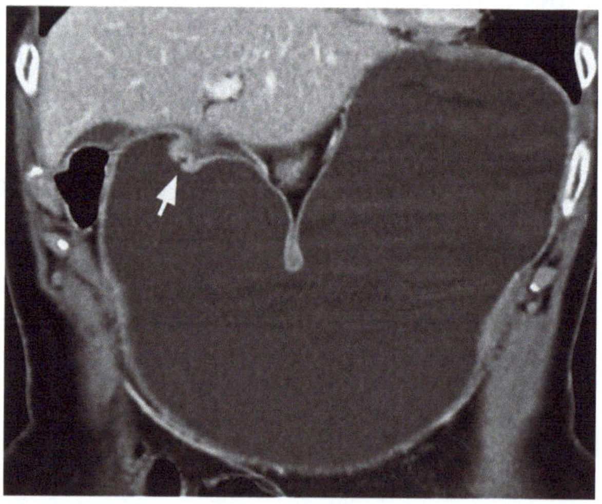

Fig. 6.2.20. Gastric ulcer. Coronal reformation shows biopsy-proven gastric ulcer (*arrow*) in the antrum with mucosal hyperaemia, wall thickening and central ulceration

6.2.7.3 Ménétrier's Disease

Ménétrier's disease is a rare chronic gastric disorder of unknown aetiology, which predisposes for gastric cancer. It occurs most commonly in middle life, more often in men than women. Grossly thickened lobulated folds of the gastric fundus and body are characteristic signs of Ménétrier's disease, with relative antral sparing. The greatest degree of fold thickening occurs on or near the greater curvature (Fig. 6.2.21). Focally enlarged folds can be mistaken for polypoid carcinomas. The most important differential diagnosis is lymphoma (Williams et al. 1978).

6.2.8 Benign Gastric Emphysema

Gas in the wall of the stomach usually occurs as a result of trauma, caused, for example, by vomiting as a result of gastric outlet obstruction (Fig 6.2.22) or volvulus of the stomach. It has also been reported following endoscopy and the passage of a nasogastric tube. This condition of gastric emphysema is of a benign self-limiting nature and has to be distinguished from emphysematous gastritis. The latter condition is associated with clostridial infection and carries a grave prognosis.

6.2.9 Gastric Outlet Obstruction

In adults, peptic ulcer disease is by far the most common cause of gastric outlet obstruction (60–65% of cases). An annular, constricting carcinoma of the distal antrum or pylorus is the second leading

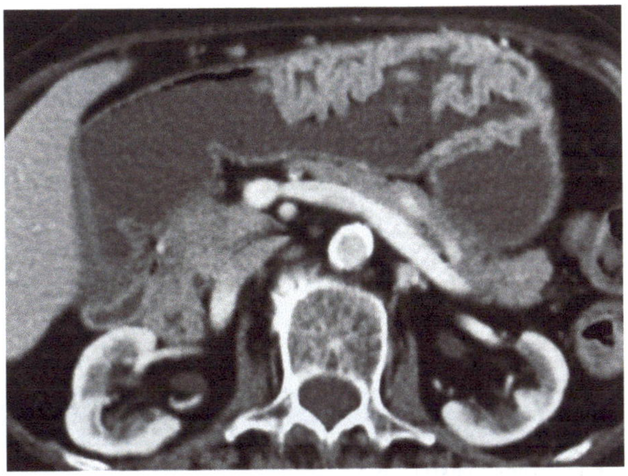

Fig. 6.2.21. Ménétrier's disease. Coronal reformation shows large, lobulated folds and preserved gastric mucosa of the fundus in a patient with biopsy-proven Ménétrier's disease

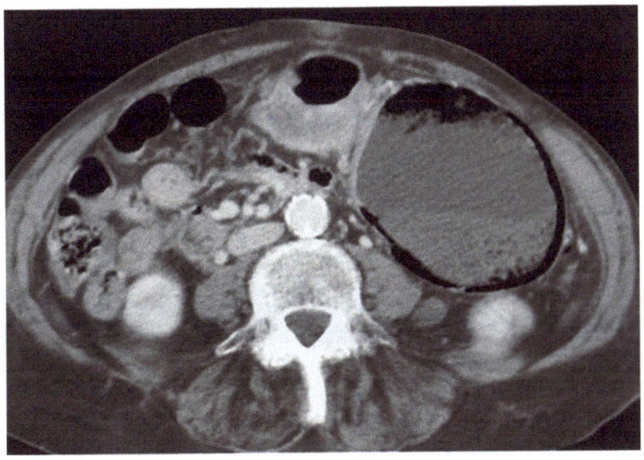

Fig. 6.2.22. Gastric emphysema. Note air in the wall of the stomach together with much gastric residue. The patient was vomiting as a result of the tumour of the distal stomach, causing gastric outlet obstruction

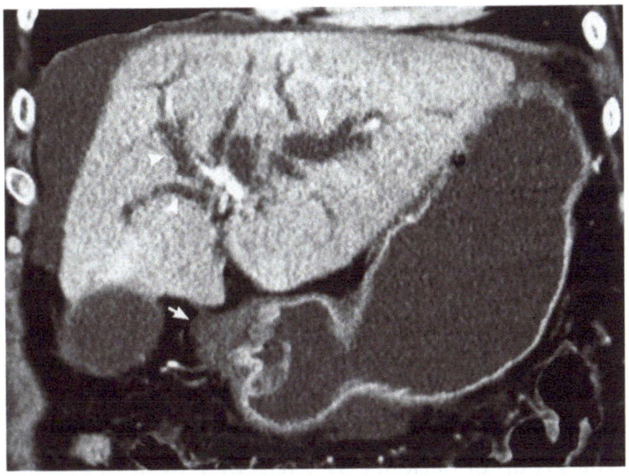

Fig. 6.2.23. Gastric outlet obstruction. Coronal reformation illustrates gastric outlet obstruction due to infiltration by a cholangiocarcinoma (*arrow*). Note the dilated intrahepatic bile ducts (*arrowheads*)

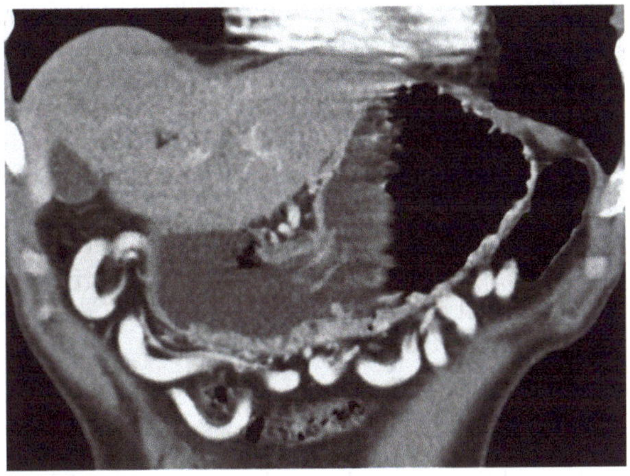

Fig. 6.2.24. Coronal reformation shows gastric varices of the small gastric veins in a patient with chronic pancreatitis and obstruction of the splenic vein

cause of gastric outlet obstruction (30–35% of cases), but other infiltrating primary malignant tumours or metastatic lesions can also produce gastric outlet obstruction (Fig. 6.2.23). Infrequently, it is caused by mural infiltration or spasm resulting from inflammatory disorders such as severe pancreatitis or cholecystitis. Fibrous scarring after ingestion of corrosive substances may cause antral narrowing. CT demonstrates an enormously dilated stomach. The differentiation between a benign and malignant cause of gastric outlet obstruction is based on the evidence of a mass in the region of the gastric outlet or by the demonstration of inflammatory disease in the vicinity of those structures.

6.2.10 Gastric Varices

Varices are commonly associated with splanchnic obstruction or portal hypertension (Balthazar et al. 1984). The presence of gastric varices without oesophageal varices has classically been considered a sign of isolated splenic vein occlusion, most commonly secondary to pancreatitis or pancreatic carcinoma.

Gastric varices appear on CT as well-defined clusters of rounded or tubular soft tissue densities within the posterior and posteromedial wall of the proximal stomach (Fig. 6.2.24). In some patients, CT may indicate the aetiology of the varices by identifying such conditions as hepatic cirrhosis, calcific pancreatitis and pancreatic carcinoma.

Table 6.2.4. The CT features of benign gastric diseases

Leiomyoma[a]
• Most common in the antrum and body
• Solid mass without areas of necrosis
• Smooth borders
• Submucosal lesion with preserved mucosal lining
• Ulceration of mucosa in the central portions of the tumour may occur
Gastritis
• Thickened gastric folds
• Wall thickening with soft tissue attenuation
• Poor gastric distension may imitate gastritis
Gastric ulcer disease
• Focal wall thickening with demonstration of a non-transmural lesion
Ménétrier disease
• Giant folds of tissue in the gastric wall
• May contain ulcers
• Most common in the fundus
Gastric varices
• Usual location: fundus and proximal gastric body
• Appearing as enhancing, tubular structures
• Collateral vessels commonly seen in the region of the gastrohepatic ligament, near the lesser omentum, along the course of the coronary vein

[a] Gastrointestinal stromal tumours

6.2.11 Clinical Value of Multislice CT

Previously, in the realm of gastric cancer most patients would undergo surgical exploration unless imaging had proven distant metastases. Multislice CT offers the opportunity to define more accurately the group of patients who will or will not be suited for primary surgical therapy. If CT shows definite transmural extension with peritoneal tumour spread, presurgical chemotherapy is used to downstage the tumour. After completion of chemotherapy, restaging of the tumour will be performed. If there is a positive response to chemotherapy, curative surgical therapy may be attempted; therefore at present, preoperative staging of gastric cancer appears to be by far the main clinical indication. In addition, multislice CT plays an important role in the evaluation of post-operative complications and the detection of tumour recurrence in patients following partial gastrectomy. Multislice CT remains an evolving method for the assessment of intra- and extraluminal processes of the gastric wall, and it is likely that its role here will increase.

Acknowledgement:
Much of the material for this chapter was originally published by the authors as an article in RadioGraphics 2003. The authors are indepted to the RSNA and the Editor of Radiographics for permission to use such material in the above chapter.

References

Baert AL, Roex L, Marchal G et al (1989) Computed tomography of the stomach with water as an oral contrast agent: technique and preliminary results. J Comput Assist Tomogr 13:633–636

Balthazar EJ, Rosenberg H, Davidian MM (1980) Scirrhous carcinoma of the pyloric channel and distal antrum. Am J Roentgenol 134:669–673

Balthazar EJ, Megibow A, Naidich D, Le Fleur RS (1984) Computed tomographic recognition of gastric varices. Am J Roentgenol 142:1121–1125

Cho KC, Baker SR, Alterman DD, Fusco JM, Cho S (1996) Transpyloric spread of gastric tumors: comparison of adenocarcinoma and lymphoma. Am J Roentgenol 167:467–469

Davis GR (1993) Neoplasms of the stomach. In: Sleisenger MH, Fordtran JS (ed) Gastrointestinal disease, 5th edn. Saunders, Philadelphia, pp 763–792

Davis G, Blanchard D, Hatch G et al (2000) Tumors of the stomach. World J Surg 24:412–420

D'Elia F, Zingarelli A, Palli D, Grani M (2000) Hydrodynamic CT preoperative staging of gastric cancer: correlation with pathological findings. A prospective study of 107 cases. Eur Radiol 10:1877–1885

DeMatteo R, Lewis J, Leung D et al (2000) Two hundred gastrointestinal stromal tumors: recurrence patterns and prognostic factors for survival. Ann Surg 231:51–58

Feczko PJ, Halpert RD, Ackerman LV (1985) Gastric polyps: radiological evaluation and clinical significance. Radiology 155:581–584

Fischback W, Kestel W, Kirchner T, Mossner H, Wilms K (1992) Malignant lymphomas of the upper gastrointestinal tract. Results of a prospective study in 103 patients. Cancer 70:1075–1080
Fishman EK, Urban BA, Hruban RH (1996) CT of the stomach: spectrum of disease. Radiographics 16:1035–1054
Fleischmann D, Rubin GD, Bankier AA, Hittmair K (2000) Improved uniformity of aortic enhancement with customized contrast medium injection protocols at CT angiography. Radiology 214:363–371
Fukuya T, Honda H, Hayashi T et al (1995) Lymph-node metastases: efficacy for detection with helical CT in patients with gastric cancer. Radiology 197:705–711
Ginsberg GG, Al-Kawas FH, Fleischer DE, Reilly HF, Benjamin SB (1996) Gastric polyps: relationship of size and histology to cancer risk. Am J Gastroenterol 91:714–717
Godwin JD (1975) Carcinoid tumors. An analysis of 2,837 cases. Cancer 36:560–569
Goodman P, Raval B, Bonmati C, Schmidt WA (1990) Leiomyoma involving the gastrocolic ligament: CT demonstration. Comput Med Imaging Graph 14:431–435
Hoare AM, Elkington SG (1976) Gastric lesions in generalized neurofibromatosis. Br J Surg 63:449–451
Jacobs JM, Hill MC, Steinberg WM (1991) Peptic ulcer disease: CT evaluation. Radiology 178:745–748
Kapeh MS, Leon L, Klimstra D, Brennan MF (2000) Lymph node staging in gastric cancer: Is location more important than number? An analysis of 1,038 patients. Ann Surg 232:362–371
Kavlie H, White TT (1972) Leiomyomas of the upper gastrointestinal tract. Surgery 71:92–104
Levine MS, Elmas N, Furth EE, Rubesin SE, Godwin MI (1996) Helicobacter pylori and gastric MALT lymphoma. Am J Roentgenol 166:85–86
Lewin KJ, Ranchod M, Dorfman RF (1978) Lymphomas of the gastrointestinal tract: a study of 117 cases presenting with gastrointestinal disease. Cancer 42:693–707
Maruyama M, Baba Y (1994) Diagnosis of the invasive depth of gastric cancer. Abdom Imaging 19:532–536
Megibow AJ, Balthazar EJ, Hulnick DH, Naidich DP, Bosniak MA (1985) CT evaluation of gastrointestinal leiomyomas and leiomyosarcomas. Am J Roentgenol 144:727–731
Merino S, Saiz A, Moreno MJ et al (1999) CT evaluation of gastric wall pathology. Br J Radiol 72:1124–1324
Miettinen M, Lasota J (2001) Gastrointestinal stromal tumors: definition, clinical, histological, immunohistochemical, and molecular genetic features and differential diagnosis. Virchows Arch 438:1–12
Miettinen M, Sarlomo-Rikala M, Lasota J (1999) Gastrointestinal stromal tumors: recent advances in understanding of their biology. Hum Pathol 30:1213–1220
Moore JR (1986) Gastric carcinoma: 30-year review. Can J Surg 29:25–28
Oiso T (1975) Incidence of stomach cancer and its relation to dietary habits and nutrition in Japan between 1900 and 1975. Cancer Res 35:3254–3258
Parker SL, Tong T, Bolden S, Wingo PA (1996) Cancer statistics. CA Cancer J Clin 4:5–27
Sato T, Sakai Y, Ishiguro S, Furukawa H (1986) Radiologic manifestations of early gastric lymphoma. Am J Roentgenol 146:513–517
Williams SM, Harned RK, Settles RH (1978) Adenocarcinoma of the stomach in association with Menetrier's disease. Gastrointest Radiol 3:387–390

Magnetic Resonance Imaging of the Stomach

7

Markus Dux

CONTENTS

7.1 Introduction

Magnetic resonance imaging (MRI) of the stomach is not a standard examination, due to inherent artefacts from peristalsis, pulsations, and respiration. Only a few groups have shown interest in this topic, as conventional MRI of the stomach does not provide the image resolution of small areas of interest that is needed for the depiction of gastric wall pathology. However, the use of surface coils has improved the signal-to-noise ratios, consequently allowing high-spatial-resolution MR imaging. There are technical limitations with respect to intracavitary coils inserted into the stomach, and clinical feasibility has not yet been proven.

MR endoscopy has been used in the rectum for imaging of rectal carcinoma, the adjacent prostate, or cervix (Schnall et al. 1994; Milestone et al. 1991). It has shown promising results, especially in tumour staging. Experimental MR studies have shown that depiction of the anatomic layers of the gastric wall is possible, and it is well accepted that endoscopic MR examinations of the stomach may have the potential for visualization of gastric disease (Auh et al. 1994; Oi et al. 1997; Yamada et al. 2001; Lubienski et al. 2002).

7.2 Indications

Although endoscopy is the method of choice for diagnosis of gastric disease, visualization is limited to surface mucosa. Endoscopic biopsy may show invasion of tumour beneath the mucosa but lesions with no superficial component, and those with infiltration of deep gastric wall layers may be difficult to diagnose. Currently, endoscopic ultrasound (EUS) is the only imaging method with which different layers of the gastric wall can be shown reliably, and it therefore enables evaluation of the extent of gastric disease beneath the mucosa (Kimmey et al. 1989; Caletti et al. 1993; Botet et al. 1991; Tio et al. 1989). The role of EUS in the depiction of gastric wall pathology is controversial. It has been performed for preoperative staging of gastric carcinoma, but it has limited value as peri-tumour inflammation of the gastric wall cannot be distinguished from tumour infiltration. In addition, EUS is highly operator-dependent and judgment of tumour infiltration may differ from sonographer to sonographer, even in the same patient.

MRI has recently been used for the visualization of gastric tumours. In gastric carcinoma tumourous infiltration of the serosa may be shown by conventional MRI (Matsushita et al. 1994; Oi et al. 1997), but accurate local staging of gastric carcinoma by MRI requires reliable interpretation of the wall layers. This may be achieved by high-spatial-reso-

M. Dux, MD, PhD
Department of Diagnostic and Interventional Radiology, Krankenhaus Nordwest, Teaching Hospital of the Johann Wolfgang Goethe University of Frankfurt, Steinbacher Hohl 2–26, 60488 Frankfurt am Main, Germany

lution MRI using endoluminal receiver coils (Inui et al. 1995; Dux et al 2001). However, endoscopic MRI of the stomach is only performed in vitro or in selected human studies, as it requires technical improvements before being used routinely.

7.3 Technique

7.3.1 Conventional MRI

Distension of the gastric wall by ingestion of 600–1000 ml of water is required prior to MR examination of the stomach. Patients are examined in the supine or prone position depending on the location of the gastric lesion. MR imaging is usually performed with a 1.5-T magnet; 20–40 mg of scopolamine butylbromide or 1 mg of glucagon is administered intravenously before the examination in order to minimize peristalsis.

The MRI technique used by Matsushita et al. (1994) includes spoiled gradient-recalled acquisition in the steady state (GRASS) with a repetition time of 33 or 45 ms, an echo time of 12 or 7 ms, a 30° flip angle, 1 NEX, matrix size of 256 × 128, and section thickness of 5 or 7 mm. Unenhanced coronal and axial images are obtained using the breath-hold technique, followed by sagittal and/or oblique images perpendicular to the tumour. Then, contrast medium-enhanced MR images are obtained with the same slice orientations. Published data from clinical studies using conventional MR techniques for visualization of the stomach wall report contradictory results on the use of T2-weighted sequences (Matsushita et al. 1994; Oi et al. 1997; Marcos and Semelka 1999).

7.3.2 Endoscopic MR

Endoscopic MR imaging is performed using a gastroscope that is MR-compatible and contains no ferromagnetic materials (De Souza et al. 1995; Inui et al. 1995; Kulling et al. 1997; Dux et al. 2001) (Fig. 7.1). The handling of the MR endoscope is similar to that of a conventional instrument. It has full endoscopic capability and measures between 12 mm and 13 mm in diameter, which equals that of a thera-

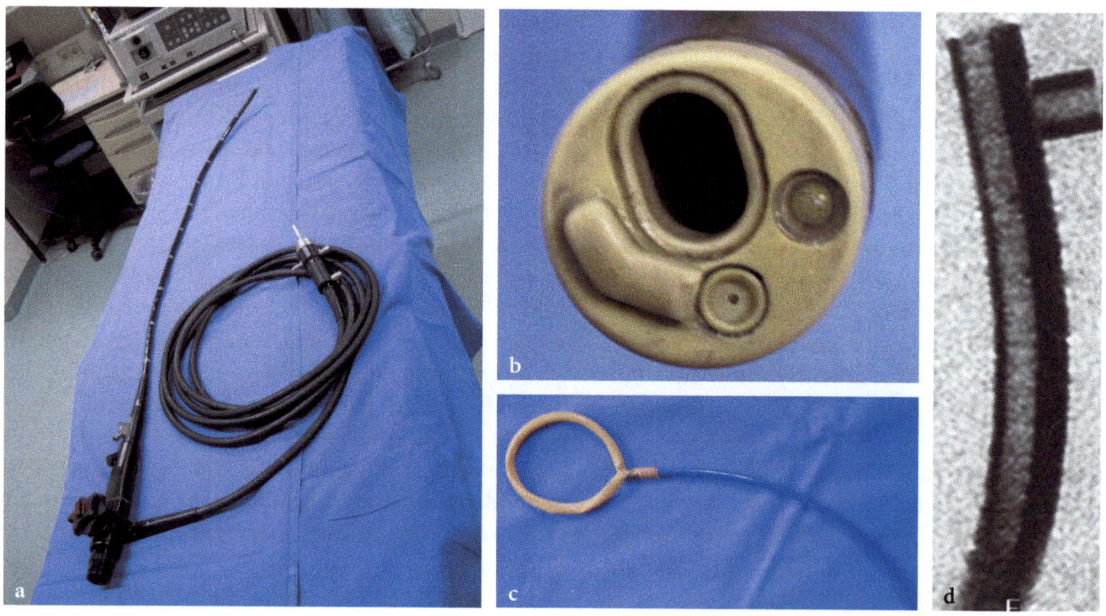

Fig. 7.1a–d. An endoscope used for endoscopic MR imaging is not very different from other gastroscopes, but it is manufactured with materials that do not produce artefacts which interfere with imaging. **a** The endoscope used by Dux et al (2001). The tip of the endoscope **b** shows the oversized biopsy channel that is used to advance the coil into the stomach. **c** The prototype of the receiver coil used nowadays. The diameter of the coil released from the endoscope is variable depending on the size of the tumour that is to be imaged. **d** shows that the endoscope is compatible with MRI, and the channel that accommodates the receiver coil is clearly depicted

peutic gastroscope. MR endoscopes that have been used in patient studies are different with respect to the construction of the tip. Olympus Optical Co. (Tokyo, Japan) has manufactured a 10 mm × 30 mm receiver coil that is attached to the tip of the instrument (Inui et al. 1995; Kulling et al. 1997). The coil is surrounded by a disposable latex balloon that is inflated with 2–20 ml of air. This is necessary to stabilize the MR coil and to keep it at a minimum distance of 2–5 mm from the mucosal surface to improve the image quality. Another MR-compatible endoscope was developed by De Souza et al. (1995) in co-operation with Endoscan (Burgess Hill, UK). It works with a 10 mm × 25 mm receiver coil that is accommodated within the biopsy channel of the endoscope and can be manoeuvred separately. It may be advanced to a certain distance from the endoscope and is maintained in the latter position for imaging of the gastric wall. The third prototype of an MR-compatible endoscope has also been manufactured by Endoscan according to the plans of Dux et al. (2001). Again the coil is accommodated within the biopsy channel of the endoscope, but the diameter of the coil released from the endoscope is variable and may be adjusted according to the lumen of the stomach or the size of the tumour. All instruments are biocompatible, easy to sterilize, and work with a specially constructed cable enabling the endoscopy cart containing the light source and other non-MR-compatible devices to be located at a safe distance from the magnet.

MR endoscopy of the stomach has been performed with a 0.5-T (De Souza et al. 1995) or a 1.5-T magnet (Inui et al. 1995; Kulling et al. 1997; Dux et al. 2001). At 0.5 T, standard T1-weighted spin echo images (TR 700–800 ms; TE 20 ms) are obtained in the transverse plane using 3-mm slice thickness and a 10-cm FOV. At 1.5 T, T1- and T2-weighted spin echo images are acquired without breath-holding whereas the gradient echo sequences are performed during breath-holding. In vitro studies (Kulling et al. 1997; Dux et al. 1997; Yamada et al. 2001) have shown that the spin echo technique is best suited to perform high-spatial-resolution MR imaging of the stomach by choosing a voxel size between 0.08 mm^3 and 2.43 mm^3. Despite the long scanning times the spin echo technique is the technique of choice at present, and is regularly applied at endoscopic MRI (Inui et al. 1995; Dux et al. 2001; Feldman et al. 1997). Usually GRASS sequences are additionally obtained. However, the gradient echo technique often produces poor-quality images, emphasizing the need for improved endoscopic ultrafast imaging techniques.

7.4 MRI Appearances of Normal Gastric Wall

Gastric wall layers cannot be distinguished at conventional MR imaging of the stomach, resulting in a major limitation of the technique (Fig. 7.2). It may be occasionally possible to depict two layers of the gastric wall at T2-weighted imaging; however, these layers are not visible throughout the whole

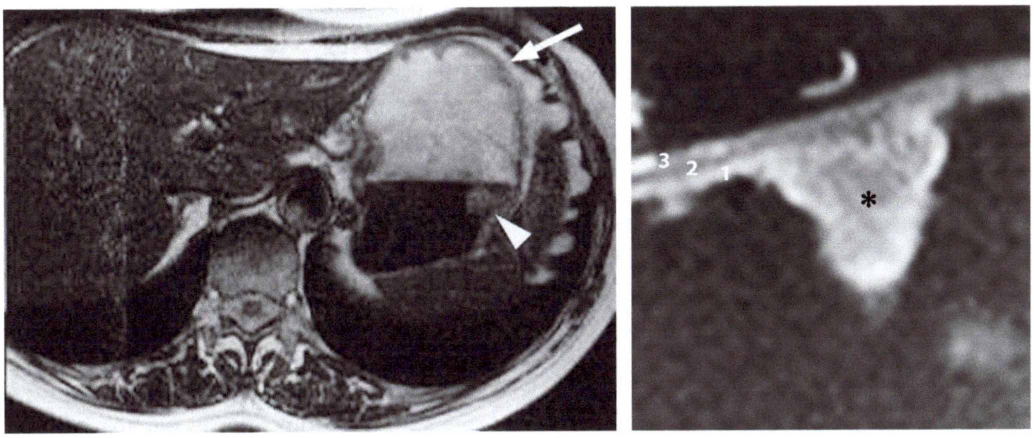

Fig. 7.2a,b. Conventional MR imaging usually reveals no gastric wall layers. Sometimes two layers may be distinguished using T2-weighted sequences (*arrow*, **a**). In addition a polypoid tumour (*arrowhead*) of the gastric wall is visible. The patient was positioned prone, and water was used for luminal distension. In contrast, experimental high-spatial-resolution MR imaging of the stomach reveals three layers of the gastric wall **b**. Opposed-phase imaging shows an early gastric carcinoma (*), type I, that does not penetrate the second/middle gastric wall layer. (*1*) mucosa, (*2*) submucosa, (*3*) muscularis propria

circumference of the gastric wall. At conventional MRI the normal gastric wall is a thin non-layered band that, depending on the degree of distension, has a maximum thickness of 5 mm (Matsushita et al. 1994; Chou et al. 1994). Endoscopic MRI reveals three layers of the gastric wall which correspond to the mucosa, submucosa, and muscularis propria (Inui et al. 1995). The subserosa and serosa cannot be distinguished from the muscularis propria and therefore belong to the third layer visible at endoscopic MRI. There is still controversy regarding which imaging sequence allows the best differentiation of gastric wall layers (Kulling et al. 1997; Dux et al. 1997; Yamada et al. 2001). Dux et al. (1997) performed in vitro imaging of gastric specimens with a 1-T magnet and succeeded in regularly depicting three to five layers of the gastric wall on T2-weighted images. Yamada et al. (2001) described four and six layers of the gastric wall at T1- and T2-weighted spin echo sequences respectively at 1.5 T. The four layers depicted on T1-weighted MR images correspond to the mucosa (low signal intensity), the submucosa (low or high signal intensity), the muscularis propria (low signal intensity), and subserosa or serosa (low or high signal intensity). On T2-weighted sequences the mucosa shows low signal intensity and the submucosa high signal intensity. The muscularis propria is depicted as three layers which correspond to the inner circular (low signal intensity) and outer longitudinal muscle layers (low signal intensity). These are separated by a thin layer of high signal intensity that corresponds to loose connective tissue. The sixth layer shows low signal intensity and is defined as subserosa or serosa. The results obtained at in vitro studies cannot be applied to clinical practice because of the very long acquisition time (over 20 min). At present, only three layers of the gastric wall are reliably depicted by endoscopic MRI of the stomach.

7.5 Gastric Carcinoma

7.5.1 Diagnosis of Gastric Carcinoma

At MRI, a focal thickening together with marked contrast enhancement and disruption of the layered pattern of the gastric wall are suspicious of gastric carcinoma (Matsushita et al. 1994; Chou et al. 1994; Oi et al. 1997). Thus CT and US criteria can be applied to MR imaging. MRI has the same limitations as CT imaging using liquids for luminal distension (Dux et al. 1999).The diagnosis of gastric carcinoma is strongly dependent on the distension of the gastric wall, the size of the tumour, and depth of penetration. Various oral contrast agents have been reported for use in gastrointestinal MR imaging (Wesbey et al. 1985; Hahn et al. 1987; Bisset 1989; Laghi et al. 2003). The water filling method is not only appropriate for CT imaging but has also been successfully applied at MR imaging (Matsushita et al. 1994). Contrast-enhanced MRI shows a thickened wall of high signal intensity compared to water, which acts as a negative contrast agent on T1-weighted images. Water does not cause susceptibility artefacts, is safe, and replaces gastric air. The latter aspect is important because gastric wall structures cannot be accurately evaluated by MRI if air is located adjacent to the gastric wall, as it produces a low-signal-intensity artefact due to magnetic field inhomogeneity. It is generally agreed that diagnosis of advanced gastric carcinoma is better achieved if luminal distension is applied. However, inappropriate distension of the gastric wall may impair the image quality due to motion artefacts, leading to failure to demonstrate even advanced gastric carcinoma. MRI may not be able to detect macroscopic early gastric cancer or tumours less than 2 cm (Dux et al. 2000). At present, no firm conclusions can be drawn on the role of MRI in diagnosis of early gastric carcinoma.

Endoscopic MRI does not have those limitations because it can be divided into two procedures. First endoscopy of the stomach is performed to locate the tumour. Endoscopy is the method of choice to diagnose gastric tumours because there are relatively few false-negative results compared with other imaging modalities (Dekker and Tytgat 1997). Once gastric carcinoma is depicted by the endoscopist the receiver coil is placed adjacent to the tumour and endoluminal MRI is performed for staging purposes.

7.5.2 Staging of Gastric Carcinoma

MRI is performed not only for local T- and N-staging of gastric carcinoma but also for M-staging of the abdomen. Endoscopic MRI is performed with the aim to improve local staging of gastric carcinoma using high-spatial-resolution MRI (Fig. 7.3). It is not aimed at M-staging because the field of view is limited to tissues and structures surrounding the stomach. However, M-staging may be accomplished

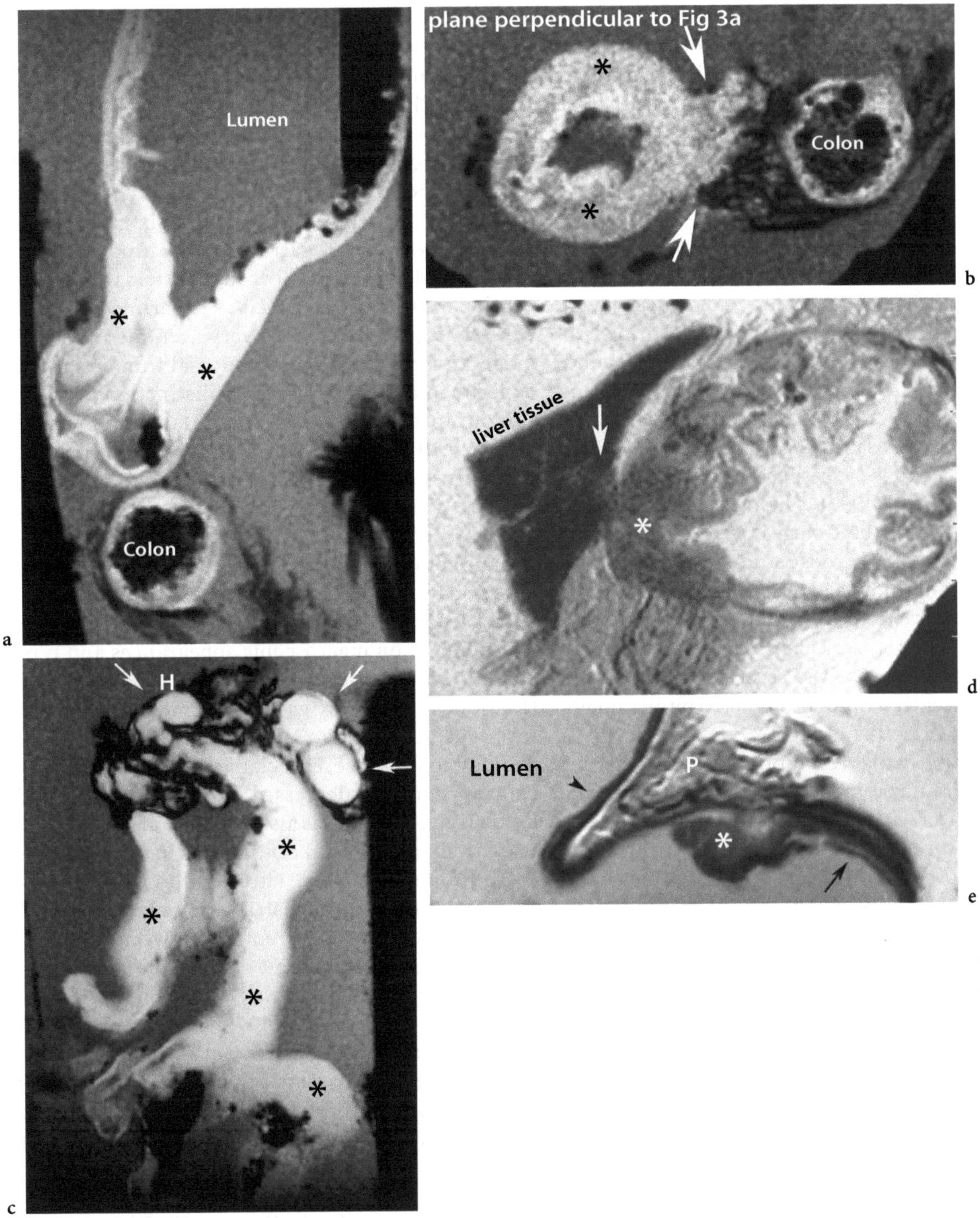

Fig. 7.3a–e. Experimental high-spatial-resolution MRI of gastric specimens depicts early and advanced gastric carcinoma. Opposed-phase imaging (**a–c**) is best suited to diagnose gastric tumours because of their high signal intensities. **a, b** show a carcinoma (*) of the gastric antrum that involves the whole circumference of the gastric wall. The tumour was suspected to have infiltrated the transverse colon that therefore was resected. At histology and MRI, mesenteric infiltration (*arrow*) was diagnosed and the tumour finally was staged pT4. **c** A signet ring cell carcinoma (*) involving more than two-thirds of the gastric wall as well as locoregional lymph node metastases (*arrows*) that have signal intensities identical to that of the primary tumour. **d** An axial view of a gastric specimen at T2-weighted imaging. The carcinoma (*) penetrates the gastric wall and infiltrates liver tissue that therefore was resected. Local invasion of the liver was correctly depicted by MRI that showed tiny areas of signal intensity changes (*arrow*) within the liver parenchyma. Compared to that of the primary tumour the areas of focal invasion have similar signal intensities. **e** A polypoid early gastric carcinoma (*) at T2-weighted imaging that allows depiction of three (*arrowhead*) or up to five gastric wall layers (*arrow*) and therefore is best suited to perform T-staging of gastric carcinoma. *P*: peritoneal fatty tissue

after removal of the endoscope using the body coil for imaging of the abdomen. Thus endoscopic MRI may be part of an *all in one procedure* that eventually may play a key role on the management of gastric carcinoma.

7.5.2.1 T-Staging

Because MRI cannot depict the fine structure of the gastric wall. T-staging accuracy of conventional MRI is limited to gastric carcinomas confined to the gastric wall (T1 or T2), those extending beyond the gastric wall (T3), and lesions invading adjacent structures (T4) Sensitivity and specificity of MRI to correctly depict serosal infiltration of gastric carcinoma are 97% and 79%, respectively (Matsushita et al. 1994; Oi et al. 1997). The overall accuracy of MRI in determining the T-stage is 88%. The majority of gastric carcinomas in those studies were stage pT3 or pT4, resulting in a selection bias towards fairly advanced gastric carcinomas that are more likely to have invaded the serosa. Diagnosis of serosal invasion is difficult because the serosa is a single cell layer that currently cannot be depicted by any imaging modality (Kimmey et al. 1989; Dux et al. 1997, 1999). Since the spatial resolution of MRI using the body coil technique is inadequate for distinguishing gastric wall layers, it can be concluded that it is inadequate for accurately diagnosing serosal infiltration as well. Endoscopic MRI can offer more accurate staging of gastric carcinomas since three layers of the gastric wall may be visualized on both T1- and T2-weighted sequences (De Souza et al. 1995; Inui et al. 1995; Kulling et al. 1997; Dux et al. 2001). In clinical practice, however, adequate visualization of gastric carcinoma is often not achieved because it may be difficult to maintain the coil in a stable position for imaging the tumour. Inui et al. (1995) managed to obtain MR images of good quality in only 58% of patients who underwent endoscopic MRI of the stomach. In patients in whom adequate visualization was achieved, accuracy to predict the T-stage of gastric carcinoma was 89%. However, only advanced gastric carcinomas (pT3 and pT4) were correctly staged, and the only early gastric carcinoma was not visible for appropriate staging on endoscopic MRI. Therefore studies that have evaluated endoscopic MRI in patients show that the procedure is still too lengthy and the image quality is still inadequate for use in clinical practice.

High-spatial-resolution MRI has been widely used in vitro for assessing the signal intensity characteristics of gastrointestinal tumours (Imai et al. 1990; Auh et al. 1994; Dux et al. 1997; Yamada et al. 2001). Interesting work has especially been performed with respect to staging of early gastric carcinoma. Yamada et al (2001) examined nine early gastric carcinomas in vitro and correctly staged all the tumours. He was able to exactly locate and determine the depth of invasion in six carcinomas confined within the gastric mucosa and in three submucosal carcinomas because gastric wall layers can be accurately visualised at experimental MRI. Auh et al. (1994) were also very accurate in distinguishing mucosal from submucosal tumours using experimental MRI. However, a distinction between tumour invasion, fibrosis, and inflammation of the gastric wall is not possible. At present, no imaging modality can distinguish gastric carcinoma from reactive changes in the surrounding tissue (Tio et al. 1989; Botet et al. 1991; Dux et al. 1999) because inflammation or fibrosis adjacent to the malignant lesion may mimic tumour invasion of the submucosa. Detection of early gastric carcinoma by MRI is dependent on macroscopic appearances and type of the tumour according to Lauren's classification (Lauren 1965). Early gastric carcinoma of the diffuse type according to Lauren classification can be difficult to visualise, especially when it macroscopically appears as a depressed (type IIc) or excavated lesion (type-III). This is also valid for large early gastric carcinoma (several centimetres in size). Despite these limitations all in vitro studies of high-spatial-resolution MRI of gastric carcinoma show that MRI can accurately differentiate between early and advanced gastric carcinoma because the layer representing the submucosa is well visible on MR images (Auh et al. 1994; Dux et al. 1997; Kulling et al. 1997; Yamada et al. 2001; Lubienski et al. 2002) (Fig. 7.4). Overstaging of early gastric carcinoma may occur if inflammatory or fibrotic changes extend beyond the submucosa, or if lymphangiomatous carcinomatosis mimics continuous tumour growth into the proper muscularis propria or even serosa. Advanced gastric carcinoma is reliably diagnosed by high-spatial-resolution MRI with an overall T-staging accuracy ranging between 65% and 93% (Auh et al. 1994; Dux et al. 1997; Yamada et al. 2001).

Clinically useful MR imaging has been obtained up to 4 cm from the coil surface (De Souza et al. 1995; Inui et al. 1995; Feldman et al. 1997) but there may be problems in large tumours or in situations where the size of the examination field is smaller than the diameter of the tumour. Consequently, advanced gastric carcinoma, i.e. large T4 tumours

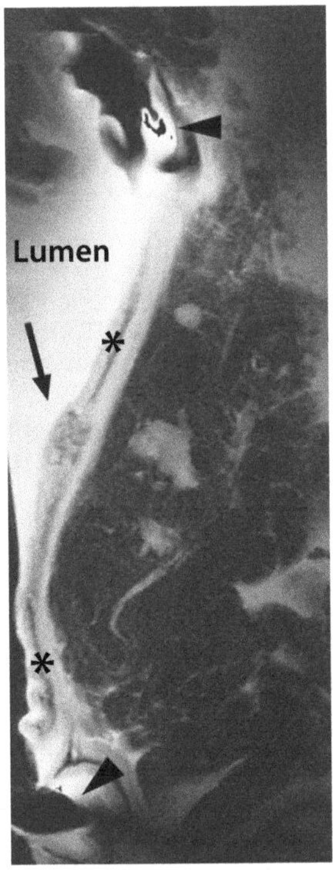

Fig. 7.4. Endoscopic MR imaging of the stomach. The receiver coil (*arrowheads*) was advanced into the lumen of the stomach and covers an area of 9–10 cm that can be used for imaging. A small early gastric carcinoma (*arrow*) is located within the gastric wall and has infiltrated the submucosa. The submucosa is represented by the middle, hypointense layer of the gastric wall (*)

may be inadequately assessed by endoscopic MRI. This limitation can be overcome by the use of expandable coils. The MR endoscope used by Dux et al. (2001) accommodates the coil within the biopsy channel. The diameter of the coil released from the endoscope is variable and may be adjusted to the lumen of the stomach or the size of the tumour. The device allows an extended FOV of 10 cm. However, this increases the complexity of device design and placement. Further evaluation of endoscopic MRI of the stomach is warranted before its use in clinical practice.

7.5.2.2
N-Staging

The presence of lymph node metastases is one of the most important prognostic factors in patients with gastric carcinoma. Although the 5-year survival rate in patients with early gastric carcinoma is significantly superior to that of patients with advanced gastric carcinoma, it decreases from almost 100% to 50%–80% in early gastric carcinomas that have already metastasized into local lymph nodes (Maehara et al. 1992; Moreaux and Bougaran 1993). As a consequence, diagnosis of perigastric lymph node metastases is essential and should be accomplished by any imaging modality used for staging a gastric carcinoma. At experimental MRI, lymph nodes as small as 4 mm are well detected (Dux et al. 1997). They appear oval with a rather sharp contour and are best visualised on T1-weighted and opposed-phase sequences. On T1-weighted images, they demonstrate low signal intensity compared to the high signal intensity of perigastric fat. Lymph nodes whose signal intensity is similar to that of the primary tumour are more easily diagnosed and indicate the presence of malignancy. However, the signal intensity characteristic of lymph nodes is not very specific, and false positive diagnoses do occur.

The sensitivity and specificity of high-spatial-resolution MRI to detect lymph nodes infiltrated by gastric carcinoma are 87% and 60% respectively (Dux et al. 1997), and N-staging accuracy of experimental MRI of gastric carcinoma is reported to be comparable to that of other imaging modalities (Tio et al. 1989; Botet et al. 1991; Caletti et al. 1993; Dux et al. 1999). These encouraging experimental results, however, cannot be translated into clinical practice because it has not been yet investigated by clinical MR studies. Conventional MRI is unlikely to be superior to CT imaging, which is often inaccurate in determining the N-staging of gastric carcinoma.

Endoscopic MRI of the stomach may provide an image resolution comparable to that of experimental MRI and thus in theory may be able to determine the N-stage of gastric carcinoma more accurately. However, in practice endoscopic MRI of perigastric lymph nodes is still at the developmental stage, and results obtained with endoscopic MRI are poor. Inui et al. (1995) were unable to depict metastatic lymph nodes located less than 3 cm from the primary tumour in four of six patients with gastric carcinoma, resulting in an overall accuracy of only 56%. At present, the data obtained from clinical trials are still too scarce to draw any firm conclusions on the role of endoscopic MRI of the stomach for the assessment of perigastric lymph node metastases. Endoscopic MRI, however, has the potential to improve N-staging accuracy of gastric carcinoma and to develop more accurate MR criteria to distinguish malignant from benign nodes. Lymphotrophic MR contrast agents may play an important role in the future (Hamm 2002).

7.5.2.3 M-Staging

Metastases from gastric carcinoma most frequently involve the liver and peritoneum. MRI is the most sensitive and specific imaging modality to detect liver metastases (Del Frate et al. 2002; Vogl et al. 2003), while peritoneal carcinomatosis is often not revealed because the peritoneal lesions are too small to visualise, and ascites may be absent. However, some studies have achieved a high sensitivity (84%) and specificity (87%) in diagnosis of malignant peritoneal disease (Chou et al. 1994; Low et al. 1997). At the moment, there is no noninvasive imaging modality that enables accurate detection of peritoneal carcinomatosis (Dux et al. 1999) whose detection would further decrease the number of futile laparotomies in patients with gastric carcinoma.

7.6 Practical Application

MRI performed for gastric imaging in vivo is associated with certain technical issues including motion artefacts (peristalsis, respiratory and patient motion) and necessity for gastric distension. For the time being there is no clinical indication for gastric MRI because there are gross limitations with respect to spatial resolution and image quality. For example, gastric wall layers cannot be reliably distinguished using conventional MR techniques, which limits accurate determination of the T-staging of gastric carcinoma. Endoscopic MRI is the most promising technique for assessing the stomach, accurately demonstrating three layers of the gastric wall, and high-spatial-resolution MRI using endoluminal receiver coils may enable staging of gastric carcinoma. Compared to other imaging modalities the high soft tissue contrast, multiplanar imaging, and contrast-enhanced studies may provide a better distinction between tumour and peri-tumour tissue changes often associated with gastric carcinoma. At present performing upper endoscopy in the MR environment must address safety issues, as it is an invasive procedure that carries an increased risk of morbidity and mortality compared to a standard upper GI endoscopy. It requires technical improvements before being used routinely, with new devices requiring proper safety testing and regulatory approval first. With further technical progress in this area, however, endoscopic MRI has the potential to overcome today's limitations regarding the staging of gastric carcinoma, which remains a major challenge.

References

Auh YH, Lim T-H, Lee DII et al (1994) In vitro MR imaging of the resected stomach with a 4,7-T superconducting magnet. Radiology 191:129–134

Bisset GS III (1989) Evaluation of potential practical oral contrast agents for pediatric magnetic resonance imaging. Pediatr Radiol 20:61–66

Botet JF, Lightdale CJ, Zauber AG et al (1991) Preoperative staging of gastric cancer: comparison of endoscopic US and dynamic CT. Radiology 181:426–432.

Caletti G, Ferrari A, Brocchi E et al (1993) Accuracy of endoscopic ultrasonography in the diagnosis and staging of gastric cancer and lymphoma. Surgery 113:14–27

Chou C.-K, Chen L.-T, Sheu R-S et al (1994) MRI manifestations of gastrointestinal wall thickening. Abdom Imaging 19:389–394

Chou CK, Liu OC, Su JH et al (1994) MRI demonstration of peritoneal implants. Abdom Imaging 19(2):95–101

Dekker W, Tytgat GN (1977) Diagnostic accuracy of fiberendoscopy in the detection of upper intestinal malignancy. A follow-up analysis. Gastroenterology 73:710–714

Del Frate C, Bazzocchi M, Mortele KJ et al (2002) Detection of liver metastases: comparison of gadobenate dimeglumine-enhanced and ferumoxides-enhanced MR imaging examinations. Radiology 225(3):766–772

De Souza NM, Gibbons AH, Coutts GA et al (1995) Magnetic resonance imaging during upper GI endoscopy: technical considerations and clinical feasibility. Mm Invasive Ther 4:277–281

Dux M, Roeren T, Kuntz C et al (1997) MRI for staging of gastric carcinoma: first results of an experimental prospective study. J Comput Assist Tomogr 21:66–72

Dux M, Richter GM, Hansmann J et al (1999) Helical Hydro-CT for diagnosis and staging of gastric carcinoma. J Comput Assist Tomogr 23:913–922

Dux M, Grenacher L, Lubienski A et al (2000) Early gastric carcinoma: CT and MR features. Eur Radiol 10:S 222

Dux M, Kuntz C, Lukas M et al (2001) Endoscopic MR imaging in the staging of gastric cancer as compared with histopathological findings. Cardiovasc Intervent Radiol 24: S191

Feldman DR. Kulling DP, Hawes RH et al (1997) MR endoscopy: preliminary experience in human trials. Radiology 202:868–870

Hahn PF, Stark DD, Saini S et al (1987) Ferrite particles for bowel contrast in MR imaging: design issues and feasibility studies. Radiology 164:37–41

Hamm B (2002) Iron-oxide-enhanced MR lymphography: just a new toy or a breakthrough? Eur Radiol 12:957–958

Imai Y, Kressel HY, Saul SH et al (1990) Colorectal tumors: an in vitro study of high-resolution MR imaging. Radiology 177:695–701

Inui K, Nakazawa 5, Yoshino J et al (1995) Endoscopic MRI: preliminary results of a new technique for visualization and staging of gastrointestinal tumors. Endoscopy 27:480–485

Kimmey MB, Martin RW, Haggitt RC et al (1989) Histologic correlates of gastrointestinal ultrasound images. Gastroenterology 96:433–441

Kulling D, Bohning DE, Kay CL et al (1997) Histological correlates to pig gastrointestinal wall layers imaged in vitro with the magnetic resonance endoscope. Gastroenterology 112:1568–1574

Laghi A, Paolantonio P, Catalano C et al (2003) MR imaging of the small bowel using polyethylene glycol solution as an oral contrast agent in adults and children with celiac disease: preliminary observations. AJR 180:191–194

Lauren P (1965) The two histologic main types of gastric carcinoma: diffuse and the so-called intestinal type carcinoma. Acta Pathol Microbiol Scand 64:31–49

Low RN, Barone RM, L.acey C et al (1997) Peritoneal tumor: MR imaging with dilute oral barium and intravenous gadolinium-containing contrast agents compared with unenhanced MR imaging and CT. Radiology 204(2):513–520

Lubienski A, Grenacher L, Reith Wet al (2002) MR-imaging of gastric wall layers in vitro: correlation to the histologic wall structure. Fortschr Rontgenstr 174:490–494

Maehara Y, Orita H, Okuyama T et al (1992) Predictors of lymph node metastasis in early gastric cancer. Br J Surg 79:245–247

Marcos HB, Semelka RC (1999) Stomach diseases: MR evaluation using combined T2-weighted single-shot echo train spin-echo and gadolinium-enhanced spoiled gradient-echo sequences. J Magn Reson Imaging 10:950–960

Matsushita M, Oi H, Murakami T et al (1994) Extraserosal invasion in advanced gastric cancer: evaluation with MR imaging. Radiology 192:87–91

Milestone BN, Schnall MD, Lenkinski RE et al (1991) Cervical carcinoma: MR imaging with an endorectal surface coil. Radiology 180:91–95

Moreaux J, Bougaran J (1993) Early gastric cancer. A 25-year surgical experience. Ann. Surg. 217:347–355

Oi H, Matsushita M, Murakami T et al (1997) Dynamic MR imaging for extraserosal invasion of advanced gastric cancer. Abdom Imaging 22(1):35–40

Schnall M, Furth EE, Rosato E et al (1994) Rectal tumor stage: correlation of endorectal MR imaging and pathologic findings. Radiology 190:709–714

Tio TL, Coene PPLO, Schouwink MH et al (1989) Esophagogastric carcinoma: preoperative TNM classification with endosonography. Radiology 173:411–417

Vogl TJ, Schwarz W, Blume S et al (2003) Preoperative evaluation of malignant liver tumors: comparison of unenhanced and SPIO (Resovist)-enhanced MR imaging with biphasic ClAP and intraoperative US. Eur Radiol 13(2):262–272

Wesbey GE, Brasch RC, Goldberg HI et al (1985) Dilute oral iron solutions as gastrointestinal contrast agents for magnetic resonance imaging: initial clinical experience. Magn Reson Imaging 3:57–64

Yamada I, Saito N, Takeshita K et al (2001) Early gastric carcinoma: evaluation with high-spatial-resolution MR imaging in vitro. Radiology 220:115–121

Endoscopic Ultrasound of the Stomach

8

Keith M. Harris

CONTENTS

8.1 Background

High-frequency ultrasound improves image resolution, but as frequency increases, depth of penetration decreases. This significantly limits the range of frequencies available for transabdominal scanning in all but the slimmest of patients. Many of the difficulties encountered with transabdominal ultrasound including adverse patient body habitus and interference from bowel gas are overcome with endoscopic ultrasound. Endoscopic ultrasound (EUS), combining endoscopy and high-frequency ultrasound, provides a unique opportunity to visualize the bowel wall and adjacent structures. The ultrasound probe mounted on the tip of a flexible endoscope can be manipulated to within close contact of the area of interest without interference from intervening bowel gas, and high frequencies can be utilised to produce images of exceptional quality. Endoscopic ultrasound has been in use since the early 1980's but has been slow to gain acceptance in certain countries.

K. M. Harris, MB, BS, FRCS, FRCR
Consultant Radiologist, Leeds General Infirmary, Great George Street, Leeds, LS1 3EX, UK

8.2 Equipment

There are two basic types of echoendoscope commercially available with either radial or linear array transducer technology. The bowel is a tube and it is the author's opinion that radial scanning is the most appropriate way to image it. A range of products is currently available from several manufacturers. The author's experience is with those made by Olympus (Olympus, KeyMed, Southend UK) and the images within this chapter are all taken using Olympus echoendoscopes. The current model the GF-UE260-AL5 ultrasonic gastrovideoscope is an electronic 360° radial scanner with variable frequencies between 5 and 10 Mhz. Colour and Power Doppler facilities allow easy demonstration of vascular structures and analysis of blood flow within. The ultrasound probe is mounted on the distal tip of the instrument and 55° forward-oblique viewing optics allow easy identification of any mucosal or submucosal abnormality and enable the endoscope to be manipulated to the area of interest under direct vision. This echoendoscope is larger than most conventional end-viewing diagnostic endoscopes that may create difficulties when attempting to negotiate stenotic oesophageal lesions and a number of gastric cancers may also prove to be non-traversable. One study that included 63 patients with oesophageal cancer and 147 with gastric cancer encountered non- traversability rates of 31.6% and 14% respectively (Grimm et al 1993). A single frequency mechanical 7.5MHz 'blind esophagoprobe' (Olympus MH-908) is also available without viewing optics and consequently considerably smaller in diameter (8.5mm) allowing negotiation of a greater proportion of oesophageal strictures. A monorail guide-wire system ensures its safe passage through stenotic tumours. This is however, as its name implies, designed primarily for use in staging stenotic oesophageal tumours and is of little value in the stomach other than for tumours at the gastro-oesophageal junction. Echoendoscopes using linear/curved array transducers provide a slightly more limited ultrasound field of view but in addition to diagnostic studies have the advantage that they enable real-time ultrasound image guided fine-needle biopsy. These instruments also have colour Doppler facilities for easier identification of blood vessels – especially useful during interventional procedures. They have working channels of up to 3.7mm maximum diameter (eg Olympus GF-UCT240) allowing a wide range of therapeutic interventions to be undertaken. Miniprobes are small high frequency transducers that can be passed down the biopsy channel of a conventional endoscope. Miniprobes can be manipulated into the biliary tree or pancreatic duct in a similar fashion that a catheter is during ERCP. Their main use within the stomach however is for staging of small superficial tumours and the assessment of small submucosal nodules.

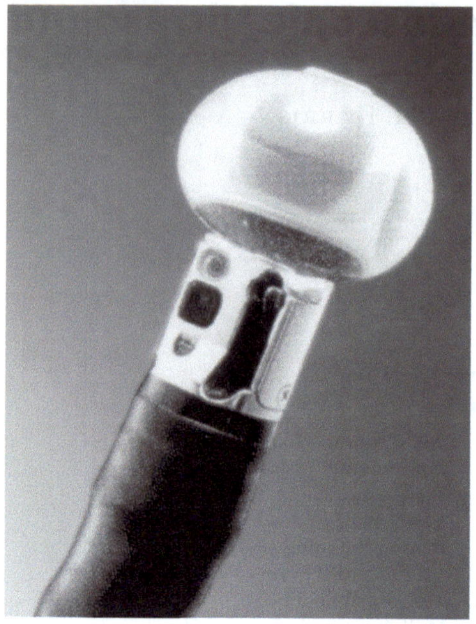

Fig. 8.1. Close-up of the tip of the Olympus GF-UM200 echoendoscope demonstrating the partially inflated water-filled balloon

8.3 Technique

Upper gastrointestinal endosonography is performed in a similar fashion to conventional endoscopy. Informed consent having been previously obtained the patient is routinely fasted. Sedation with midazolam (with or without additional opiate analgesia) and topical pharyngeal anaesthesia are most commonly used in the UK. General anaesthesia is rarely required for examination of the oesophagus or stomach. More time consuming examinations, particularly those of the pancreaticobiliary tree, will occasionally however be undertaken more easily and acceptably by a fully anaesthetised patient. The larger diameter and slightly longer inflexible tip of the echoendoscope can make intubation a little more difficult than with a conventional end-viewing endoscope. The oesophagus, stomach, and duodenum are negotiated under direct vision. At the area of interest air is aspirated from the lumen of the bowel to achieve acoustic coupling between the transducer and the adjacent bowel wall. Inflation of the water-filled balloon (Fig. 8.1) and / or instillation of water into the bowel lumen facilitate contact, the choice dependent upon the area under inspection. Care must be taken to protect the airway when using large volumes of water to fill the lumen of the stomach, recognising the risk of aspiration. The use of contrast-enhanced EUS has been discussed and may in selected cases add further additional information (Nomura et al. 1999).

8.4 Bowel Wall Anatomy

The normal anatomy of the bowel wall is consistently well demonstrated (Fig. 8.2)–from the luminal side: (1) an echogenic layer representing the interface between the transducer and the superficial mucosa, (2) a hypoechoic layer representing the deeper mucosa including the muscularis mucosae, (3) an echogenic layer comprising the submucosa, (4) a hypoechoic layer representing the muscularis propria, and an outermost echogenic layer (5) the serosa (where present). Higher-frequency probes are able to identify up to nine distinct layers including the circular and longitudinal muscle components of the muscularis propria. Certain areas such as the gastric fundus in particular present significant problems for EUS. The more limited manoeuvrability and reduced retroflexion of the tip of the echoendoscope render some small fundal lesions beyond the reach of the echoendoscope. Overall however this is a minor limitation, as the vast majority of the stomach is easily accessible and good views routinely achieved. Changing the position of the patient during the examination from the routine left lateral to prone or supine may improve visualisation a

b

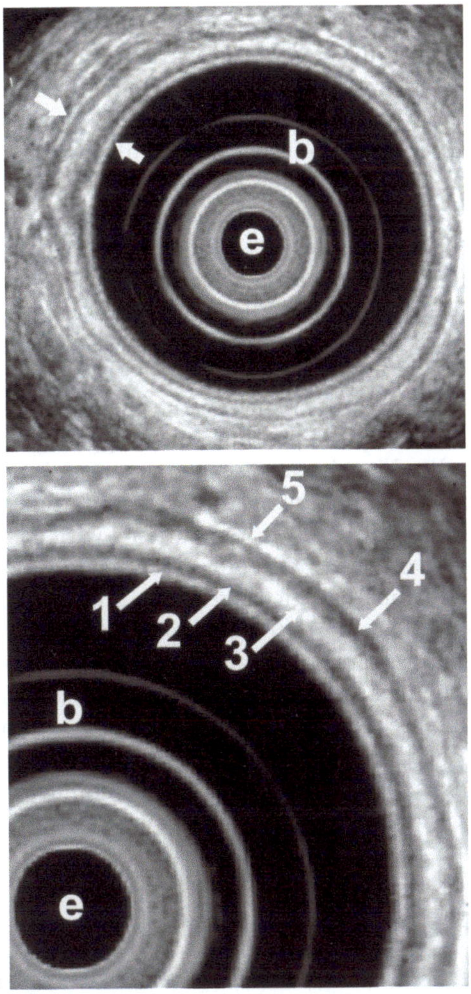

Fig. 8.2. a The normal stomach wall at 12 Mz. The five layers, between arrows, are well demonstrated. *E*= echoendoscope, *b*= water-filled balloon and associated ring-artefacts. **b** Close-up of image **a**. *1*= an echogenic layer representing the interface between the balloon (b) and the superficial mucosa, *2*= a hypoechoic layer representing the deeper mucosa including the muscularis propria, *3*= an echogenic layer comprising the submucosa, *4*= a hypoechoic layer, the muscularis propria, and *5*= the echogenic serosa

of certain areas and/or allow better utilisation of the intraluminal water. Miniprobes are ideal for evaluation of small superficial mucosal lesions. The probe can be guided precisely onto the lesion under direct endoscopic vision, and the higher frequencies used significantly improve image resolution. More gentle pressure minimises the risk of compression of the component layers of the stomach wall. The submucosal layer in particular is so readily compressible it can be spuriously obliterated by the pressure exerted by a larger echoendoscope with, for example, the risk of overstaging a T1 tumour as T2. The coeliac trunk (Fig. 8.3) with its common hepatic and splenic artery branches are useful landmarks with significant importance for tumour staging.

8.5 Benign Pathology

8.5.1 Submucosal Lesions

EUS can accurately define the anatomical location of bowel wall indentations and differentiate between extrinsic compression and intramural masses. Knowledge of the exact layer of origin within the bowel wall helps limit the differential diagnosis, but as in other areas it must be emphasised that EUS is not histology. A paper by Kawamoto et al. (1997) includes a very useful diagrammatic representation of the various submucosal masses encountered. More recently EUS has been utilized to direct endoscopic mucosal resection of a number of submucosal tumours with a low complication rate (Waxman et al. 2002). Gastrointestinal stromal tumours (GISTs) have a characteristic appearance and usually arise from the fourth hypoechoic layer (Fig. 8.4) corresponding to the muscularis propria, although they occasionally are based upon the second layer (muscularis mucosae). The natural history of such

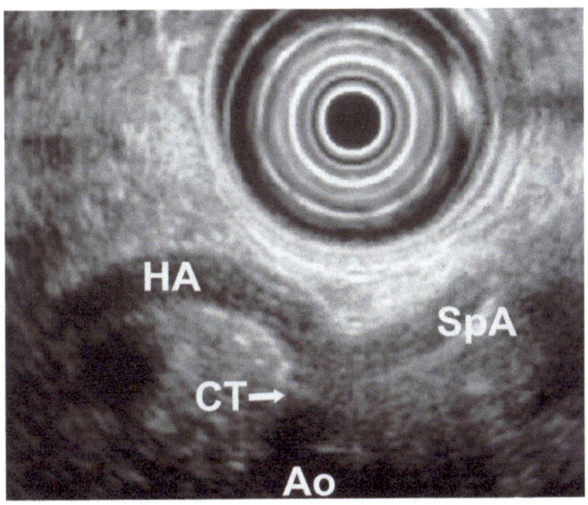

Fig. 8.3. Coeliac trunk and its major divisions likened to a "whale's tail". *Ao*= aorta, *CT*= coeliac trunk, *SpA*= splenic artery, *HA*= hepatic arteryt

tumours is variable, though EUS has been used to predict the likelihood of malignant change. Certain EUS features predictive of the possibility of malignant change have been identified (Palazzo et al. 2000). Those authors published the results of the EUS evaluation of 56 histological proven stromal cell tumours. Irregular extraluminal margins, cystic spaces, and malignant-looking lymph nodes were most predictive of malignant or borderline stromal cell tumours. Of these characteristics the presence of cystic spaces and irregular margins were considered to be independently the most worrisome. Conversely, tumours less than 30 mm with regular margins and a homogeneous echo pattern are usually benign. Interobserver agreement between experts in EUS in interpreting these features has been shown to be fair to moderate (Chak et al. 1997). There are similar data (Gress et al. 2001) supporting good interobserver agreement for characterising a wider range of submucosal masses. On the basis of these cumulative data, an expectant policy with EUS review can be employed for small asymptomatic lesions with no sinister features. Lack of interval change as judged by serial EUS assessment adds further confidence to the suggested benign nature of the lesion. Standard fine-needle biopsy of stromal cell tumours is usually unrewarding, though EUS-guided fine-needle aspiration with immunohistochemical analysis has been usefully employed to provide further information regarding the nature and malignant potential of the tumour (Ando et al. 2002). Lipomas are another commonly observed submucosal swelling and can be indistinguishable endoscopically from a suspected stromal cell tumour. EUS however reveals very different appearances; a lipoma is seen as a well-defined mass, more echogenic than a GIST, usually confined to the submucosal layer displacing adjacent muscle layers (Fig. 8.5). Pancreatic rests (aberrant or heterotopic pancreas) can present a diagnostic challenge, as whilst the endoscopic appearance may suggest such an abnormality, biopsies are often too superficial and unrewarding. A comparative study was undertaken (Matsushita et al. 1999) in ten patients with gastric aberrant pancreas undergoing resection to allow subsequent histopathologic correlation. Endoscopic biopsies failed to confirm the diagnosis in all cases. The EUS features are indistinct margin, heterogeneous echotexture (mainly hypoechoic with small scattered hyperechoic areas), and location within the either the third and fourth layers (submucosa and muscularis propria) or within the submucosa alone. The lesions are mostly accompanied by thickening of the muscularis propria. With such vari-

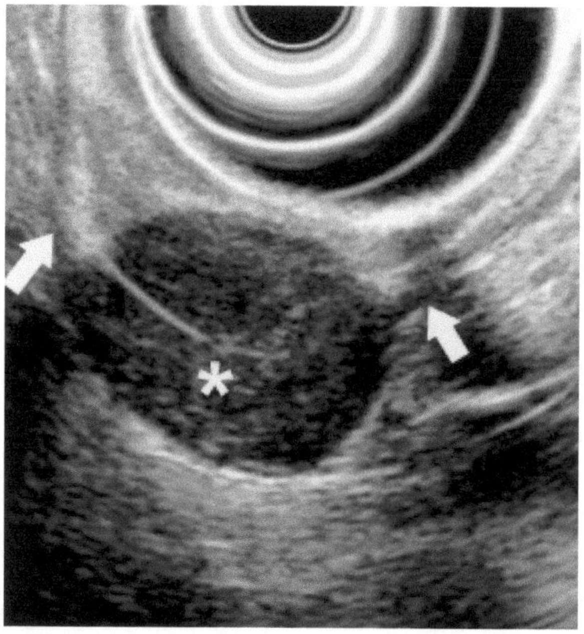

Fig. 8.4. A stromal tumour (*) clearly arising from the muscularis propria (*arrows*) of the stomach wall. Imaging features suggest an entirely benign lesion

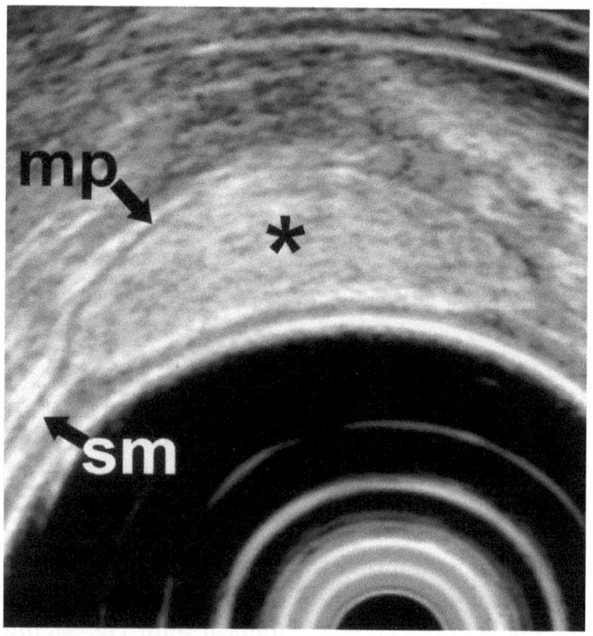

Fig. 8.5. A lipoma (*) arising from the submucosal layer (*sm*) of the stomach wall. The muscularis propria (*mp*) is displaced but not directly involved

able EUS features, a precise diagnosis by imaging alone may be difficult, and again it must be stressed that whenever there is diagnostic doubt or concern, resection for histology is required (Fig. 8.6). Some nodules that are considered endoscopically to be submucosal are in fact extrinsic, and indentations into the stomach from the gallbladder and liver are not uncommon. EUS allows easy identification of such structures, often without the requirement for further imaging or intervention.

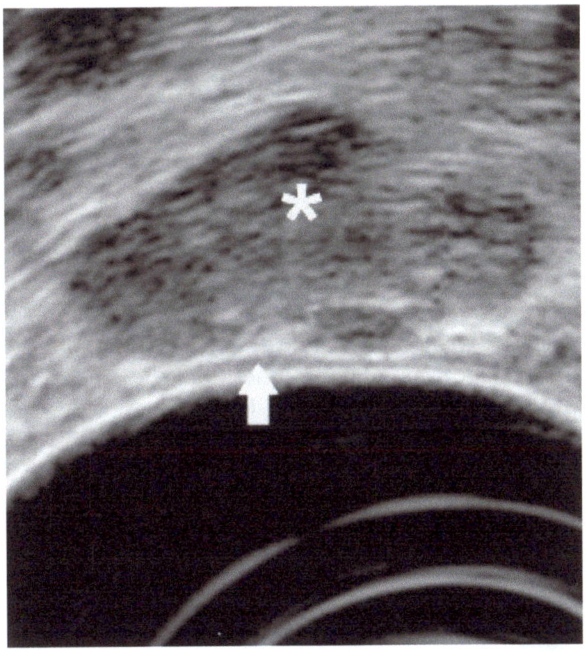

Fig. 8.6. An intramural gastric lesion (*) with indeterminate EUS imaging features. The precise layer of origin deep to the muscularis mucosa (*arrow*) is unclear. Diagnostic uncertainty and noncontributory biopsies necessitated surgical resection. Aberrant pancreas proven histologically

8.5.2 Thickened Folds

When gastric folds are thickened, EUS can demonstrate which wall layers are causing the thickening and whether or not the layered structure is preserved. Thickening of the mucosa is seen in various types of gastritis, Ménétrier's disease, and some patients with early lymphoma. More generalized thickening with loss of the layer structure suggests malignancy, such as advanced lymphoma or linitis plastica. Whilst subtle features may help differentiate these pathologies (Caletti et al. 1993), the true diagnosis can often not be made with EUS alone; more that EUS is of help in suggesting the diagnosis and identifying the need for further biopsies–endoscopic or surgical. Enlarged intramural vessels (Fig. 8.7), varices, and excess collateral extramural vessels are all well seen with EUS. Colour Doppler is not usually required to identify these vessels, though it may be helpful when selecting a site for EUS-guided intervention minimising the risk of haemorrhagic complications.

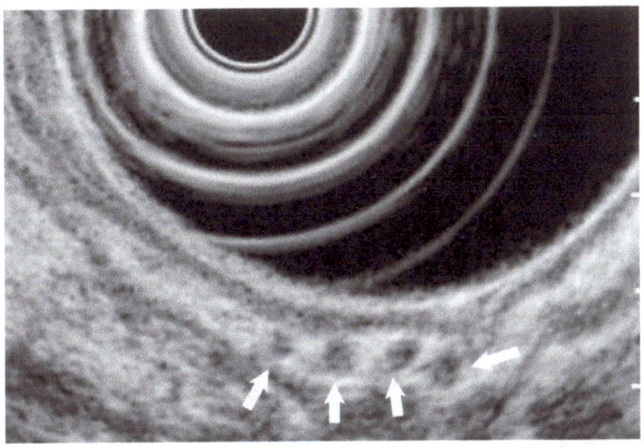

Fig. 8.7. Enlarged submucosal gastric vessels (*arrows*). Identification of intramural and adjacent vessels clearly important if trans-gastric biopsy or drainage is being considered

8.6 Malignant Pathology

8.6.1 Gastric Cancer

Accurate staging of gastro-oesophageal cancer is essential to allow a well-informed decision to be made to plan appropriate treatment. Such precise stage-dependent management will limit the incidence of unnecessary exploratory surgical interventions. Accurate tumour staging is also clearly important when comparing outcomes of various non-surgical interventions, as there is no pathological gold standard. Small superficial early gastro-oesophageal cancers can sometimes be removed endoscopically but knowledge of the precise depth of tumour penetration and exclusion of more distant spread are essential prerequisites. The ability to identify the component layers of the bowel wall provides the basis for tumour staging within the widely accepted TNM classification. The ability to identify the component layers of the bowel wall provides the basis for tumour staging within the widely accepted TNM / AJCC classification (Greene et al. 2002, and see 6.1.4.1). This defines the extent of malignant tumours and allows easy correlation of results from more than one centre. The revised classification in the sixth edition contains some important changes relating to gastric cancer. (Table 8.1 & Fig. 8.9). The omental reflections around the stomach are not clearly seen with EUS and this classification raises important issues for EUS staging of gastric carcinomas. It is difficult or impossible to know if a carcinoma has penetrated the muscularis propria into the greater or lesser omenta but not breached the visceral peritoneum beyond i.e.? T2b or? T3 (Ziegler et al 1993). There is therefore a significant risk, in particular, of overstaging T2b tumours as T3 (Fig. 8.9). Tumours with histological confirmation of true T stage are illustrated (Figs. 8.10–8.13). EUS is superior to computed tomography (CT) for the local staging of gastric carcinoma (Akahoshi et al. 1991; Ziegler et al. 1993; Greenberg et al. 1994; Perng et al. 1996) and is more accurate in predicting resectability, though the complementary nature of these imaging techniques must be emphasised (Botet et al. 1991; François et al. 1996). A comprehensive literature review in 1998 (Harris et al. 1998) extracted data from 27 studies addressing the performance of endoscopic ultrasound for the pre-

Table 8.1. TNM classification of gastric cancer (Greene et al. 2002)

T1	Tumour invades lamina propria or submucosa
T2	Tumour invades muscularis propria or subserosa * **T2a:** Tumor invades muscularis propria **T2b:** Tumor invades the subserosa
T3	Tumour penetrates serosa (visceral peritoneum) without invasion of adjacent structures
T4	Tumour invades adjacent structures
N0	No regional lymph node metastasis
N1	Metastasis in 1 to 6 regional nodes
N2	Metastasis in 7 to 15 regional nodes
N3	Metastasis in > 15 regional nodes
M0	No distant metastasis
M1	Distant metastasis

* Tumour penetration through the muscularis propria extending into the greater or lesser omentum but without penetration of the overlying visceral peritoneum is classified as T2.

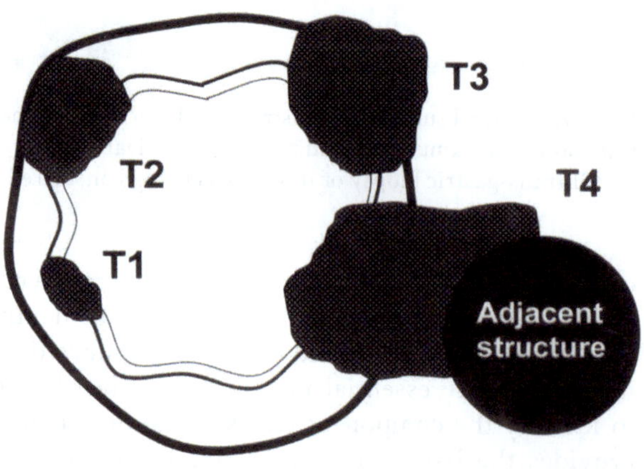

Fig. 8.8. Diagrammatic representation of the T stages of gastric cancer

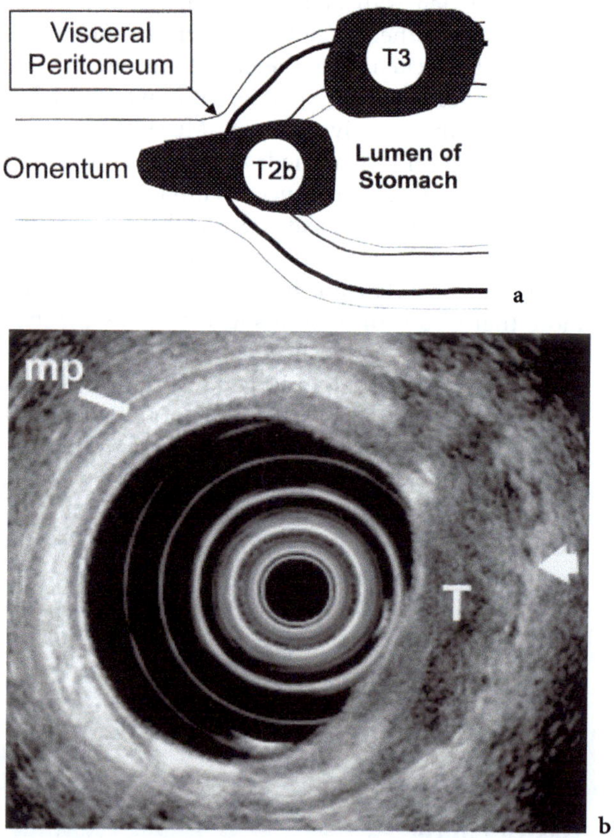

Fig. 8.9. a Diagram demonstrating the potential for incorrectly staging T2b and T3 tumours of the stomach. The omental reflections are not seen with EUS. b. Gastric tumour (T). There is definite localised breach of the muscularis propria (white arrow), suggesting T3, but pathology indicated T2b as the visceral peritoneum, not visible on EUS, had not been breached. Muscularis propria (mp) elsewhere intac **b** Gastric tumour (*T*). There is definite localised breach of the muscularis propria (*white arrow*), suggesting T3, but pathology indicated T2 as the visceral peritoneum, not visible, had not been breached. Muscularis propria (*mp*) elsewhere intact

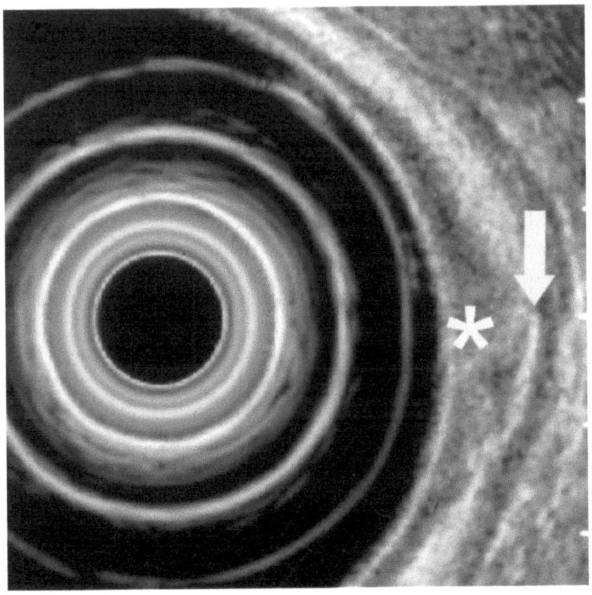

Fig. 8.10. T1 gastric cancer (*). Note preservation of the underlying deep submucosa (*arrow*)

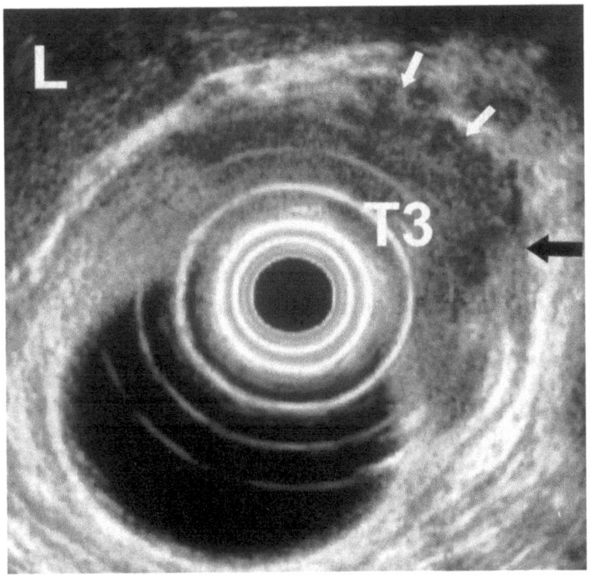

Fig. 8.12. *T3* gastric cancer. The muscularis propria and serosa are clearly breached (*white arrows*). Elsewhere the muscularis propria is intact (*black arrow*). *L* = liver

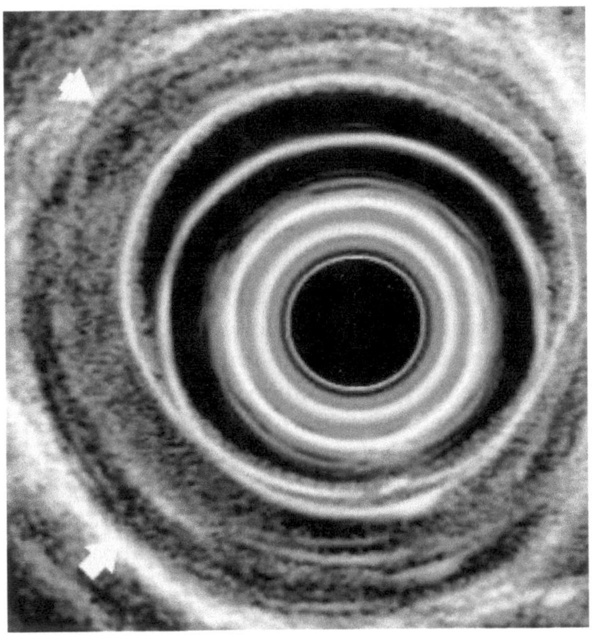

Fig. 8.11. T2 gastric cancer. The deep muscularis propria is not breached throughout the circumference of the tumour (*arrows*)

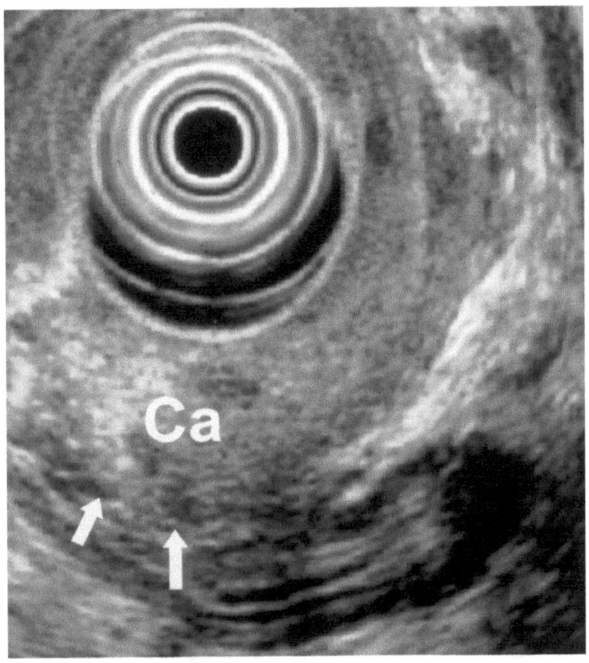

Fig. 8.13. T4 gastric cancer. The cancer (*Ca*) has invaded (*arrows*) adjacent transverse colon (TC)

operative staging of gastro-oesophageal cancer. The paucity of randomised controlled trials necessitated the acceptance of evidence from other study designs. Staging performance results (sensitivity, specificity, positive predictive value, negative predictive value, accuracy, and odds ration) were synthesised, and receiver operator characteristic curves for the differentiation of tumour stages T1 and T2 from T3 and T4 were plotted. A summary statistic (Q*, balancing sensitivity and specificity) was calculated, Q* for gastric cancer T stage = 0.93 and for gastric cancer N staging = 0.76. A more recent analysis however suggests that the accuracy for T staging in clinical practice may be lower than previously reported, with blinded analysis producing poorer results (Meining et al. 2002). These data however further support the fact that EUS is a complimentary investigation, the results of which should not be used in isolation from other available information. EUS is useful in being able to predict a complete resection for gastric cancer, with one study (Dittler and Siewert 1993) demonstrating almost identical predicted and actual RO resection rates. Recent guidelines (Allum et al. 2002) suggest that "in the absence of metastatic disease, assessment of operability is preferably made by endoscopic ultrasound." The presence of direct invasion into adjacent structures (T4) can be difficult to establish on both CT and EUS. Using CT, the suggestion of invasion is often based solely upon the area of contact with the contiguous organ, but EUS also allows evaluation in real-time, and free movement between the tumour and the adjacent organ (particularly the liver) excludes direct invasion (Fig. 8.14). Lymph nodes are well seen, and certain features correlate well with malignant infiltration: Nodes greater than 1 cm diameter, with well-defined margins, rounded and hypoechoic are likely to be involved (Fig. 8.15) (Catalano et al. 1991). Malignant nodes unfortunately may not demonstrate all four features, and large benign, reactive nodes are well recognised. Whilst other imaging modalities are required to demonstrate the whole of the liver and more distant lymph node groups, the left lobe of the liver is well seen with EUS, and small previously undetected metastases can be easily identified. Small-volume ascites, frequently undetected by other imaging modalities, (Fig. 8.16) can also be demonstrated with EUS, and will alert the surgeon to the possibility of peritoneal spread. EUS has a limited depth of penetration, and whilst it is well suited to the evaluation of local invasion, it is of limited usefulness in the overall assessment of more distant spread. Unfortunately patients with gastro-oesophageal cancer often present late in the course of the disease, and CT remains an essential part of the staging process for evaluation of the presence of distant metastases. Even state-of-the-art multi-slice CT is however unable to resolve the component layers of the bowel wall and therefore cannot discriminate between T1 and T2 tumours. EUS is more accurate than CT for all T stages. EUS N-staging is less accurate than EUS T-staging, but here again better than CT. The complimentary nature of EUS and CT has been described, but in addition there is a similar combined role for EUS and endoscopy in the evaluation of early gastric cancer when assessing the potential for endoscopic resection (Yanai et al. 1997, 1999). EUS cannot reliably discriminate between a benign or

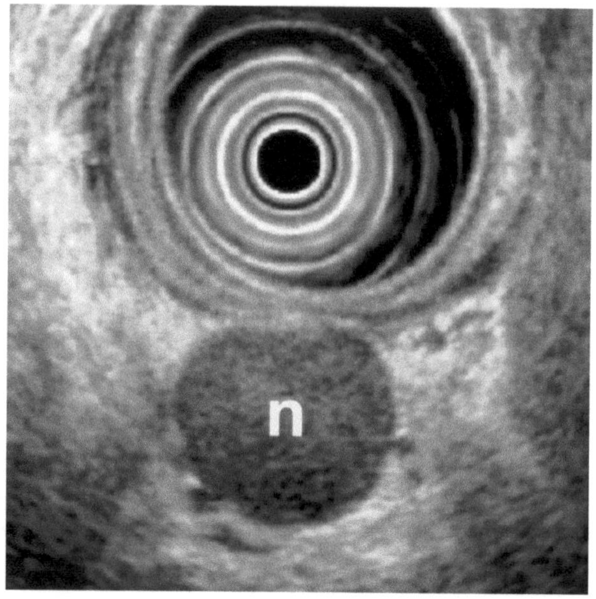

Fig. 8.15. A perigastric lymph node (*n*) measuring 14 mm in diameter with imaging features suggesting metastatic involvement

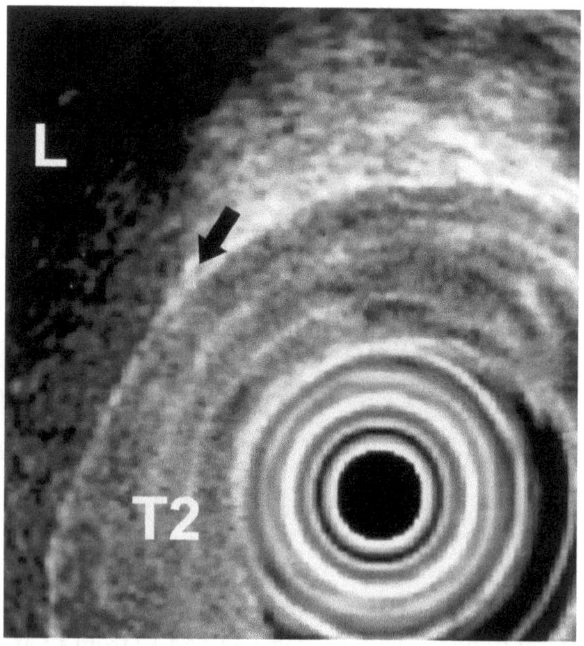

Fig. 8.14. Sizeable *T2* gastric tumour. *Arrow* demonstrates clear line of separation from the adjacent liver (*L*). Real-time scanning demonstrated obvious movement between the tumour and the liver, making invasion unlikely

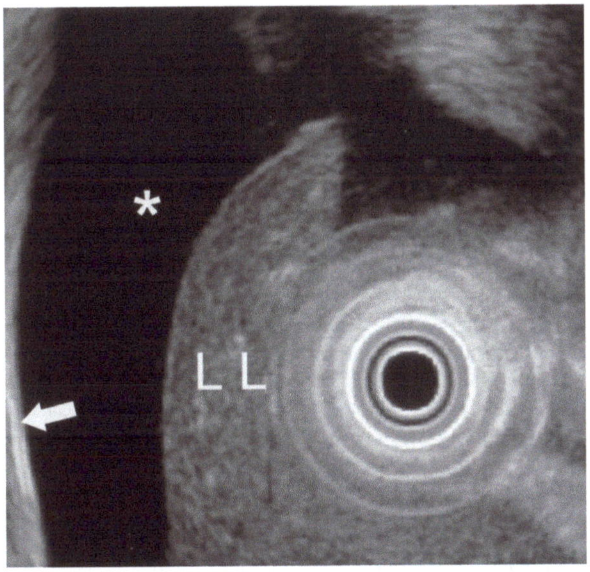

Fig. 8.16. Ascites (*) between the free edge of the left lobe of liver (*LL*) and the left hemi-diaphragm (*arrow*)

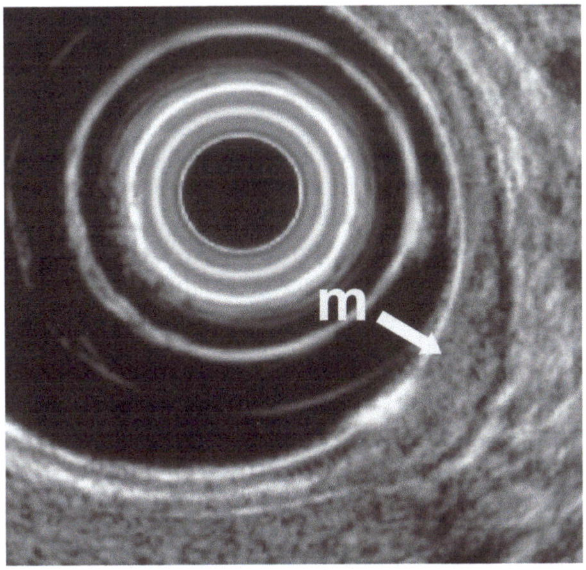

Fig. 8.17. Patient with biopsy-proven maltoma following a course of *H. pylori* eradication. Post-treatment biopsies suggested disease-free, but EUS demonstrates persistent abnormality (*m*). Further targeted biopsies confirmed persistent disease

malignant gastric ulcer such that surgery would be based upon the EUS findings alone. Repeated biopsies are essential, and whilst EUS may add helpful information it is not a reliable replacement for histology. Large reactive nodes are well recognised with aggressive-looking though benign ulcers.

8.6.2 Gastric Maltoma

Mucosa-associated lymphoid tissue (MALT) lymphoma can be assessed with EUS. EUS has been shown to be more sensitive than endoscopy or CT for accurate staging and crucial for predicting tumour response to bacterial eradication (Ruskoné-Formestraux et al. 2001). Gastric MALT lymphoma may regress completely after *H. pylori* eradication, and pretreatment EUS staging can predict outcome, assess response to nonsurgical therapy, and may avoid unnecessary surgery. A study of 15 patients with proven MALT lymphoma indicated that EUS could differentiate superficial from infiltrative types that may have prognostic significance and confirm remission or persistence of the disease with medical treatment during follow-up (Lévy et al. 1997). When the gastric wall remains thick, even if histology is negative, repeated biopsies should be performed as persistent disease is likely (Fig. 8.17). The addition of EUS-guided fine-needle aspiration (FNA) of suspicious lymph nodes may also increase the accuracy of EUS staging. Interobserver agreement for staging gastric MALT lymphoma by EUS is however suboptimal both before and after treatment of *H. pylori* infection. This evidence suggests that gastric EUS may in fact be more technically difficult compared with EUS of other areas, possibly due to the size of the stomach and the uncertainty that all areas have been fully assessed.

8.7 Interventional EUS

Endoscopic ultrasound has been used to provide accurate guidance for injection, biopsy, aspiration, and drainage in a wide range of settings. Fine-needle aspiration biopsy of the suspected primary tumour or of lymph node masses is well established and may become more important with improvements in chemo-radiotherapeutic regimes. Such regimes will require a cytological or histological diagnosis that may be most easily achieved by EUS. The limitations of a negative biopsy due to sampling error and the associated risks (principally haemorrhage) must however always be borne in mind.

8.8 Impact and outcomes

EUS is a safe, useful imaging modality, helpful in improving diagnostic certainty and altering patient management (Jafri et al. 1996; Nickl et al. 1996; Allescher et al. 1999). There are however currently very few good data regarding the influence of EUS on patient outcome. A study from Leeds UK (Preston et al. 2000) demonstrated that EUS was an extremely useful tool aiding management decision-making in the majority of 100 consecutive patients with oesophageal and junctional cancers. The addition of EUS to the staging of patients with cancer of the oesophagus and oesophago-gastric junction resulted in an altered management strategy for between one in three to one in six patients.

References

Akahoshi K, Misawa T, Fujishima H et al (1991) Preoperative evaluation of gastric cancer by endoscopic ultrasound. Gut 32:479-482

Allescher H-D, Rösch T, Willkomm G et al (1999) Performance, patient acceptance, appropriateness of indications and potential influence on outcomes of EUS: a prospective study in 397 consecutive patients. Gastrointest Endosc 50:737-745

Allum WH, Griffin SM, Watson A et al (2002) Guidelines for the management of oesophageal and gastric cancer. Gut 50 [Suppl V]:v1-v23

Ando N, Goto H, Niwa Y et al (2002) The diagnosis of GI stromal tumors with EUS-guided fine needle aspiration with immunohistochemical analysis. Gastrointest Endosc 55:37-43

Botet JF, Lightdale CJ, Zauber AG et al (1991) Preoperative staging of gastric cancer: comparison of endoscopic ultrasound and dynamic CT. Radiology 181:426-432

Caletti G, Ferrari A, Brocchi E et al (1993) Accuracy of endoscopic ultrasonography in the diagnosis and staging of gastric cancer and lymphoma. Surgery 113:14-27

Catalano MF, Sivak Jr MV, Rice T et al (1994) Endosonographic features predictive of lymph node metastasis. Gastrointest Endosc 40:442-446

Chak A, Canto MI, Rösch T et al (1997) Endosonographic differentiation of benign and malignant stromal cell tumours. Gastrointest Endosc 45:468-473

Dittler HJ, Siewert JR (1993) Role of endoscopic ultrasonography in gastric carcinoma. Endoscopy 25:162-166

François E, Peroux J-L, Mouroux J et al (1996) Preoperative endosonographic staging of cancer of the cardia. Abdom Imaging 21:483-487

Greenberg J, Durkin M, Van Drunen M et al (1994) Computed tomograpahy or endoscopic ultrasonography in preoperative staging of gastric and esophageal tumours. Surgery 116:696-702

Greene FL, Fritz, AG, Balch CM, Haller DG, Page DL, Fleming ID, Morrow M (eds) (2002) AJCC Cancer Staging Handbook, 6th edn. Springer, New York

Gress F, Schmitt C, Savides T et al (2001) Interobserver agreement for EUS in the evaluation and diagnosis of submucosal masses. Gastrointest Endosc 53:71-76

Grimm H, Binmoeller KF, Hamper K et al (1993) Endosonography for preoperative locoregional staging of esophageal and gastric cancer. Endoscopy 25:224-230

Harris KM, Kelly S, Berry E et al (1998) Systematic review of endoscopic ultrasound in gastro-oesophageal cancer. Health Technol Assess 2 53-62

Jafri IH, Saltzman JR, Colby JM et al (1996) Evaluation of the clinical impact of endoscopic ultrasonography in gastro-intestinal-disease. Gastrointest Endosc 44:367-370

Kawamoto K, Yamada Y, Utsunomiya T et al (1997) Gastrointestinal submucosal tumours: evaluation with endoscopic ultrasound. Radiology 205:733-740

Lévy M, Hammel P, Lamarque D et al (1997) Endoscopic ultrasonography for the initial staging and follow-up in patients with low-grade gastric lymphoma of mucosa-associated lymphoid tissue treated medically. Gastrointest Endosc 46:328-333

Matsushita M, Hajiro K, Okazaki K et al (1999) Gastric aberrant pancreas: EUS analysis in comparison with the histology. Gastrointest Endosc 49:493-497

Meining A, Dittler HJ, Wolf A et al (2002) You get what you expect? A critical appraisal of imaging methodology in endosonographic cancer staging. Gut 50:599-603

Nickl NJ, Bhutani MS, Catalano M et al (1996) Clinical implications of endoscopic ultrasound: the American Endosonography Club Study. Gastrointest Endosc 44:371-377

Nomura N, Goto H, Niwa Y et al (1999) Usefulness of contrast-enhanced EUS in the diagnosis of upper GI tract diseases. Gastrointest Endosc 50:555-560

Palazzo L, Landi B, Cellier C et al (2000) Endosonographic features predictive of benign and malignant gastrointestinal stromal cell tumours. Gut 46:88-92

Perng D-S, Jan C-M, Wang W-M et al (1996) Computed tomography, endoscopic ultrasound and intraoperative assessment in TN staging of gastric carcinoma. J Formos Med Assoc 95:378-385

Preston SR, Clark GWB, Martin IG et al (2000) The effect of endoscopic ultrasound on the management of 100 consecutive cases of oesophageal and junctional carcinoma. Endoscopy 32:A4

Ruskoné-Formestraux A, Lavergne A, Aegerter PH et al (2001) Predictive factors for regression of gastric MALT lymphoma after anti-Helicobacter pylori treatment. Gut 48:297-303

Waxman I, Saitoh Y, Raju GJ et al (2002) High-frequency probe EUS-assisted endoscopic mucosal resection: a therapeutic strategy for submucosal tumours of the GI tract. Gastrointest Endosc 55:44-49

Yanai H, Matsumoto Y, Harada T et al (1997) Endoscopic ultrasonography and endoscopy for staging depth of invasion in early gastric cancer: a pilot study. Gastrointest Endosc 46:212-216

Yanai H, Noguchi T, Mizumachi S et al (1999) A blind comparison of the effectiveness of endoscopic ultrasonography and endoscopy in staging early gastric cancer. Gut 44:361-365

Ziegler K, Sanft C, Zimmer T et al (1993) Comparison of computed tomography, endosonography, and intraoperative assessment in TN staging of gastric carcinoma. Gut 34:604-610

CT of the Duodenum

9

Rivka Zissin

CONTENTS

9.1 Introduction

CT provides superb anatomic detail and offers a high diagnostic specificity for various gastrointestinal tract (GIT) pathological processes, as it allows direct imaging of the intestinal wall, secondary signs of bowel disease within the surrounding mesentery, and abnormal findings in adjacent structures (Freeman 2001). In clinical practice and in the radiological literature, most emphasis is placed on CT imaging of the colon, the stomach, and the distal small bowel. The current widespread use of abdominal CT, however, has also resulted in the detection of various duodenal abnormalities (Jayaraman et al. 2001; Zissin et al. 2002). This chapter reviews the CT findings of a spectrum of different common and uncommon pathological entities affecting the duodenum.

9.2 Anatomy

The duodenum is the shortest and most fixed part of the small intestine, about 25 cm long, extending in the retroperitoneum as a C-shaped loop. It begins at the pylorus, passes to the right of the midline, and courses in an incomplete circle to its union with the jejunum at the level of the ligament of Treitz. This is situated to the left of the midline at the level of the transpyloric plane opposite the second lumbar vertebra. Descriptively, the duodenum is divided into four parts: the superior (including the duodenal bulb), the descending (containing the duodenal papilla with the opening of the biliary and pancreatic ducts at the ampulla of Vater), the horizontal part, and the ascending part.

Except for the duodenal bulb, which is an intraperitoneal segment, the duodenum is a retroperitoneal structure, partially covered with peritoneum over its anterior aspect, and located within the anterior pararenal space. At this location it bears a close relation with important contiguous viscera such as the pancreatic head, the hepatic flexure, the right kidney, and the gallbladder, as well as with major vascular structures [the inferior vena cava, (IVC), the abdominal aorta, and the superior mesenteric vessels] (Gray 1995). A variety of pathological processes in these structures may have a secondary effect on the duodenum.

R. Zissin, MD
Head of CT Unit, Department of Diagnostic Imaging, Meir General Hospital, Sapir Medical Center, Tchernichovsky St., Kfar Saba 44281, Israel; affiliated with the Sackler Faculty of Medicine, Tel-Aviv University, Tel-Aviv, Israel

9.3 CT Technique

Standard abdominal CT imaging is usually obtained following the administration of dilute water-soluble contrast medium by mouth, as well as an intravenous injection of contrast medium. Optimized imaging of the duodenum depends on the prospective acquisition of thin-section helical CT (slice collimation of 5 mm or less), dynamically enhanced imaging of the upper abdomen, and good distension of the duodenum by the ingestion of a large amount of oral contrast medium (Jayaraman et al. 2001). Changing the patient's position may be further required for optimal demonstration of various parts of the duodenum.

CT-angiography with the use of a multislice helical scanner, with faster scanning speeds and narrow collimation following dynamic contrast injection on both axial images and multiplanar reformats, allows for high-quality demonstration of the surrounding vasculature.

When histologically proven duodenal cancer is demonstrated by endoscopy, helical image acquisition, following the ingestion of water as a negative contrast medium together with drug-induced hypotonia and dynamic intravenous contrast injection, may be the best combination for tumor staging (Rossi et al. 1999). This technique is optimal for evaluating local tumour invasion, as filling the duodenum with water reduces beam-hardening artifacts caused by the oral contrast agent.

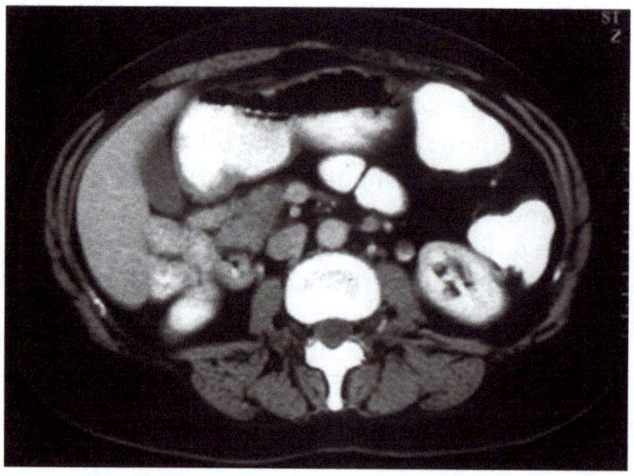

Fig. 9.1. Nonrotation type of intestinal malrotation. CECT at the level of the pancreatic head shows right-sided contrast-filled small bowel loops, left-sided colon, and absence of the horizontal duodenum. Note an abnormal relationship of the superior mesenteric vessels and aplasia of the uncinate process of the pancreas

9.4 Congenital Anomalies

9.4.1 Intestinal Malrotation

Midgut malrotation refers to a spectrum of congenital anomalies of the position of the intestine resulting from inadequate rotation of the primitive intestinal loop around the axis of the superior mesenteric artery during the 6th–11th weeks of fetal life. There are numerous anatomical variations of abnormal intestinal rotation. The type of malrotation, either nonrotation or any subtype of incomplete rotation, relate to the embryological stage of development at which arrest or error of the normal rotation occurred. The most common type of intestinal malrotation is Type Ia, which is rarely associated with complications, and is often found incidentally in adult life by imaging studies, on abdominal surgery, or at autopsy (Fig. 9.1). It is defined by nonrotation of the colon and the duodenum, whereas Type IIa is defined by nonrotation of the duodenum only. In Type IIb, the duodenum and colon show reversed rotation. In Type IIc, the duodenum passes anteriorly to the superior mesenteric vessels, and the large bowel passes in a normal position in front of both of them, features that are clearly demonstrated on CT (Fig. 9.2) (Zissin et al. 1999). In Type IIIa, the duodenal-jejunal flexure lies in the midline to the right of the left-side pedicle of the lumbar spine. Type IIIb is characterized by incomplete fixation of the hepatic

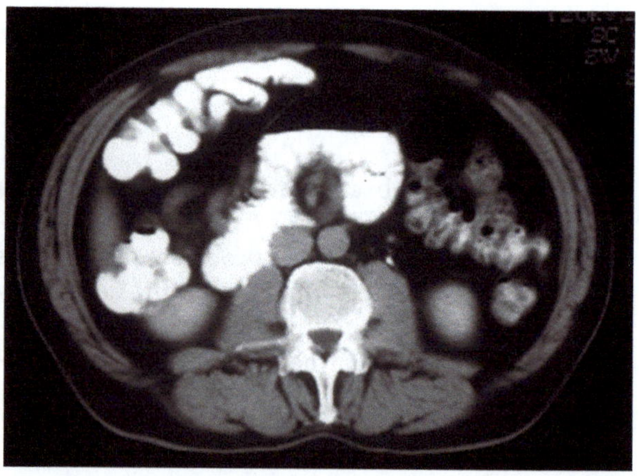

Fig. 9.2. Type IIc of intestinal malrotation: The horizontal duodenum passes anteriorly to the vertically oriented superior mesenteric vessels with a normally located colon in front of it. (Reprinted with permission from Zissin et al. 1999)

flexure. In Type IIIc, incomplete attachment of the cecum is seen. Type IIId is characterized by an internal hernia near the ligament of Treitz (Stringer and Babyn 2000). Intestinal malrotation may occur as an isolated congenital anomaly in patients with situs solitus or as a component of situs anomalies, which may be associated with IVC anomalies, polysplenia, short pancreas, and preduodenal portal vein (PPV) (Gayer et al. 1999; Zissin et al. 1999; Pickhardt and Bhalla 2002).

The characteristic CT findings of intestinal nonrotation include abnormal orientation of the superior mesenteric vessels, aplasia or hypoplasia of the uncinate process of the pancreas, right-sided small bowel loops, a left-sided colon, and the absence of the horizontal part of the duodenum. Vertical or reversed location of the superior mesenteric vessels is, however, not specific for intestinal malrotation.

Complications of intestinal malrotation after childhood are rare but include small intestinal obstruction due to internal hernia and midgut volvulus. The latter may have a clinical presentation of recurrent episodes of colicky abdominal pain associated with vomiting or sometimes with diarrhea and malabsorption. On CT there may be signs of small bowel obstruction, or more typically there is the "whirlpool" sign. This is caused by the swirling appearance of twisted bowel loops and mesentery around the superior mesenteric vessels, which together with abnormally placed bowel help in establishing the diagnosis (Pickhardt and Bhalla 2002).

9.4.2 Duodenal Diverticulum

Duodenal diverticulum is a frequent incidental finding, found in up to 10% of upper GIT barium studies. The most common site is at the mesenteric border of the descending and horizontal parts of the duodenum, particularly near the ampulla of Vater. Indeed the ampulla may be situated within a diverticulum so that the common bile duct drains into such a periampullary diverticulum. On CT, the diverticulum is seen as an air-filled pocket, or it may demonstrate an air-fluid level with contrast medium and food debris in the dependent part (Fig. 9.3) (Stone et al. 1989; Jayaraman et al. 2001; Zissin et al. 2002).

Intraluminal duodenal diverticulum (ILDD) is a rare congenital duodenal anomaly caused by an incomplete congenital web of membrane in which a sac-like fluid collection is forced into the duodenal lumen. It may be associated with other congenital abnormalities such as annular pancreas, intestinal malrotation, situs inversus, and congenital heart anomalies (Tasu et al. 1999). On CT, the ILDD is usually seen as a small fluid collection within the contrast-filled duodenum, but it may enlarge when distended with food. A large ILDD can lead to episodes of recurrent pancreatitis, partial duodenal obstruction, or upper GIT hemorrhage.

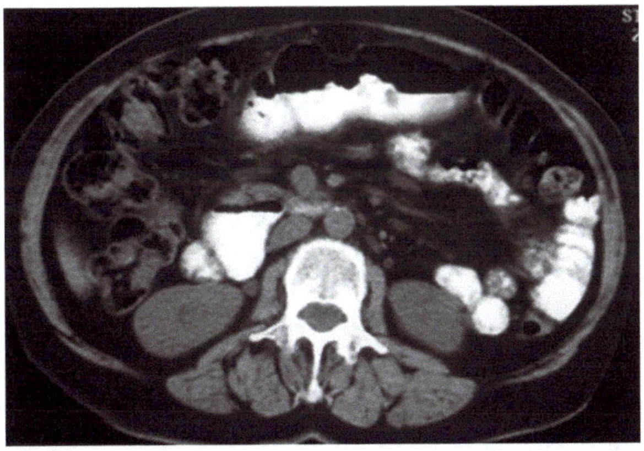

Fig. 9.3. Duodenal diverticulum. A large rounded collection of the oral contrast medium with an air-fluid level seen medially to the duodenal loop

9.4.3 Duodenal Duplication

Duodenal duplication is a rare congenital anomaly, accounting for only 5% of all GIT duplications. It has a 1–2-mm-thick wall composed of functional mucosa and a muscular layer of smooth muscle, which in most cases connects with the muscular layer of the normal intestinal wall. The lumen of the cyst, however, does not usually communicate with the duodenal lumen. A duplication cyst is often found along the mesenteric side of the first and second portions of the duodenum (Macpherson 1993; Berrocal et al. 1999). On CT, it appears as a cystic, fluid-filled lesion in the concavity of the duodenal C-loop, indenting and displacing the lumen laterally (Fig. 9.4). It may contain mobile enteroliths within the fluid content. The differential diagnosis of duodenal duplication includes a choledochocele (cystic dilatation of the intraduodenal portion of the common bile duct), a pancreatic pseudocyst, and an ILDD (Fidler et al. 1998). Sonography, particularly endoscopic, has proved to be helpful in establish-

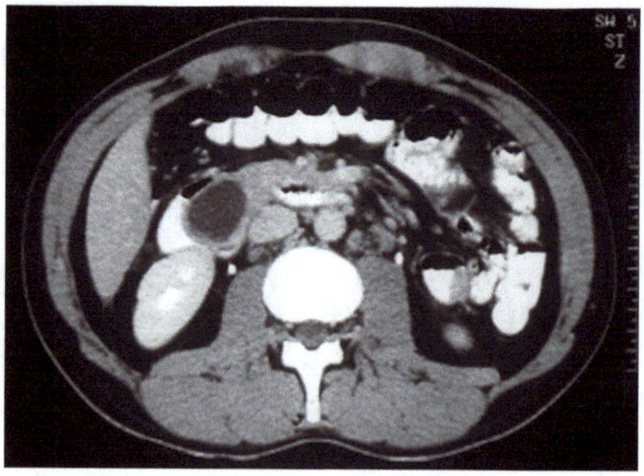

Fig. 9.4. Duodenal duplication. CECT shows a cystic structure in the medial portion of the descending duodenum. This is narrowing and displacing its lumen

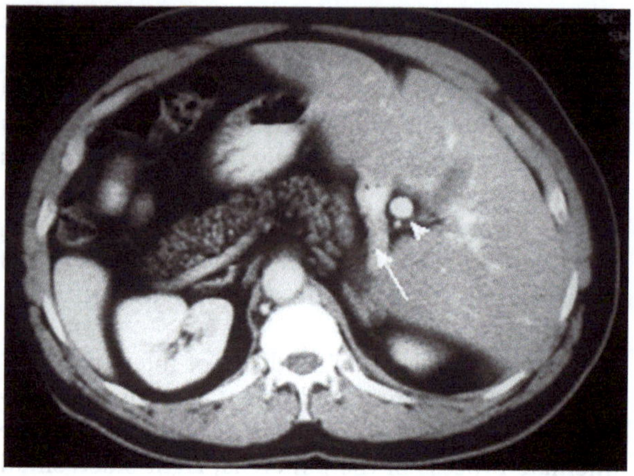

Fig. 9.5. Preduodenal portal vein (*arrowhead*) is seen crossing laterally to the descending part of the duodenum (*arrow*) in a patient with associated congenital anomalies of situs inversus and interrupted IVC (Reprinted with permission from Gayer et al. 1999)

ing the correct diagnosis of duodenal duplication by demonstrating the pathognomonic sign of a layered wall of hyperechoic mucosa surrounded by a thin hypoechoic halo representing the muscular layer.

Duodenal duplication and diverticulum are usually asymptomatic lesions, often diagnosed incidentally by imaging. They may, infrequently, become symptomatic owing to complications such as acute inflammation, perforation, hemorrhage, acute pancreatitis, intussusception, or biliary obstruction (Oshimoa et al. 1998; Rao 1999).

9.4.4 Preduodenal Portal Vein

Preduodenal portal vein (PPV) is a rare congenital anomaly associated with additional various anomalies, including intestinal malrotation, situs anomalies, IVC anomalies, polysplenia, pancreatic anomalies, duodenal atresia, and cardiac anomalies (Tsuda et al. 1991; Gayer et al. 1999). On CT, the preduodenal and prepancreatic localization of the portal vein is demonstrated, as well as any associated anomalies (Fig. 9.5). The diagnosis of a PPV before surgical intervention in the upper abdomen is important to prevent its inadvertent ligation or transection (Tsuda et al. 1991).

Duodenal atresia, midgut volvulus, and annular pancreas are other congenital anomalies which affect the duodenum and may lead to duodenal obstruction during the neonatal period. Abdominal plain radiography is often diagnostic and specific, demonstrating a "double bubble sign", and further imaging studies are rarely required (Berrocal et al. 1999).

9.5 Inflammatory Diseases

9.5.1 Peptic Disease and Its Complications

Most duodenal ulcers are found within the duodenal bulb, usually diagnosed by endoscopy or by barium meal on an upper GIT series (Hwang et al. 1998; Darrah and Nolan 1999). Yet, abdominal CT, often performed for nonspecific upper abdominal complaints, may demonstrate marked thickening of the duodenal wall, sometimes even with an ulcer crater (Fig. 9.6), suggesting the diagnosis of peptic ulcer disease. Duodenal wall thickening is, however, not a specific finding and may be seen in other forms of duodenitis apart from that associated with *Helicobacter pylori*. These include Zollinger-Ellison syndrome and acquired immunodeficiency syndrome (Jayaraman et al. 2001). Clinical evaluation and additional imaging or endoscopic procedures are often needed to establish the correct diagnosis.

Acute complications of duodenal ulcer are commonly diagnosed by CT, as it is frequently the first imaging modality performed for acute abdominal conditions. A perforated duodenal ulcer is suggested by the presence of pneumoperitoneum (the most common finding) and intraperitoneal extravasation of the oral contrast medium, particularly if it is seen leaking from a thick-walled duodenum (Figs. 9.7, 9.8). A penetrating duodenal ulcer is demonstrated

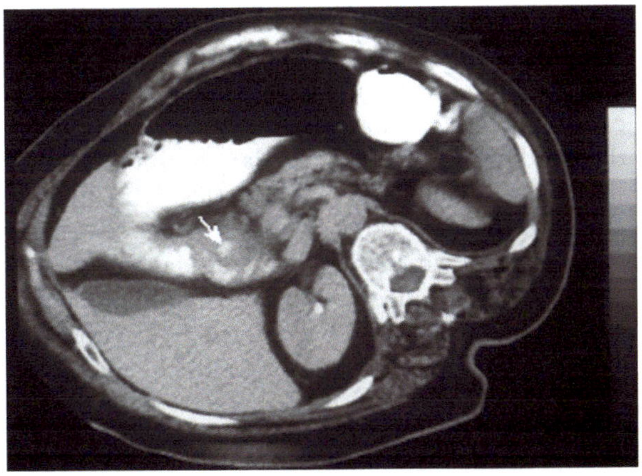

Fig. 9.6. Duodenal ulcer. Mural thickening of the proximal duodenum with an ulcer crater (*arrow*) in a patient with peptic ulceration. (Reprinted with permission from Zissin et al. 2002)

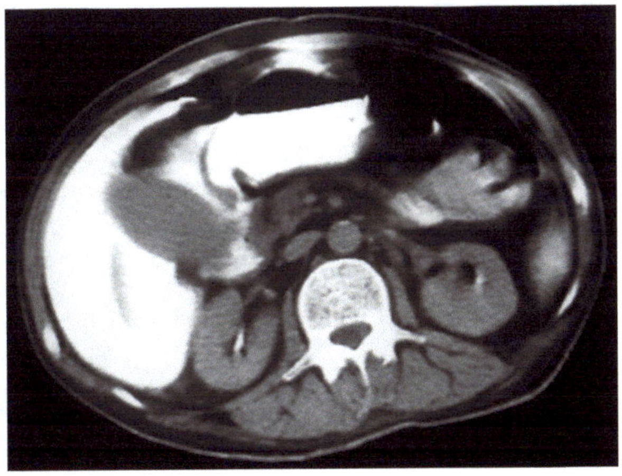

Fig. 9.8. Perforated duodenal ulcer. CT shows leakage of the orally ingested contrast medium, seen around the gallbladder due to intraperitoneal perforation. Note the thick-walled duodenum

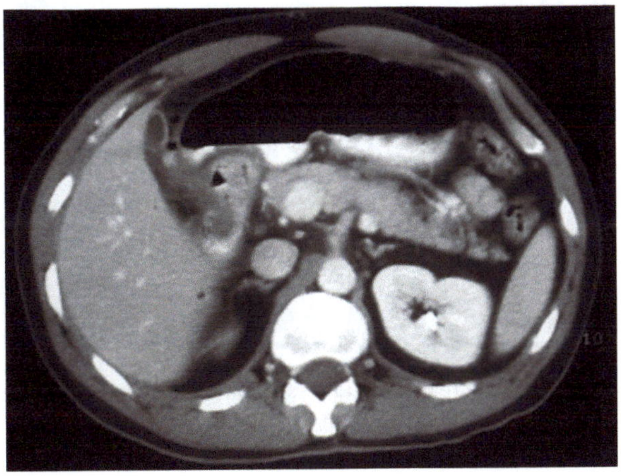

Fig. 9.7. Perforated duodenal ulcer. CECT shows free air bubble and a small extraluminal air-fluid level of the orally ingested contrast together with irregular mural thickening of the proximal duodenum due to a perforated duodenal ulcer

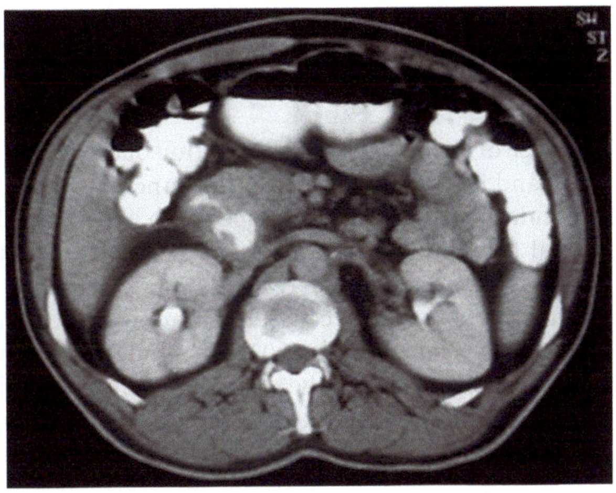

Fig. 9.9. Penetrating duodenal ulcer. CECT shows a round collection of the orally ingested contrast medium protruding from the posterior wall of the descending portion of the thickened-wall duodenum and associated thickening of the right Gerota's fascia

as a localized pocket filled with the oral contrast medium, which usually projects from the posterior aspect of the post-bulbar part of the duodenum. The surrounding inflammatory changes differentiate from a diverticulum (Fig. 9.9) (Fultz et al. 1991). Chronic duodenal ulceration may be complicated by a fistula to the biliary tree, mainly to the adjacent common bile duct.

9.5.2 Crohn's Disease

Crohn's disease, generally a chronic ileocolonic inflammatory disease, may affect the entire GIT. Aphthous ulcers in the upper GIT mucosa may be detected in 20%–40% of patients with established disease in the ileum and/or colon, but imaging evidence of Crohn's disease in the duodenum is found in about 4% (Wagtmans et al. 1997; Darrah and Nolan 1999). CT features range from nonspecific thickening of the valvulae conniventes to a tubular stricture with associated mesenteric lymphadenopathy in more advanced disease, similar to the findings seen in the distal ileum, which is nearly always concomitantly affected (Fig. 9.10).

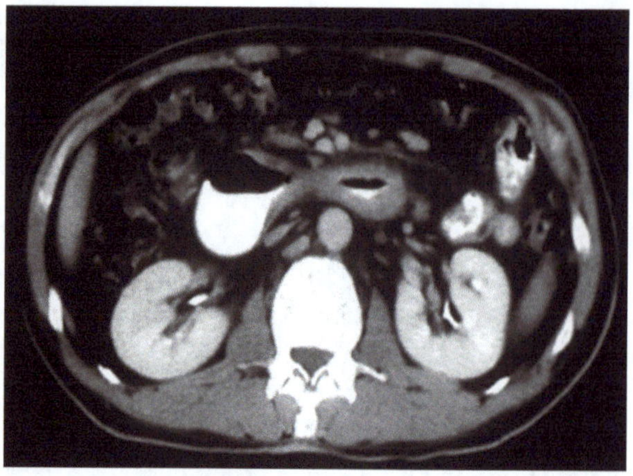

Fig. 9.10. Crohn's disease. CECT shows mural thickening of the horizontal portion of the duodenum with tubular stricture, causing prestenotic duodenal dilatation. Note the slightly enlarged mesenteric nodes

9.5.3 Extrinsic Inflammatory Diseases Affecting the Duodenum

Because of the retroperitoneal location of the duodenum and its close proximity to the pancreatic head, secondary inflammatory changes with oedema and mural thickening of the duodenal loop may result from adjacent acute pancreatitis (Fig. 9.11). Severe pancreatitis can also cause intramural duodenal hematoma (Abbas et al. 2002), and indeed in this situation thickening of the duodenal wall may lead to symptoms of bowel obstruction. Pancreatic pseudocyst following acute pancreatitis may also cause obstructive symptoms (Fig. 9.12) (Jayaraman et al. 2001; Zissin et al. 2002).

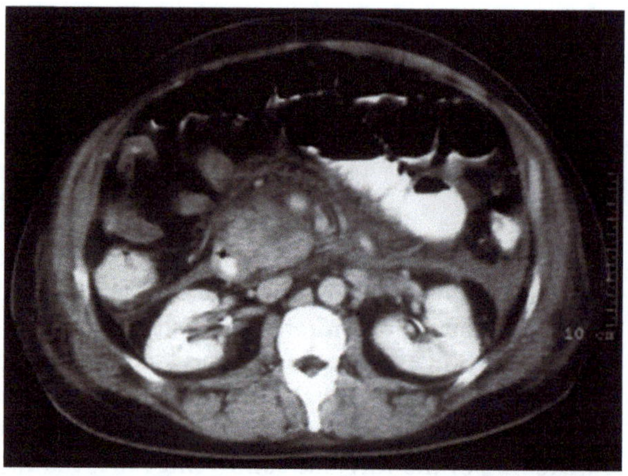

Fig. 9.11. Duodenal edema and acute necrotizing pancreatitis. CECT shows enlarged, nonhomogeneous pancreatic head with thickening of both Gerota's fascias and associated peripancreatic fat strandings

Gallbladder inflammation is another frequent cause of reactive changes on the lateral aspect of the duodenal loop with secondary mural thickening seen in acute severe cholecystitis (Fig. 9.13). Chronic cholecystitis may rarely cause a cholecystoduodenal fistula, in which a gallstone erodes through the chronically inflamed gallbladder wall into the adjacent duodenum. The CT findings of gas-fluid level within the gallbladder abutting a thickened duodenal wall and an air-filled fistulous tract are suggestive of a cholecystoduodenal fistula (Figs. 9.14a,b,

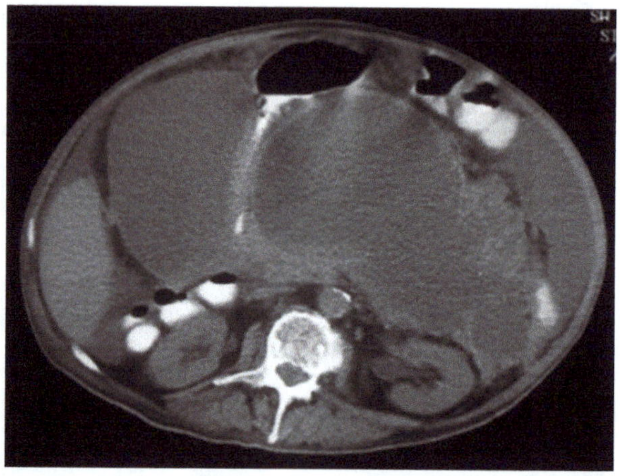

Fig. 9.12. Pancreatic pseudocysts compress the descending portion of the duodenum on both sides

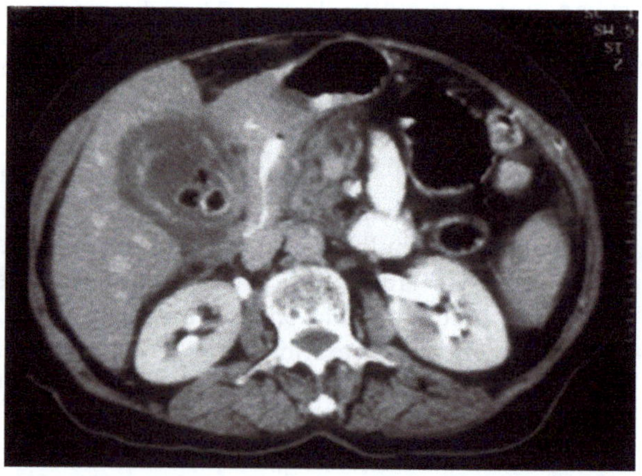

Fig. 9.13. Acute cholecystitis. CECT shows a distended gallbladder with gas-containing gallstones and marked mural thickening with interrupted mucosa compatible with acute, necrotizing cholecystitis. Note the reactive thickening of the adjacent duodenal wall. (Reprinted with permission from Zissin et al. 2003)

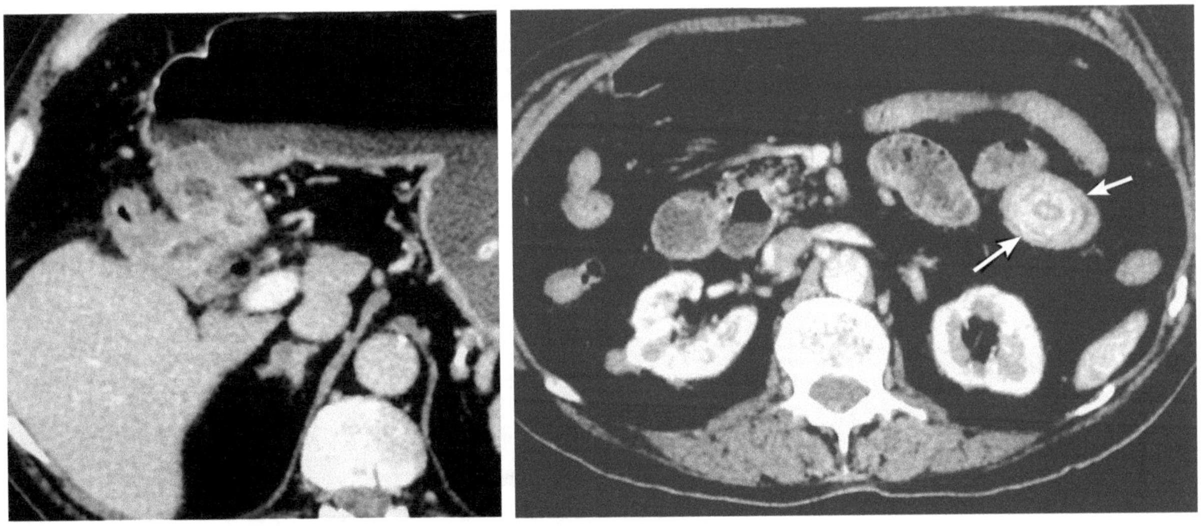

a b

Fig. 9.14a,b. Gallstone ileus. CECT showing (a) marked thickening of the wall of the proximal duodenum due to inflammatory change following passage of a gallstone. Note the thick walled gallbladder containing a fleck of air. (b) gallstone demonstrated in the proximal jejunum

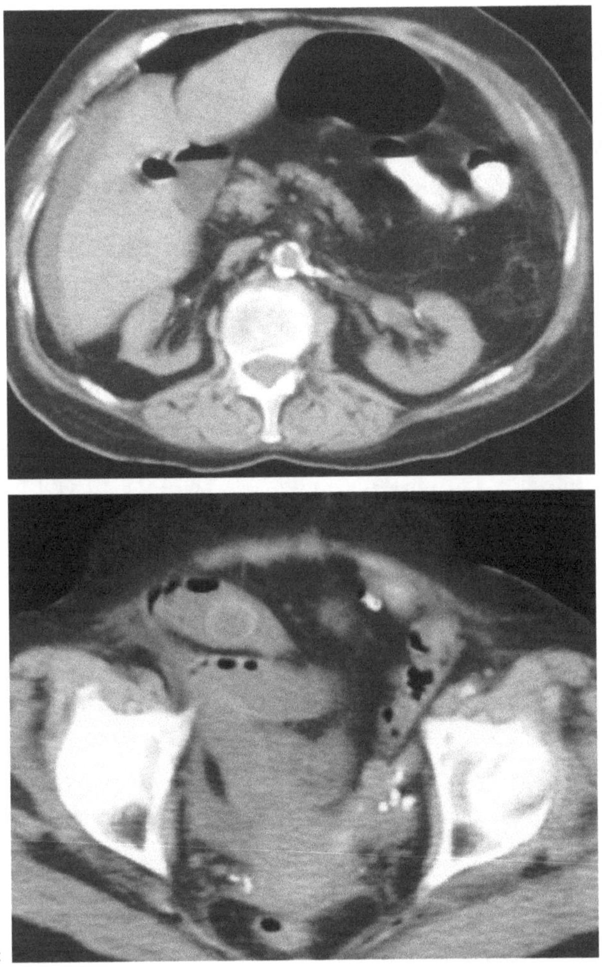

a c

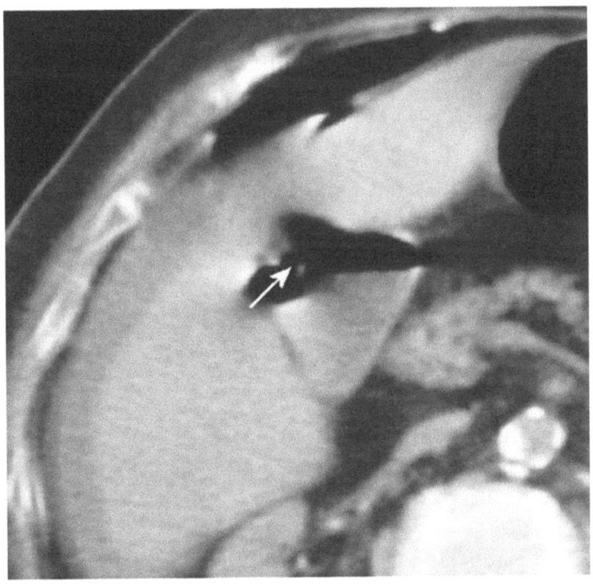

b

Fig. 9.15a–c. Gallstone ileus. CECT showing (a) an air filled gallbladder. Note the adjacent air filled duodenal cap and also evidence of a pneumoperitoneum. (b) An air-filled fistulous track between the gallbladder and duodenal cap (*arrow*) and (c) the gallstone in the distal ileum

9.15a–c). The complications of such a fistula are gallstone ileus, small bowel obstruction due to a gallstone migrating through the fistula distally into the bowel lumen (Jayaraman et al. 2001), and Bouveret's syndrome, gastric outlet obstruction caused by a large gallstone obstructing the duodenal bulb (Darrah and Nolan 1999).

9.6 Duodenal Neoplasms

9.6.1 Primary Duodenal Neoplasms

Duodenal tumours are rare. They account for about one-third of all small bowel neoplasms, which in turn represent approximately 5%–6% of all GIT neoplasms (Kazerooni et al. 1992). Benign tumours include adenoma, adenomatous polyp, lipoma, and leiomyoma. The latter is a benign gastrointestinal stromal tumor (GIST) of smooth-muscle type. A lipoma is the only tumour that can be diagnosed by certainty on CT as a well-circumscribed, homogeneous intraluminal mass with characteristic fat density, based on negative attenuation numbers (Fig. 9.16).

An intraluminal mass lacking associated mural thickening or evidence of extraduodenal disease is a useful criterion to predict its benignity (Fig. 9.17a), although small polypoid adenocarcinomas may occur (Kazerooni et al. 1992). Duodenal adenomatous polyps have been observed in 24%–33% of

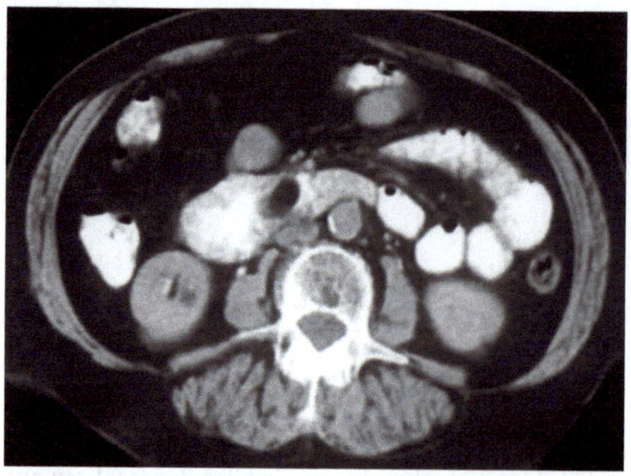

Fig. 9.16. Duodenal lipoma. An intraluminal filling defect with low attenuation values of fat density is seen within the horizontal part of the duodenum

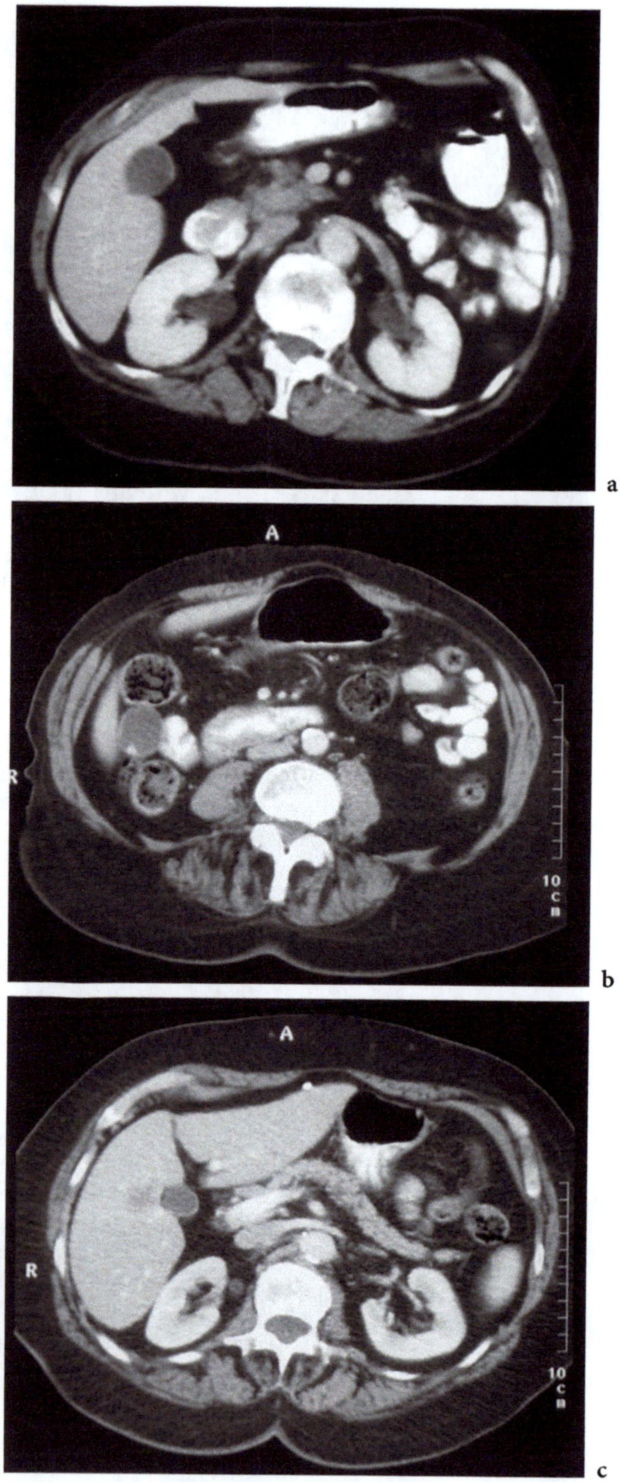

Fig. 9.17. a Intraluminal villous adenoma. CECT shows a soft-tissue polypoid mass with a small pedicle, arising from the medial aspect of the descending duodenum, with no mural thickening or extraduodenal disease. b Malignant villous tumor of the duodenum. Note the extensive carpet-like lesion involving most of the inferior duodenal flexure as well as the liver metastasis (c)

patients with Gardner's syndrome, mainly in the periampullary region. An adenoma-carcinoma sequence of these lesions has been observed, and periampullary carcinomas have been reported in 4%–12% of these patients (Williams and Peller 1994). Villous adenomas also occur in the duodenum, and around one-third are likely to be malignant (Fig. 9.17b,c) (Pezet et al. 1995)

Primary malignant tumors include mainly adenocarcinoma, leiomyosarcoma, and lymphoma (Kazerooni et al. 1992; Hwang et al. 1998; Darrah and Nolan 1999; Zissin et al. 2002). Primary adenocarcinoma of the duodenum comprises about 80%–90% of all primary malignant duodenal neoplasms. They are usually found in the periampullary region as either a polypoid mass or as an irregular, annular constricting lesion with mural thickening (>1 cm thickness) causing deformity of the lumen (Fig. 9.18). Associated CT findings of extraduodenal involvement, such as invasion of the retroperitoneal fat planes or surrounding organs, lymphadenopathy, vascular encasement, and distant metastases help in predicting the malignancy of a tumour and its resectability (Kazerooni et al. 1992).

Duodenal leiomyosarcoma, a subtype of GISTs composed of malignant smooth-muscle elements, account for about 10% of all duodenal malignancies. Similar to GISTs in other segments of the GIT, these tumours typically have a large extraluminal component usually with tumour necrosis, ulceration, or haemorrhagic changes (Fig. 9.19). The tumour is usually greater than 5 cm, and metastatic spread may be seen at the time of diagnosis. A leiomyoma may, however, have the same morphological features of a marked exophytic mass with necrosis and ulceration. Only the presence of extraduodenal involvement is highly accurate in predicting malignancy (Kazerooni et al. 1992).

Most duodenal lymphomas result from contiguous spread of gastric non-Hodgkin's lymphoma, while primary duodenal lymphoma is rare. CT findings include asymmetric mural thickening that seldom causes obstruction or a large polypoid mass with necrosis or cavitation, similar to leiomyosarcoma (Figs. 9.20, 9.21). Aneurysmal dilatation of the affected segment is a diagnostic clue, as well as visceral or retroperitoneal lymphadenopathy and splenomegaly.

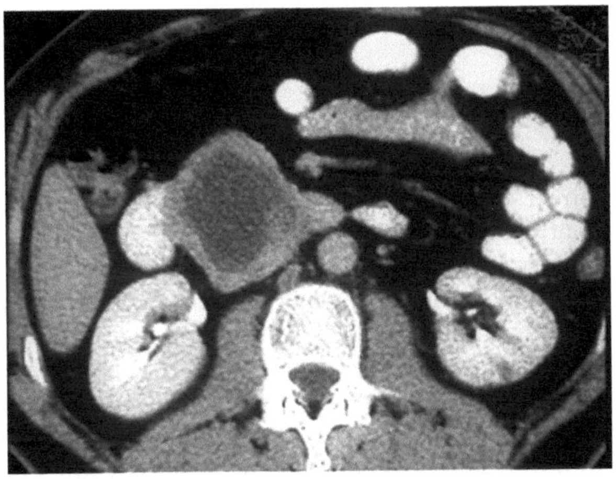

Fig. 9.19. Duodenal leiomyosarcoma. CECT shows a low-attenuation mass arising from the horizontal portion of the duodenal loop

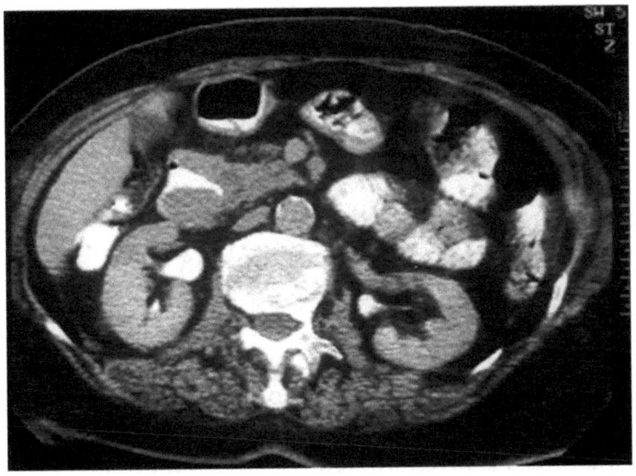

Fig. 9.18. Duodenal adenocarcinoma. Circumferential thickening of the descending duodenal wall causing irregular luminal narrowing

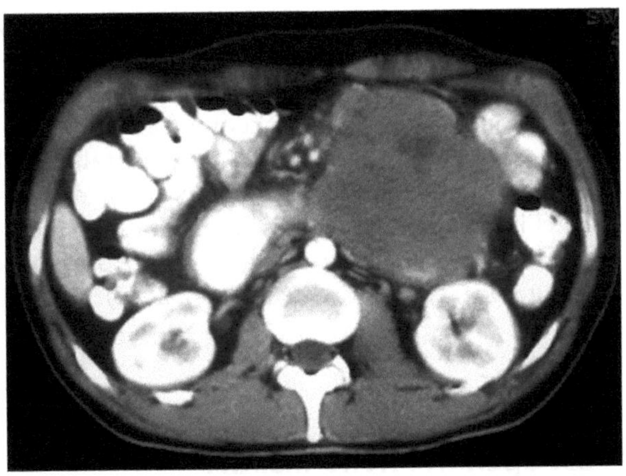

Fig. 9.20. Lymphoma. CECT shows a large extramural mass in the distal horizontal duodenum causing luminal narrowing and proximal dilatation

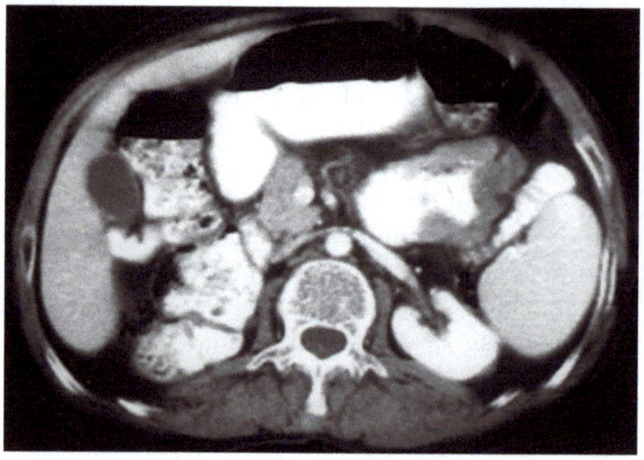

Fig. 9.21. Lymphoma. Irregular mural thickening at the level of the ligament of Treitz with an associated irregular central ulcer. (Reprinted with permission from Zissin et al. 2002)

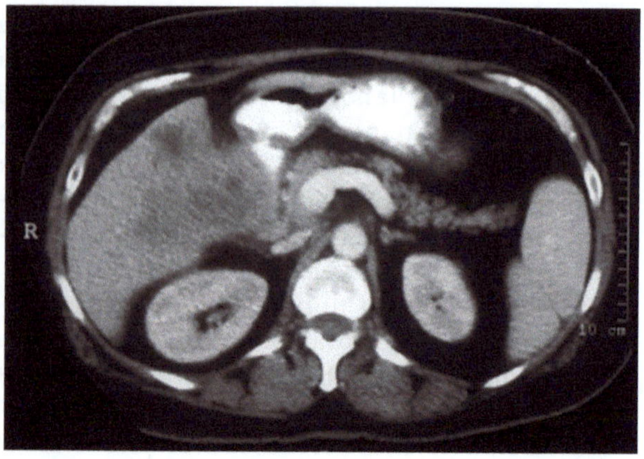

Fig. 9.22. Direct extension of a gallbladder tumour. A large inhomogeneous mass replaces the gallbladder, directly involving the liver and lateral portion of the proximal duodenum

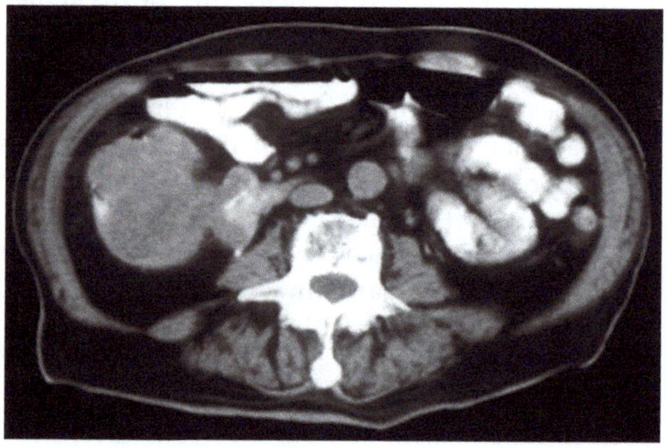

Fig. 9.23. Local involvement by a right colonic tumour. CECT shows a large tumor of the ascending colon directly invading the descending part of the duodenum

9.6.2 Metastases

Direct extension from primary neoplasms from contiguous organs is the commonest route of secondary involvement of the duodenum. Pancreatic, gallbladder (Fig. 9.22), and right renal tumours may directly invade the medial or lateral aspect of the duodenal wall, while gastric tumours may spread into the duodenum across the pylorus. Tumours of the right colon may spread through the mesocolon, which extends between the hepatic flexure and the descending duodenum (Fig. 9.23), or via lymphatic drainage to the mesenteric nodes surrounding the duodenum. Enlarged periduodenal lymph nodes from lymphoma or metastatic lung and breast cancer can encase the duodenum as well.

Hematogenous spread from various primary tumours, mainly malignant melanoma, bronchogenic and breast carcinoma, may metastasize to the duodenum or diffuse wall thickening (see Fig. 6.1.24). A metastasis may be seen on CT as an intraluminal soft tissue mass. Larger metastases often demonstrate intratumoral necrosis or cavitation, indistinguishable from lymphoma or leiomyosarcoma (Jayaraman et al. 2001; Zissin et al. 2002).

9.7 Post-operative Abnormalities

Afferent loop syndrome (ALS), caused by obstruction of the duodenum and jejunum proximal to a gastrojejunal anastomosis, is an uncommon complication after Billroth II subtotal gastrectomy. It occurs in approximately 0.3% of patients (Wise 2000; Gayer et al. 2002), and may rarely occur following gastrectomy with Roux-en-Y procedure (Wada et al. 2000). Most cases of ALS are due to mechanical obstruction of the afferent loop by internal hernia, adhesions, kinking at the anastomosis, and anastomotic stenosis by inflammatory or malignant changes (Gale et al. 1982; Gayer et al. 2002). The obstructive symptoms may occur acutely within days after surgery or may become manifest as a chronic syndrome, years later. The clinical diagnosis is often difficult, as the symptoms of this syndrome are nonspecific, including postprandial fullness, intermittent epigastric or right upper quadrant pain relieved by bilious vomiting, and rarely obstructive biliary disease. The appearance of ALS on CT is quite characteristic. Normally, an uncomplicated afferent loop appears as a tubular structure, sometimes with recognizable mucosal folds, in the anatomic location of the duodenum with surgical metallic sutures seen at its over-sewn end. It usually contains a small amount of air bubbles and fluid (Fig. 9.24a,b), and it may be on occasion be opacified with oral contrast medium. In ALS, the dilated afferent loop is seen on CT in the anatomic location of the horizontal part of the duodenum, between the aorta and the superior mesenteric vessels, displacing the latter anteriorly. It appears as a U-shaped fluid-filled tubular structure, non-opacified with oral contrast medium, with an approximately equal diameter of 4–8 cm throughout (Gayer et al. 2002). A few stretched valvulae conniventes are usually seen within it (Fig. 9.25a,b), as well as dilatation of the biliary system due to back pressure from the obstructed afferent loop.

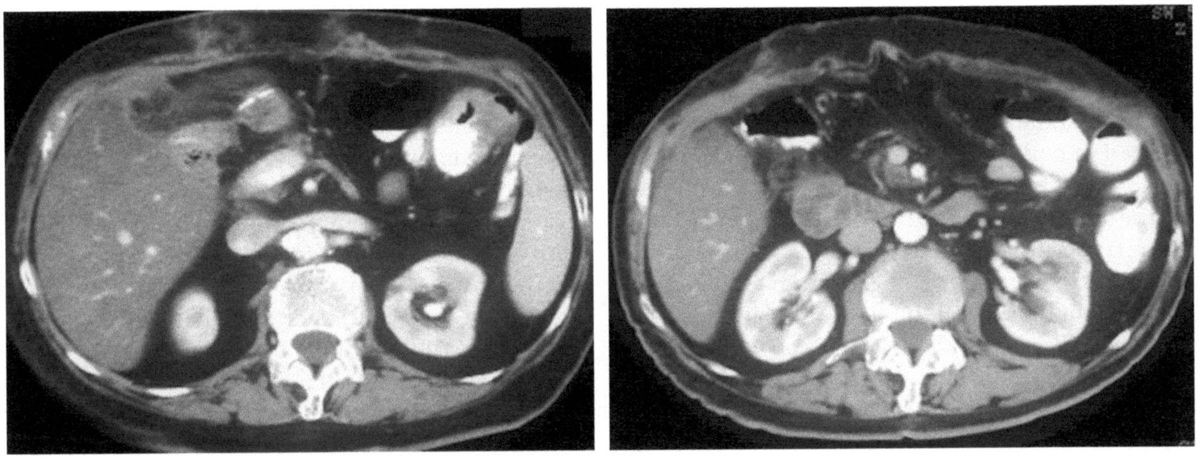

a b

Fig. 9.24a,b. A normal afferent loop following a Billroth II gastrojejunostomy anastomosis. **a** The duodenal stump, which is the blind end of the collapsed afferent loop, is noted in the right subhepatic space, closed off with metallic surgical clips. **b** An image obtained 2 cm caudally shows recognizable mucosal folds in the region of the inferior duodenal flexure

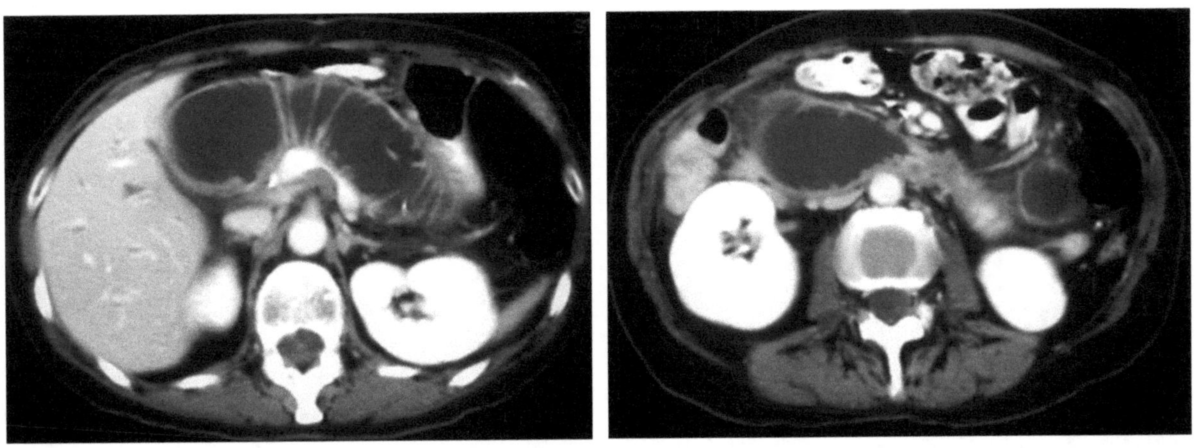

a b

Fig. 9.25a,b. Afferent loop syndrome. **a** CECT of the upper abdomen shows a markedly distended fluid-filled tubular structure with identifiable valvulae conniventes compatible with a dilated afferent loop. Note the dilated intrahepatic bile ducts. **b** A more caudal image demonstrates that the dilated afferent loop is obstructed by a recurrent tumoral mass at the level of the horizontal part of the duodenum

9.8 Duodenal Trauma

9.8.1 Blunt Duodenal Trauma

Blunt duodenal injury occurs rarely, with a reported rate of 0.2% in a retrospective study of 22,163 blunt trauma patients (Allen et al. 1998), and results in either perforation of the duodenum or an intramural hematoma. Typical causes include seat belt injuries and kicks from a horse. Blunt duodenal injury may be isolated or associated with pancreatic or spinal injuries (i.e. Chance flexion/destruction fracture of L1/ L2) (Degiannis and Boffard 2000). On CT, thickening of the duodenal wall with luminal narrowing and the presence of periduodenal fluid in the anterior right pararenal space may be seen in both types of duodenal injury. Only the presence of free gas and/or oral contrast medium in the right anterior pararenal space, adjacent to the retroperitoneal duodenum, are specific signs of perforation (Kunin et al. 1993). Increased attenuation within the wall of the thickened duodenum in an unenhanced CT examination is characteristic of an acute intramural hemorrhage (Fig. 9.26) (Katz et al. 1999). High attenuation is seen during the first two weeks and gradually decreases due to clot lysis (Abbas et al. 2002).

9.8.2 Penetrating Duodenal Trauma

Penetrating duodenal injury occurs in areas with a high incidence of civilian violence. Due to the anatomic location of the duodenum and the close relation to adjacent vital viscera and vascular structures, isolated penetrating duodenal trauma is rare and is often diagnosed during exploratory laparotomy performed for the evaluation of associated injuries (Degiannis and Boffard 2000).

9.8.3 Iatrogenic Duodenal Trauma

Iatrogenic duodenal injuries are rare complications of endoscopy. Perforation rarely occurs during routine endoscopy but may result from incorrect mucosal biopsy. Duodenal perforation is much more likely to follow endoscopic retrograde cholangiopancreatography (ERCP) and sphincterotomy. The latter procedure involves a diathermy cut through the muscular sphincter of Oddi in a cranial direction. The line of the cut should ideally run in a twelve o'clock direction to the papilla, and retroperitoneal perforation is much more likely to occur if there is significant deviation from this approach. The reported incidence is 0.5%–2% (Zissin et al. 2000). On CT,

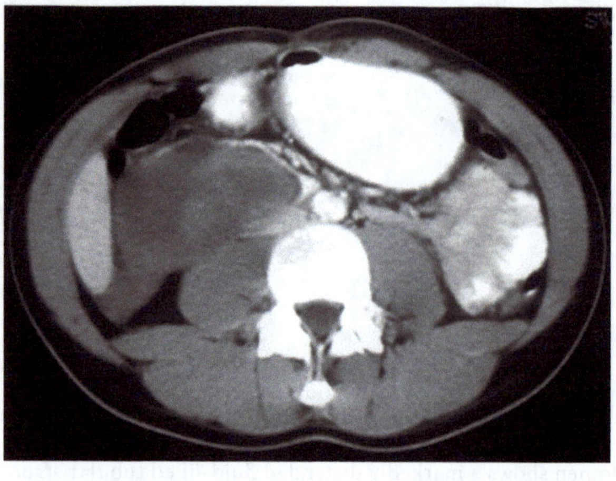

Fig. 9.26. Acute intramural duodenal hemorrhage with characteristic mixed attenuation is demonstrated. (Reprinted with permission from Zissin et al. 2002)

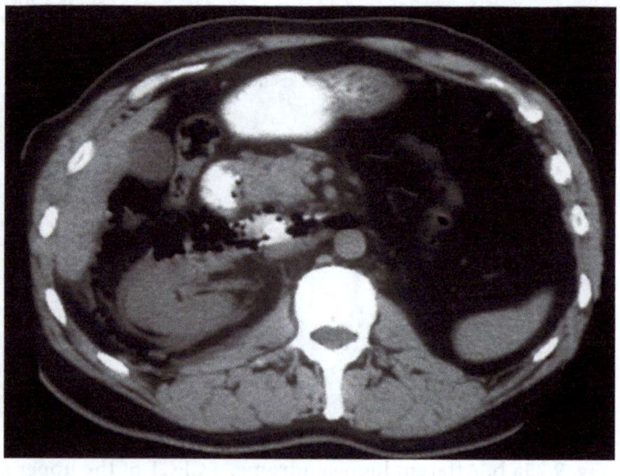

Fig. 9.27. A duodenal perforation following a diagnostic endoscopic US. CT scan shows retroperitoneal air bubbles and extravasation of the orally ingested contrast medium

dissection of air through anatomic retroperitoneal compartments is characteristic of a retroperitoneal perforation. Leakage of oral contrast medium is diagnostic of duodenal perforation (Fig. 9.27). Inadvertent duodenal perforation after laparoscopic cholecystectomy has also been rarely reported (Croce et al. 1999).

9.9 Miscellaneous

9.9.1 Spontaneous Haematoma

Spontaneous intramural hematoma was once considered rare; it is now seen more frequently, mainly in association with anticoagulant treatment and coagulopathies. Other rare causes of intramural duodenal hematoma include alcoholism, pancreatitis, duodenal ulcer, and iatrogenic complications following duodenal biopsy and endoscopic treatment of a bleeding duodenal ulcer (Lane et al. 1997; Abbas et al. 2002). The clinical presentation varies from vague abdominal complaints to partial duodenal obstruction with epigastric pain and vomiting. On CT, spontaneous intramural hematoma has an identical CT appearance as posttraumatic hemorrhage.

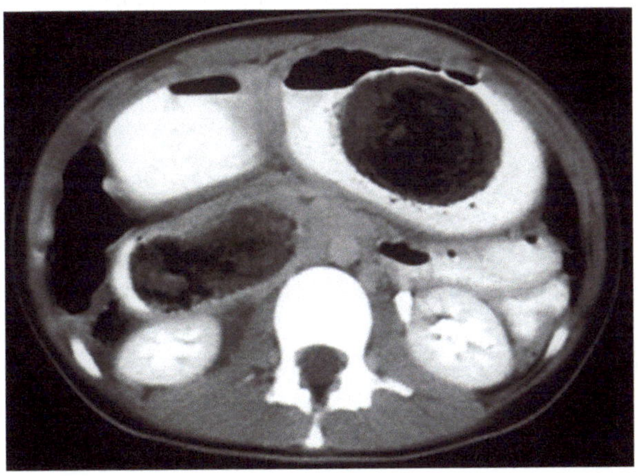

Fig. 9.28. Trichobezoar. A large intraluminal heterogeneous mass, with mottled gas is seen within the stomach, surrounded by the orally ingested contrast. A similar lesion is seen within the horizontal part of the duodenum, displacing its contrast-filled lumen. (Reprinted with permission from Zissin et al. 2002)

9.9.2 Bezoar

Bezoar is a concentration of ingested material within the GIT. Trichobezoars (a concentrated ingested ball of hair) and phytobezoars (a concentration of poorly digested fibres, fruit seeds and pulpy fruits) are the two most common bezoars. Trichobezoar occurs mainly in children and young women who masticate and swallow their hair. It usually fills the stomach and the first portion of the duodenum but may extend through a long segment of the small bowel and even reach the ileo-caecal valve. The clinical presentation includes epigastric discomfort or pain, symptoms of gastric outlet obstruction, weight loss and anemia, or an asymptomatic palpable epigastric mass. The CT appearance of a trichobezoar is characteristic of a large inhomogeneous intraluminal mass occupying nearly the entire intestinal lumen. The mottled gas pattern of entrapped air within the mass is a helpful diagnostic sign (Fig. 9.28) (Gayer et al. 1999).

References

Abbas MA, Collins JM, Olden KW (2002) Spontaneous intramural small-bowel hematoma: imaging findings and outcome. Am J Roentgenol 179:1389–1394

Allen GS, Moore FA, Cox CS Jr et al (1998) Delayed diagnosis of blunt duodenal injury: an avoidable complication. J Am Coll Surg 187:393–399

Berrocal T, Torres I, Gutierrez J et al (1999) Congenital anomalies of the upper gastrointestinal tract. Radiographics 19:855–872

Croce E, Golia M, Russo R et al (1999) Duodenal perforations after laparoscopic cholecystectomy. Surg Endosc 13:523–525

Darrah ERA and Nolan DJ (1999) Radiology of the duodenum. Hosp Med 60:10–18

Degiannis E, Boffard K (2000) Duodenal injuries. Br J Surg 87:1473–1479

Fidler JL, Saigh JA, Thompson JS et al (1998) Demonstration of intraluminal duodenal diverticulum by computed tomography. Abdom Imaging 23:38–39

Freeman AH (2001) CT and bowel disease. Br J Radiol 74:4–14

Fultz PJ, Skucas J, Weiss SL (1991) CT in upper gastrointestinal perforation secondary to peptic ulcer disease. Gastrointes Radiol 17:5–8

Gale ME, Gerzof SG, Kiser LC et al (1982) CT appearance of afferent loop obstruction. Am J Roentgenol 138:1085–1088

Gayer G, Apter S, Jonas T et al (1999) Polysplenia syndrome detected in adulthood: report of eight cases and review of the literature. Abdom Imaging 24:178–184

Gayer G, Jonas T, Apter S et al (1999) Bezoars in the stomach and small bowel - CT appearance. Clin Radiol 54:228–232
Gayer G, Barsuk D, Hertz M et al (2002) CT diagnosis of afferent loop syndrome. Clin Radiol 57:835–839
Gray H (1995) Gray's anatomy, 38th edn. Churchill Livingstone, New York
Hwang JI, Chiang JH, Yu C et al (1998) Pictorial review: Radiological diagnosis of duodenal abnormalities. Clin Radiol 53:323–332
Jayaraman MV, Mayo-Smith W, Movson JS et al (2001) CT of the duodenum: an overlooked segment gets its due. Radiographics 21:S147–S160
Katz DS, Lane MJ, Mindelzum RE (1999) Unenhanced CT of abdominal and pelvic hemorrhage. Semin Ultrasound CT MRI 20:94–107
Kazerooni EA, Quint LE, Francis IR (1992) Duodenal neoplasms: predictive value of CT for determining malignancy and tumor resectability. Am J Roentgenol 159:303–309
Kunin JR, Korobkin M, Ellis JH et al (1993) Duodenal injuries caused by blunt abdominal trauma: value of CT in differentiating perforation from hematoma. Am J Roentgenol 160:1221–1223
Lane MJ, Katz DS, Mindelzum RE et al (1997) Spontaneous intramural small bowel haemorrhage: Importance of non-contrast CT. Clin Radiol 52:378–380
Macpherson RI (1993) Gastrointestinal tract duplication: clinical, pathologic, etiologic and radiologic considerations. Radiographics 13:1063–1080
Oshimoa K, Suzuki N, Ikeda H et al (1998) Infected duodenal duplication with unusual clinical and radiological manifestations: a case report. Pediatr Radiol 28:518–520
Pezet D, Rotman N, Slim K, Bondet MJ, Chipponi J, Faigniez PL (1995) Villous tumours of the duodenum: a retrospective study of 47 cases by the French Associations for surgical research. J Am Coll Surg 180:541–544
Pickhardt PJ, Bhalla S (2002) Intestinal malrotation in adolescents and adults: spectrum of clinical and imaging features. Am J Roentgenol 179:1429–1435
Rao PM (1999) Case 11: perforated duodenal diverticulitis. Radiology 211:711–713
Rossi M, Broglia L, Graziano P et al (1999) Local invasion of gastric cancer: CT findings and pathologic correlation using 5-mm incremental scanning, hypotonia, and water filling. Am J Roentgenol 172:383–388
Stone EE, Brant WE, Smith GB (1989) Computed tomography of duodenal deverticula. J Comput Assist Tomogr 13:61–63
Stringer DA and Babyn PS (2000) Chapter 9 Small Bowel. In: Pediatric Gastrointestinal Imaging and Intervention. 2nd Edition BC Decker Inc Hamilton London
Tasu JP, Rocher L, Amouyal P et al (1999) Intraduodenal diverticulum: radiological and endoscopic ultrasonography findings of an unusual cause of acute pancreatitis. Eur Radiol 9:1898–1900
Tsuda Y, Nishimura K, Kawakami S et al (1991) Preduodenal portal vein and anomalous continuation of inferior vena cava: CT findings. J Comp Assist Tomogr 15:585–588
Wada N, Seki M, Saikawa Y et al (2000) Jejunal limb obstruction caused by a cholesterol stone 15 years after a total gastrectomy and 20 years after cholecystectomy: report of a case. Surg Today 30:181–184
Wagtmans MJ, van Hogezand RA, Griffioen G et al (1997) Crohn's disease of the upper gastrointestinal tract. Neth J Med 50:S2–S7
Williams SC, Peller PJ (1994) Gardner's syndrome. Case report and discussion of the manifestations of the disorder. Clin Nuc Med 19:668–670
Wise SW (2000) Case 24: afferent loop syndrome. Radiology 216:142–145
Zissin R, Rathaus V, Oscadchy A et al (1999) Intestinal malrotation as an incidental finding on CT in adults. Abdom Imaging 24:550–555
Zissin R, Shapiro-Feinberg M, Oscdachy A et al (2000) Imaging findings of retroperitoneal perforation during endoscopic sphincterotomy. Abdom Imaging 25:279–282
Zissin R, Osadchy A, Gayer G et al (2002) CT of duodenal pathology. Br J Radiol 75:78–84
Zissin R, Osadchy A, Shapiro-Feinberg M et al (2003) CT of a thickened-wall gallbladder. Br J Radiol 76:137–43

Radionuclide Imaging of the Stomach

10

Kottekkattu Balan

CONTENTS

10.1 Introduction

Radionuclide imaging, first introduced by Griffith et al. (1966), has been used to measure gastric emptying for more than 35 years. The method provides a simple, noninvasive means of quantifying gastric motor function and is presently considered the "gold standard" for this purpose. Recent years have witnessed a renewed interest in the use of gastric emptying scintigraphy, attributed mainly to pharmacotherapeutic advances in the management of gastric motility disorders.

Several nonradionuclide methods are available to evaluate gastric emptying, but they all have serious limitations. Intubation methods require frequent aspiration of gastric contents at various time intervals following the ingestion of known quantities of test meal. The tests are cumbersome for both the patient and investigator, and the complexity of the methods restrict their use. Furthermore, the indwelling tubes may affect the normal function of stomach. Radiological techniques using liquid barium sulphate have been used extensively to study gastric emptying. Similarly, meals impregnated with barium granules may be used to demonstrate an impaired emptying of solids. However, these methods are nonphysiological, nonquantitative, and may involve substantial radiation exposure to the patient. Other modalities such as ultrasound, CT, and MR (Maughan and Leiper 1996; Kunz et al. 1998) are also available to estimate gastric emptying, but they have not been accepted widely in clinical practice.

10.2 Physiology of Gastric Emptying

The stomach can be divided into two functional regions. The proximal stomach consists of the fundus and proximal one-third of the corpus. The distal stomach includes the remainder of the body, the antrum, and the pylorus. The proximal stomach acts as a reservoir that undergoes "receptive relaxation" (Jahnberg 1977) to receive food from the oesophagus, and this is followed by more sustained "adaptive relaxation" in response to gastric distension. Tonic contractions of the proximal stomach are responsible for maintaining the intragastric pressure and gastroduodenal pressure gradient, the emptying of liquids from the stomach being dependent on the latter. The proximal stomach does not, however, play any significant role in the gastric emptying of solids. The distal stomach, on the other hand, is responsible for the mixing and grinding of solids into a form and size (<2 mm) required for emptying (Meyer et al. 1979). The contractile activities of the distal stomach originate from the pacemaker, located in the upper body of the stomach on the greater curvature.

Neural mechanisms responsible for gastric motor function involve vagal and sympathetic fibres. In addition, small intestinal receptors for acid, carbohydrate, lipids, amino acids, and osmolality are

K. Balan, MD
Consultant Physikan in Nuclear Medicine, Department of Nuclear Medicine, Addenbrooke's Hospital, Box 170, Hills Road, Cambridge, CB2 2QQ, UK

known to exert feedback control on the rate of gastric emptying by releasing hormones such as gastrin, CCK, secretin, GIP, glucagon, VIP, and somatostatin.

10.3 Radiopharmaceutical Meals

A variety of radiolabelled meals are available to estimate gastric emptying, but no single meal is universally accepted. Solid, liquid, or semisolid meals may be labelled according to the indication for the test. Although simultaneous solid (^{99m}Tc-tin colloid in scrambled egg) and liquid (^{111}In-DTPA in water) emptying tests using the dual isotope technique (Heading et al. 1976) are available, to obtain maximum information from a single tracer, the radiolabelled meal should be a solid meal because of its greater sensitivity in detecting gastric motility disorders. As liquids are emptied faster than solids, it is important that elution of isotope from the solid meal is kept to a minimum by firm binding. This is accomplished by techniques such as cooking the meal with the label or by the addition of metal chelators (EDTA or DTPA). The radiopharmaceuticals used for gastric emptying must be nonabsorbable, as this will reduce the radiation dose outside the GI tract.

10.4 Factors Influencing Gastric Emptying

The composition of the test meal plays an important part in gastric emptying. Increasing the calorific content of the solid or liquid meals (Velchik et al. 1989) and their volume (Hunt and Spurrell 1951) slows down gastric emptying. Similarly, very hot or very cold meals (Sun et al. 1988), cigarette smoking, and alcohol consumption are known to delay emptying, whereas irritants such as chilli may hasten gastric motility. Standing and sitting are associated with faster emptying than the recumbent position.

10.5.1 Indications

Radionuclide gastric emptying can be used to evaluate patients presenting with symptoms of gastroparesis and diffuse gastrointestinal dysmotility. Gastric emptying scintigraphy is of particular clinical importance in the follow-up of patients who have undergone various surgical procedures for peptic ulcer and other GI abnormalities. Gastric emptying studies are also useful in quantifying the effect of medical and therapeutic interventions and have played a pivotal role in drug development in recent years.

10.5.2 Patient Preparation

The patient should fast overnight. The use of all drugs known to influence gastrointestinal motility should be discontinued for 24 hours. Patients should also refrain from smoking and consuming caffeine-containing drinks on the morning of the test.

10.5.3 Procedure

A large-field-of view gamma camera with a low-energy, all-purpose parallel-hole collimator connected to a digital computer system for data storage and analysis is used to acquire the data. For ^{99m}Tc, the photo-peak is set at 140 keV with a 20% window. Appropriate settings are required for dual-isotope studies and single-tracer studies using ^{111}In.

The patient is encouraged to ingest the test meal within 5 minutes to ensure data acquisition prior to any significant gastric emptying. The meal may be taken in a sitting or inclined position, but the imaging position, as with the meal, must be standardised for each department. In our department, patients remain in the erect position during acquisition, and 1-minute anterior and posterior images (64×64 pixel matrix in word mode) of the stomach are obtained every 20 minutes for 2 hours after completion of the meal (Fig. 10.1).

10.5.4 Data Processing

At the conclusion of the study, computer images are displayed and two regions of interest (ROI) are drawn on each image, one defining the stomach content and the other a background region. Total gastric counts are corrected for background and isotope decay. The geometric means of anterior and posterior (Tothill et al. 1978) views are then plot-

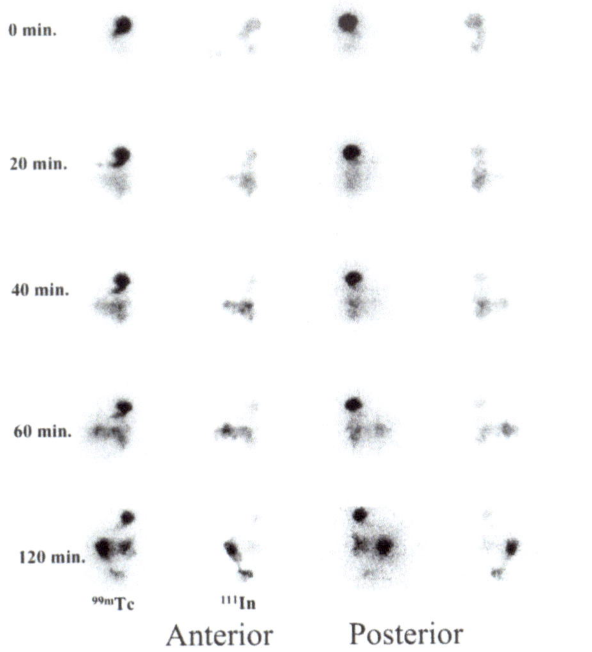

Fig. 10.1. Dual-isotope gastric emptying study using solid (^{99m}Tc-scrambled egg) and liquid (^{111}In-DTPA in water) meals. Images were acquired immediately, 20, 40, 60, and 120 minutes after meal ingestion

ted as percentage retention versus time. The activity retained or emptied (e.g. half-emptying time) at different time intervals is used to express the gastric emptying rate. For solids, another important parameter is the 'lag phase' (demonstrable only in continuous acquisition), which provides insight into antral function.

Visual inspection of sequential images provides important information about gastric activity in the time-lapse mode. This permits rapid estimation of the quality and rate of gastric emptying and also demonstrates changes in distribution of the meal within the stomach. Furthermore, information about oesophageal retention of activity or reflux and anatomical variations, especially following previous surgery, may add to the diagnostic yield.

10.6 Liquid Gastric Emptying

It is generally known that the emptying pattern of liquids (Fig. 10.2) is exponential (Hunt and Spurrell 1951), although there is some evidence (Hopkins 1966) suggesting that the pattern is more accurately described by relating the square root of the volume (the main determinant of the rate of liquid gastric emptying) remaining to time. Liquids of high nutrient density empty more slowly than liquids of low nutrient density.

10.7 Solid Gastric Emptying

The emptying of solid food is characterised by an early lag phase before the food enters the duodenum (Sheiner et al. 1980), followed by a linear pattern (Fig. 10.2). The emptying of a semi-solid food is generally intermediate between liquid and solid patterns, but may also depend on the volume and nutrient content of the meal.

10.8 Disorders of Gastric Emptying

The causes of abnormal gastric emptying can be divided into two main groups: conditions associated with delayed emptying, and conditions associated with rapid emptying (Table 10.1). As the symptoms of gastroparesis are nonspecific, mechanical causes of obstruction must be excluded in relevant cases.

In clinical practice, diabetes mellitus is probably the most common cause of delayed gastric emptying. Delayed emptying of both solids and liquids in this condition is attributed mainly to impaired neural

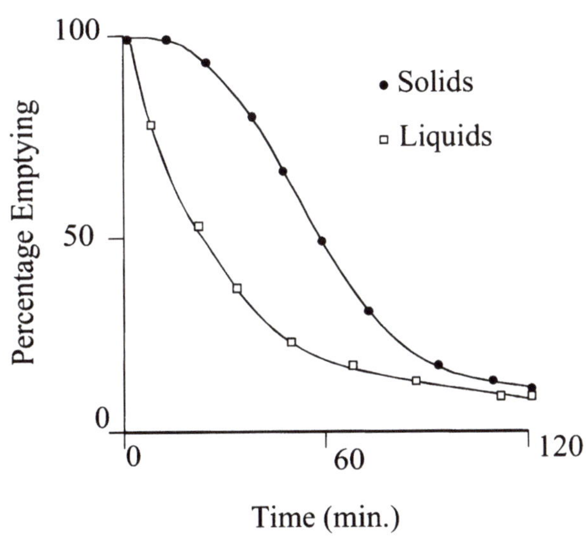

Fig. 10.2. Gastric emptying curves for solids and liquids in normal subjects

Table 10.1. Abnormal gastric emptying

Delayed	Rapid
Idiopathic	Idiopathic
Gastric outlet obstruction	Gastrectomy
Diabetic gastroparesis	Duodenal ulcer
Vagotomy	Zollinger-Ellison syndrome
Scleroderma	Thyrotoxicosis
Drugs (narcotic analgesics, anticholinergics, prokinetic drugs, antidepressants etc)	

control. Idiopathic gastroparesis has been described in patients, predominantly premenopausal women, who exhibit symptoms and signs of gastric stasis without any previously recognised causes of delayed gastric emptying. Gastroparesis is a frequent complication of gastric surgery. Vagotomy, antral resection, and Roux-en-Y gastrojejunostomy predispose patients to gastric stasis. Finally, a variety of pharmaceutical agents including narcotic analgesics, anticholinergics, L-dopa, tricyclic antidepressants, and somatostatin are known to retard gastric emptying.

Rapid gastric emptying is commonly associated with dumping syndrome resulting from vagotomies and various gastric outlet operations. Duodenal ulcer disease, Zollinger -Ellison syndrome, and thyrotoxicosis cause faster emptying. Gastric emptying has been found to be faster in patients with portal hypertension (Balan et al. 1996). Drugs such as erythromycin, metoclopramide, and domperidone have been used successfully to relieve symptoms of gastroparesis.

References

Balan KK, Grime S, Sutton R et al (1996) Abnormalities in gastric emptying in portal hypertension. Am J Gastroenterol 91:530–534

Griffith GH, Owen GM, Kirkman S et al (1966) Measurement of rate of gastric emptying using chromium-51. Lancet 1:1244–1245

Heading RC, Tothil P, McLoughlin GP et al (1976) Gastric emptying rate measurement in man. A double isotope scanning technique for simultaneous study of liquid and solid component of a meal. Gastroenterology 71:45–50

Hopkins A (1966) The pattern of gastric emptying: a new view of old results J Physiol 182:144–149

Hunt JN, Spurrell WR (1951) The pattern of emptying of the human stomach. J Physiol 113:157–168

Jahnberg T (1977) Gastric adaptive relaxation. Scand J Gastroenterol 12 [Suppl]:1–32

Kunz P, Crelier GR, Schwizer W et al (1998) Gastric emptying and motility: assessment with MR imaging-preliminary observations. Radiology 207:33–40

Maughan RJ, Leiper JB (1996) Methods for the assessment of gastric emptying in humans: an overview. Diabet Med 13:S6–S10

Meyer JH, Thomson JB, Cohen MB (1979) Sieving of solid food by the canine stomach and sieving after gastric surgery. Gastroenterology 76:804–813

Sheiner HJ, Quinlan MF, Thompson MF (1980) Gastric motility and emptying in normal and post-vagotomy subjects. Gut 21:753–759

Sun WM, Houghton LA, Read NW et al (1988) Effect of meal temperature on gastric emptying of liquids in man. Gut 29:302–305

Tothill P, McLoughlin GP, Heading RC (1978) Techniques and errors in scintigraphic measurements of gastric emptying. J Nucl Med 19:256–261

Velchik MG, Reynolds JC, Alavi A (1989) The effect of meal energy content on gastric emptying. J Nucl Med 30:1106–1110

Radiological Intervention in the Stomach and Duodenum

11

DERRICK F. MARTIN and HANS-ULRICH LAASCH

CONTENTS

D. F. MARTIN, FRCP, FRCR
Professor of GI-Radiology, Academic Dept. of GI-Radiology, South Manchester University Hospitals NHS Trust, Southmoor Road, Wythenshawe, Manchester M23 9LT, UK

H.-U. LAASCH, MD, MRCP, FRCR
Consultant Radiologist, Christie Hospital NHS Trust, Wilmslow Road, Manchester M20 4BX, UK

11.1 Introduction

Until recently interventional procedures for lesions of the gastro-oesophageal junction, the stomach and the duodenum have been the domain of the endoscopist. However, difficult or failed endoscopic cases are frequently referred for radiological management, which has led to a growing understanding amongst radiologists that such interventions can be performed as a primary procedure under fluoroscopy without the use of an endoscope. It is not the purpose of this chapter to promote fluoroscopically guided over endoscopic intervention. Instead we hope to give the reader an understanding of the full spectrum of treatment options in various benign and malignant conditions affecting the stomach from the gastro-oesophageal junction to the pylorus and duodenum.

Some therapeutic manoeuvres can clearly only be undertaken with endoscopic guidance. Polypectomy and endoscopic mucosal resection (EMR) of tumours of the oesophagus and stomach, papillectomy for tumours of the Papilla of Vater, photodynamic therapy (PDT) for the management of Barrett's oesophagus and oesophageal tumours do not have radiological equivalents and will not be considered. However, for the management of benign and malignant obstructive lesions, as well as for the provision of gastrostomy, appropriate endoscopic and non-endoscopic alternatives exist.

11.1.2 Patient Preparation

For all interventional procedures in the upper gastrointestinal tract patient preparation prior to the procedure is of considerable importance. Difficulties with consent may be encountered because of impaired ability on the patient's behalf to comprehend either the problem that requires treatment or the method of treatment itself. Gastrostomy insertion in particular presents significant ethical issues regarding the appropriate use of the procedure and it is crucial that the responsible radiologist is directly involved in discussions regarding the appropriateness of each case.

Whatever the interventional procedure, it is vital that the patient comes to the interventional room in the best possible state to reduce risk and ensure success. Care should be taken to ensure adequate hydration to maintain renal function, and anaemia and clotting abnormalities need to be corrected. As a guide the following values should be regarded as desirable: haemoglobin > 100 g/l, platelets > 50.000/µl, PT-ratio (international normalised ratio, INR) and APTT ratio ≤ 1.3.

Proper assessment of sedation risk, particularly in patients with neuro-muscular disorders (e.g. motor neurone disease) and large oro-pharyngeal tumours is essential as are adequate management of anxiety, pain or discomfort.

In some countries interventional procedures are performed routinely under general anaesthesia and the responsibility for the management and the monitoring of the patient lies with an anaesthetist. However, in most departments procedures are undertaken under conscious sedation administered by the radiologist. Guidelines exist to advise and assist radiologists in these circumstances and it is important that these are followed. Adequate monitoring and resuscitation facilities must be available. Only properly trained staff in sufficient numbers can ensure patients' safety before, during and after the procedure. UK guidelines recommend separation of the role of the sedationist from the role of the primary operator (RCR 2003). Increasingly this role is being taken on by interventional nurses, and the decision making process in drug delivery can be objectified by the use of EEG monitoring (Bell et al. 2004). Problems with sedation and analgesia contribute significantly to post procedural morbidity and will only be avoided by careful attention to detail.

11.2 Gastro-oesophageal Junction

11.2.1 Gastro-oesophageal Reflux Disease

Gastro-oesophageal reflux disease is an extremely common problem. Dyspeptic symptoms are one of the most frequent reasons patients consult their primary care physician. A trip to the local pharmacy to view the range of over-the-counter medications available for dyspepsia gives a clear measure of the problem. Indeed one recent review article described gastro-oesophageal reflux disease as being ubiquitous in the adult population of the United States (Cappell 2005). Complications of gastro-oesophageal reflux disease include Barrett's oesophagus, Barrett's ulcer, peptic stricture and adenocarcinoma of the gastro-oesophageal junction (Falk 2001; Sharma and Sidorenko 2005). With the falling incidence of squamous cell carcinoma of the oesophagus, adenocarcinoma is now the predominant tumour and its incidence in the Western world is still rising fast (DeMeester 2006). Both benign and malignant distal oesophageal lesions can present with increasing dysphagia to solid food with associated weight loss and endoscopy is mandatory for assessment and biopsy.

11.2.2 Benign Oesophageal Strictures

11.2.2.1 Peptic Strictures

Good evidence-based guidelines from the British Society of Gastroenterology (BSG) exist, summarising the approach to the patient with a benign distal oesophageal stricture requiring dilatation (Riley and Attwood 2004). A number of points from these endoscopic guidelines are relevant to the radiologist undertaking oesophageal dilatation. The use of fluoroscopy during endoscopic oesophageal dilatation is not advised as a routine, but recommended for tight, difficult or complex strictures where the endoscopic placement of a guidewire or through-the-scope (TTS) balloon is used. Complications mostly consist of perforation and are reported in 1%–2% with a mortality of 0.5% (NCEPOD 2004; Riley and Attwood 2004). The guidelines comment that there is little to choose between bougie and balloon dilation, controlled studies showing no clear benefit of one over the other.

The radiological method of benign stricture dilatation addresses two points of technique, which logically improve the safety and quality of the procedure although it must be said that evidence for this is lacking. Passing a catheter and guidewire through the stricture under fluoroscopic control invariably allows confirmation of correct guidewire position.

The inadvertent perforation of the stricture by the guidewire and the subsequent dilatation of the perforation can be entirely avoided with correct radiological technique, as it is always possible to demonstrate that the guidewire is properly placed with its distal end in the stomach. Secondly radiologists use balloons for dilatation of strictures and whilst there is no evidence that balloon dilatation is preferable to bougie dilatation in terms of outcome, the fact that with balloon dilatation only a 5-Fr balloon catheter need pass through the patient's pharynx rather than the full diameter of the solid bougie makes the procedure less uncomfortable for the patient and potentially requires less sedation.

Balloon dilatation only exerts radial force on the stricture. Pushing a rigid bougie through the stricture also contributes shearing forces, which intuitively would suggest a higher risk of rupture, but again there is no evidence for this at present.

11.2.2.1.1
Technique

Dilatation is performed after pharyngeal anaesthesia and under conscious sedation with the patient lying either in the left lateral position or preferably prone on the fluoroscopy table. A torque controlled angled catheter (e.g. Headhunter 1) is negotiated through the pharynx and the upper oesophageal sphincter into the lower oesophagus with the help of a 0.035-in. (0.89-mm) hydrophilic guidewire (Fig. 11.1). The level of the stricture can be determined by withdrawing the guidewire into the catheter during advancement. When the catheter meets the stricture, onward advancement is impeded. The wire is withdrawn, contrast medium is injected and the upper margin of the stricture marked by placement of radiopaque markers on the patient's skin (Fig. 11.2). Attaching markers to the patient's clothes should be avoided as they may be moved inadvertently during the procedure. The guidewire is reinserted and passed through the stricture followed by the catheter. At this point withdrawal of the guidewire and contrast injection allows delineation of the distal margin of the stricture, which is again indicated with skin markers. The hydrophilic guidewire is reinserted and the catheter and guidewire negotiated into the antrum of the stomach. The guidewire is withdrawn and replaced with a 0.035-in. stiff J-tipped 180-cm long guidewire. A 5-Fr, 60-cm long angiographic balloon catheter carrying a 4-cm long, 15- to 18-mm diameter balloon is passed over the guidewire and positioned with the mid-point of the balloon at the mid-point of the stricture. Inflation of the balloon with dilute contrast medium is then straightforward, but a dedicated inflation syringe with integrated manometer should be used routinely. This makes inflation easier, more controlled and avoids exceeding the burst pressure of the balloon.

The distal part of the balloon tends to inflate first, pushing the balloon forward. Slippage of the balloon

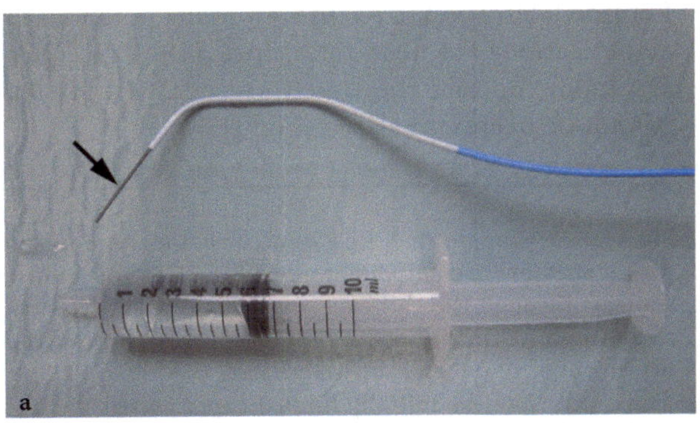

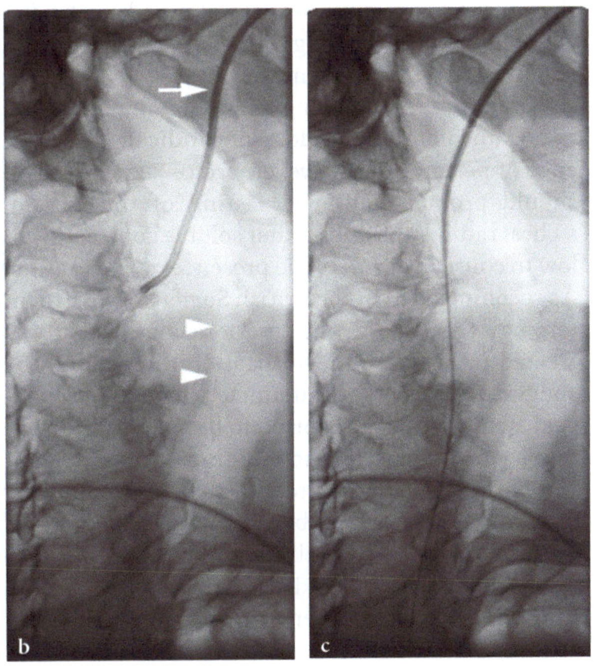

Fig. 11.1. **a** A 5-Fr Headhunter 1 catheter with hydrophilic wire (*arrow*). **b** Lateral view of the neck: the catheter (*arrow*) has been passed into the hypopharynx with help of the wire and is rotated to point posteriorly towards the upper oesophageal sphincter, avoiding the trachea anteriorly (*arrowheads*). **c** The wire is advanced into the oesophagus and followed with the catheter

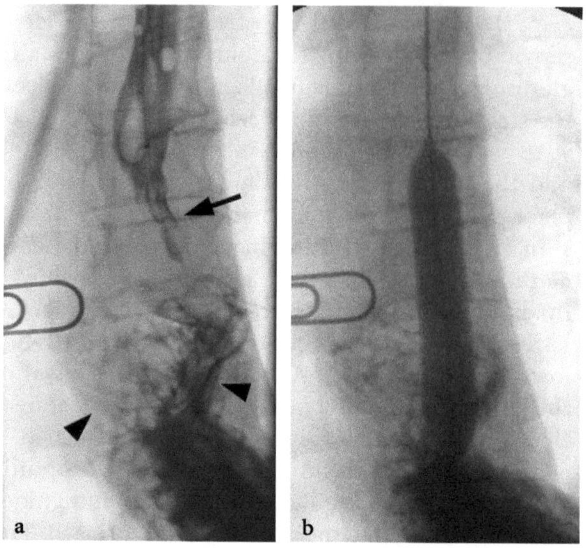

Fig. 11.2. a A short peptic stricture (*arrow*) is seen above an axial hiatus hernia (*arrowheads*). The level of the stricture is indicated by a paperclip on the patient's skin. b Successful dilatation with a 15-mm balloon

during dilatation can be controlled by partly inflating the balloon and then applying traction to the catheter to hold the balloon in position across the stricture whilst completing inflation. Radiological opinion is divided regarding the necessary duration of balloon dilatation but it seems unnecessary to continue to apply dilatation beyond the time when full dilatation and the disappearance of any waist on the balloon has been achieved. Once fully recovered the patient can be given sips of water and can be discharged when swallowing semi-solids without pain, usually later on in the same day.

Some chest pain during and following dilatation is not uncommon and does not indicate the presence of perforation. However, prolonged chest pain should prompt continued fasting of the patient, a chest radiograph and a water soluble contrast swallow to confirm or refute the presence of perforation. As recommended in the British Society of Gastroenterology (BSG) guidelines, perforation needs to be treated urgently and a surgical opinion should be sought. The use of large diameter covered oesophageal stents has been reported to be successful in the management of perforation (Siersema et al. 2003).

The BSG guidelines report that approximately 90% of patients treated by dilatation achieve relief of symptoms. Some require repeat dilatation procedures and patients should all be treated with proton pump inhibitors in order to reduce the risk of re-stenosis.

11.2.2.2 Other Benign Strictures

Strictures of other aetiology such as radiation or caustic ingestion can be treated in exactly the same way as described above. Complication rates are probably higher and success rates definitely lower.

11.2.2.3 Stents for Benign Strictures

There is a small but growing literature describing the effective use of removable stents in patients with refractory benign strictures. Some strictures are resistant to dilatation or recur very quickly so that frequent procedures are necessary. In these patients it is often tempting to place a metal oesophageal stent but the use of permanent stents almost invariably leads to long-term complications, such as erosion of the oesophagus, bleeding and further stricture formation (Song et al. 1997; Wadhwa et al. 2003). The arrival of removable stents has allowed their temporary short term use (4–8 weeks) (Evrard et al. 2004). Theoretically gentle dilatation by a slowly expanding stent, which is subsequently maintained whilst the trauma from the dilatation resolves, may allow a longer symptom free period after stent removal. Some promising results even in patients with caustic strictures have been reported. Most stents require endoscopic removal, although the first system for radiological removal has been launched in 2005 (TaeWoong Medical, Seoul, Korea; Pyramed, Surbiton, UK). In view of the potential for complications the need for a close, multi-disciplinary follow-up and the timely removal of the stent cannot be overemphasised (Fig. 11.3).

Fig. 11.3. a Complicated treatment of a therapy-resistant peptic stricture (same patient as in Fig. 11.2): injection of contrast through the catheter (*arrow*) shows the recurrent stricture above the sliding hernia (*arrowheads*). b Successful placement of a Boubella anti-reflux stent (UK Medical, Sheffield, UK). Note the initially limited expansion at the level of the stricture. c–e Planned removal after 6 weeks: Treatment had been so successful that – unbeknown to patient – the stent had migrated into the stomach. The patient was eating a normal diet. Endoscopic removal using a pair of forceps (*arrow*) was uneventful. Note the hiatus hernia outlined by air (*arrowheads*). f–h On extraction it was noticed that the stent had ruptured. The lowermost segment (*arrow*) had migrated into the sigmoid colon and impacted in an area of diverticular disease. Due to symptoms of subacute obstruction the basket had to be removed endoscopically. The patient remains asymptomatic 2 years later

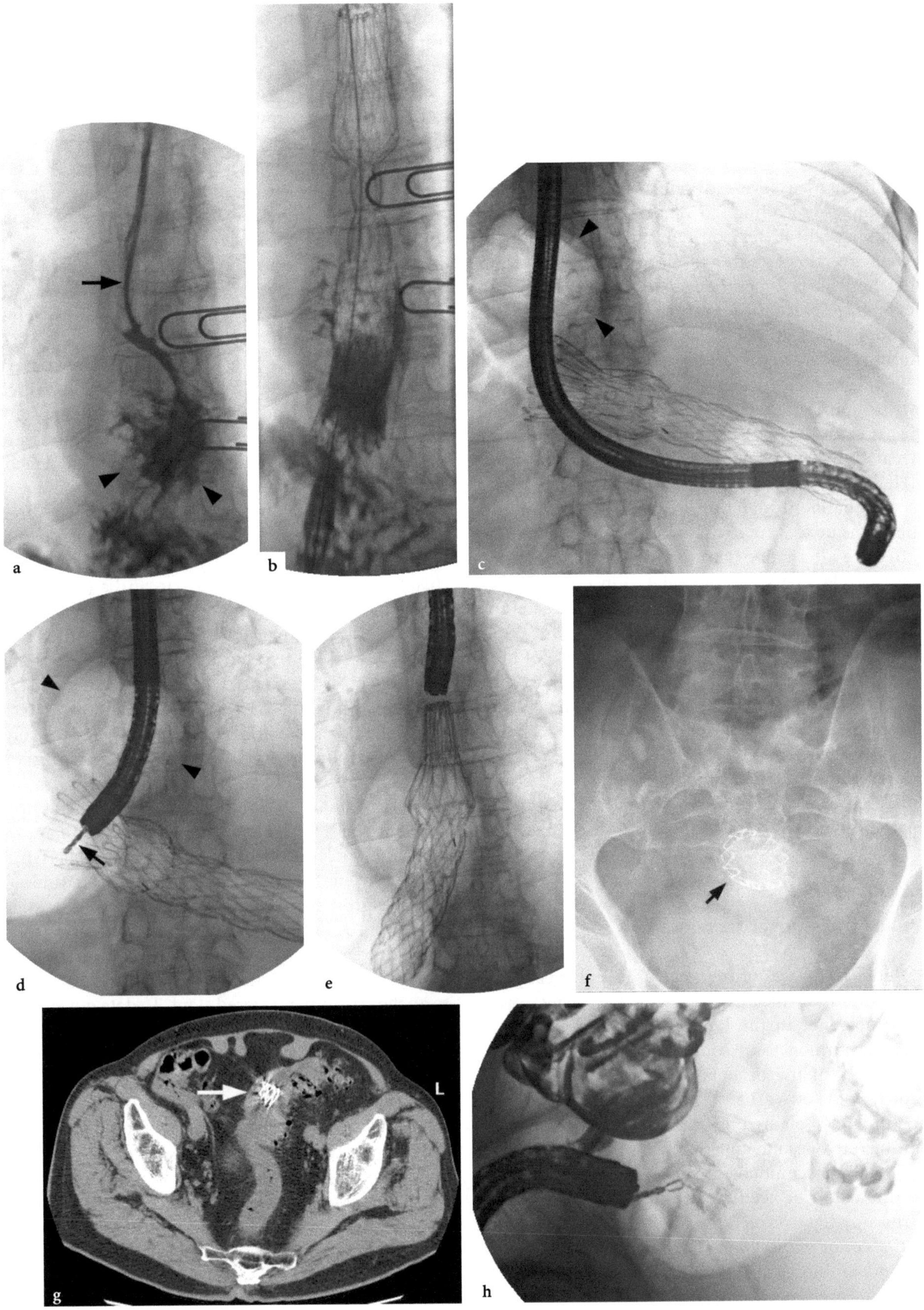
a
b
c
d
e
f
L
g
h

Bio-degradable stents may provide an interesting alternative in the future.

11.2.3 Achalasia

Achalasia is a severe dysmotility disorder of the oesophagus leading to chest pain, dysphagia, oesophageal distension, mega-oesophagus and even overflow with aspiration. The underlying mechanism is a neurodegenerative process of the myenteric plexus leading to a failure of the lower oesophageal sphincter to relax. However the precipitating causes are still under debate (Park and Vaezi 2005). The incidence of achalasia increases with age with significant variation across different countries (Mayberry 2001). In the past achalasia has been treated by surgical distal oesophageal myotomy (Heller's procedure) (Gockel et al. 2004). Endoscopic balloon dilatation of the oesophagus using balloons up to 3 cm in diameter is reported to be an effective alternative (Chan et al. 2004; Dobrucali et al. 2004). This balloon dilatation can of course be undertaken without an endoscope in the manner described above.

There is a growing literature on the use of botulinum toxin injections for the management of achalasia (Mikaeli et al. 2004) and clearly this needs to be administered under endoscopic control. There is some evidence that balloon dilatation together with Botox improves the symptom free period between procedures. Surgery nowadays should be reserved for patients with failed dilatation or injection therapy.

11.2.4 Junctional Adenocarcinoma

Adenocarcinoma at the gastro-oesophageal junction is one of the tumours with the fastest growing incidence in the Western world and it is now more common than squamous cell carcinoma of the body of the oesophagus (Botterweck et al. 2000; Bollschweiler et al. 2001). The increase has mainly been blamed upon the increasing incidence of Barrett's oesophagus (Marsman et al. 2005).

Staging techniques using CT, endoscopic ultrasound with fine needle aspiration cytology and laparoscopy have refined the identification of patients suitable for surgery but the 5-year survival rate for adenocarcinoma still remains less than 20%. Many patients present with inoperable disease and whilst a course of chemotherapy may downstage the tumour rendering it operable, palliative treatment is often the only option.

For the purpose of palliation many endoscopic techniques have come and gone over the last 20 years. Endoscopic placement of Atkinson tubes with the Nottingham introducer replaced the surgical insertion of Celestin and similar tubes. Subsequently endoscopic laser therapy had its day but most other endoscopic therapies have now declined in use in the face of self-expanding oesophageal stents. The role of brachytherapy for palliation of patients with a better long-term prognosis is currently being debated (Homs et al. 2004a).

Over the last decade oesophageal stents have developed from being simple uncovered tubes, which are open at either end, into an array of different stent designs each with its own advantages and weaknesses. At this point in the development of stent technology the benchmark stent for the management of a distal oesophageal tumour is a removable covered stent with an anti-reflux valve and which is flexible enough to align comfortably along the curve of the distal oesophagus and the gastric cardia (Fig. 11.4f). Valved stents certainly make a difference to the frequency of symptomatic reflux after stenting and should always be used in preference to open stents (Kocher et al. 1998; Lee et al. 2005; Shim et al. 2005), although this is still disputed by some authors (Homs et al. 2004b). The benefit extends well beyond the control of heartburn to the prevention of frank regurgitation of gastric content and potentially fatal aspiration (Laasch et al. 2002; Homs et al. 2004b). A membrane covering the stent skeleton, usually made from polyurethane, polyethylene or increasingly polytetrafluoroethylene (PTFE) reduces the risk of tumour through-growth but carries an increased risk of stent migration. A number of anti-migration designs are being developed ranging from barbs, bulges and collars to double stents with an outer uncovered portion to anchor the inner covered stent. To date not enough evidence is available to prove one design to be superior and as yet we do not have the perfect stent for the palliation of distal oesophageal tumours.

The fact that some oesophageal stents are now removable both with and without endoscopy has brought certain advantages to practice. A stent which has displaced proximally above a tumour can be easily removed prior to the placement of a further stent. Stents which displace distally into the stomach, either spontaneously or after a period of chemo- and/or radiotherapy can usually be pulled back into position endoscopically or completely removed. In the

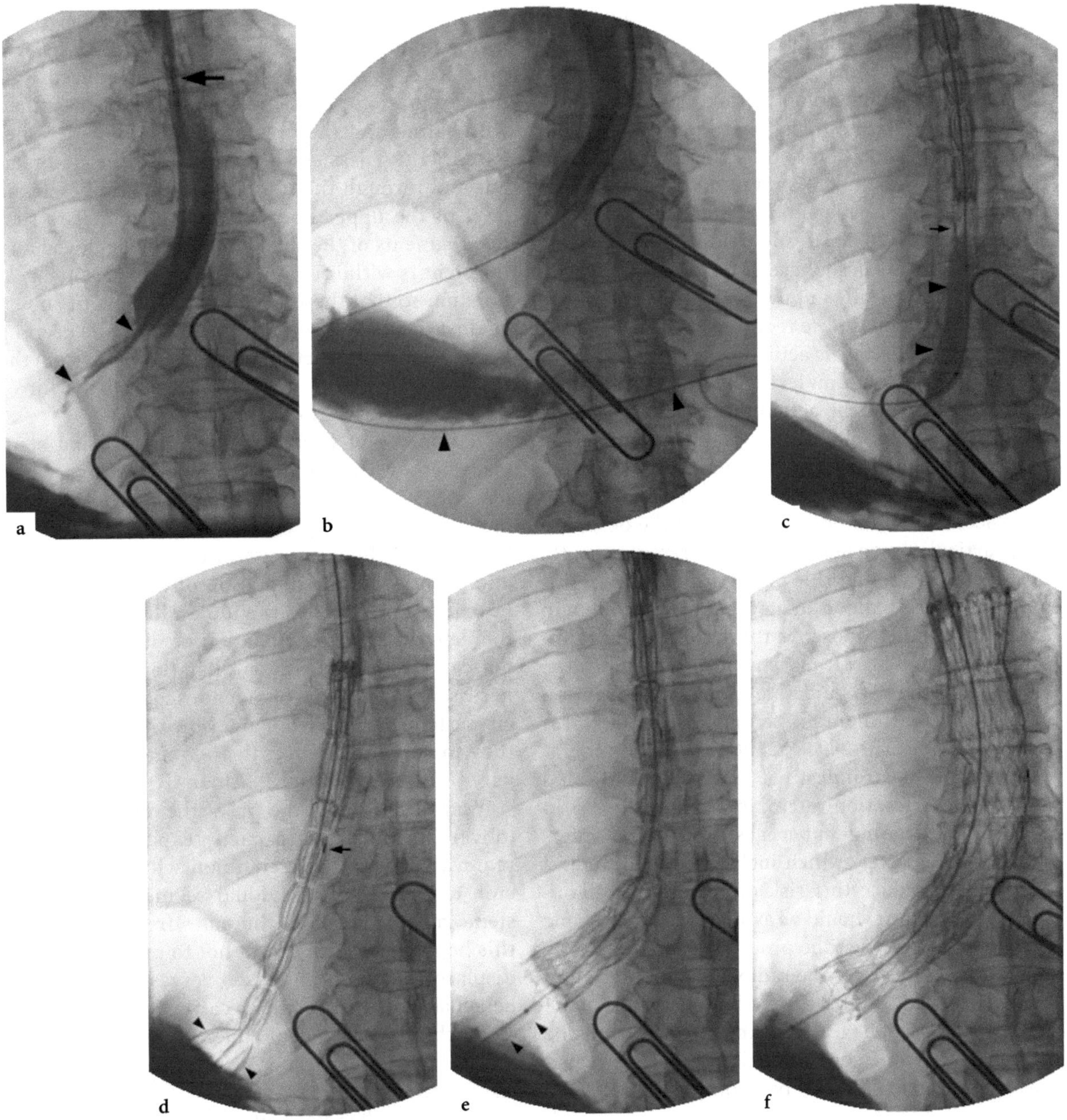

Fig. 11.4. a Oesophageal adenocarcinoma: Injection of contrast through the catheter (*arrow*) shows the typical distal oesophageal stricture (*arrowheads*). The extent is indicated by paperclips on the patient's skin. **b** A stiff wire has been inserted deep into the stomach (arrowheads) and the catheter is removed. **c** A Boubella anti-reflux stent with a balloon tip inflated with contrast (*arrowheads*) is inserted. Note the gap in the delivery sheath between the balloon and the distal end of the stent, which contains the anti-reflux valve and a retrieval string with a metal marker (*arrow*). **d** The stent is inserted a little too far and the distal basket deployed (*arrowheads*). Note the middle stent marker (*arrow*), which needs to be above the upper end of the stricture. **e** The part-deployed stent is then pulled back into final position. The deflated balloon tip is just seen in the stomach (*arrowheads*). **f** Immediate appearance after stent release

past such distally migrated stents could only be left in the stomach. Although reports of complications from this are rare, onward migration of the stent into the small bowel and colon can occasionally occur. Some of these stents simply pass into the toilet but perforation or small bowel obstruction is a potential complication and, wherever possible, migrated stents should not be left in the stomach (Kim et al. 2000; Lees et al. 2003; Ho and Ong. 2004).

The majority of oesophageal stents world-wide are placed endoscopically but unless further biopsies to confirm the diagnosis are required at the time of the procedure, endoscopy is actually superfluous. Additionally there is some low level evidence that suggests that endoscopy might actually be a disadvantage. As with dilatation of a distal oesophageal stricture blind endoscopic passage of a guidewire through the tumour without fluoroscopic control may lead to misplacement and even perforation of the oesophagus, particularly if a hiatus hernia is present beneath. In order to get round this problem the endoscopist may undertake balloon dilatation of the tumour in order to pass the endoscope through into the stomach and ensure correct placement of the guidewire. However, as the BSG guidelines point out, dilatation of oesophageal tumours is complicated by perforation in 6%–7%. The 2004 NCEPOD report on therapeutic upper gastrointestinal endoscopy indicated an overall perforation rate of approximately 4% in patients undergoing upper gastrointestinal interventional endoscopy which included dilatation and stenting. To reduce this risk of perforation dilatation of the tumour should be avoided. If fluoroscopic guidance is used then the procedure can be exactly as described above for the radiological dilatation of benign oesophageal strictures. The 2004 report of the Registry of Oesophageal Stenting (ROST) from the British Society of Interventional Radiology revealed no perforation in 445 stent procedures (BSIR 2004).

11.2.4.1 Technique

Under pharyngeal anaesthesia and intravenous sedation a catheter and guidewire are passed to the level of the tumour as described above for benign oesophageal strictures. After injection of non-ionic contrast medium, the upper and lower margins of the tumour are indicated with external skin markers and catheter and guidewire negotiated into the antrum (Fig. 11.4a–f). A 180-cm long 0.035-in. (0.89-mm) diameter stiff guidewire is placed with its tip in the antrum of the stomach. For some older stent introducer systems the 180-cm long guidewire is insufficient and it may be necessary to use a 260-cm guidewire. The delivery system is introduced over the wire after its guidewire channel has been flushed with saline and the outside lubricated with water based jelly. The stent is passed into the oesophagus and through the tumour until its tip lies at the level of the upper body of the stomach. The first two segments of the stent can then be deployed and the stent is withdrawn into the gastro-oesophageal junction so that these deployed segments fit snugly against the distal end of the tumour. While keeping gentle backward traction on the delivery system the remainder of the stent is deployed and the introducer system and guidewire removed.

A number of problems can arise during stent placement. Although the slim modern delivery systems of 18- to 24-Fr can be easily advanced through most tumours, very occasionally the stricture is too tight to allow the system to pass. In this situation gentle balloon dilatation of the stricture to 5 or 6 mm (= 15- to 18-Fr) should allow insertion of the delivery system. Dilatation of this nature does not carry the same risk as dilatation up to 15 mm necessary for passage of an endoscope. Some delivery systems benefit from an even stiffer guide than the Amplatz wire, such as the 185-cm Back-up Meier wire (Boston Scientific, St. Albans, UK).

Very occasionally the tip of the delivery system (olive) can impact in a partly expanded stent on removal. This is more common with a stent skeleton consisting of individual segments than with stents made from a continuous wire mesh. Should this happen, it is important not to pull, as this will displace the stent. Some delivery systems have a detachable distal olive which can be released into the stomach after stent deployment (Fig. 11.5) or even a deflatable balloon tip (Fig. 11.4c,e). If the olive is fixed to the delivery system, this can be dis-impacted by advancing the retracted outer sheath of the delivery system back into the narrowed part of the stent above the olive. Pushing the sheath forward, whilst applying traction to the olive prevents proximal displacement of the stent and usually allows the olive to be withdrawn. A gentler alternative is to leave the stent for 5 min to expand, if patient and operator are relaxed enough for this. This will allow removal of the delivery system in most cases.

If all this fails a second guidewire can be passed through the stent alongside the impacted system followed by a small dilatation balloon. Gentle dilatation of the narrowed segment to no more than 8 mm will allow the olive to be withdrawn.

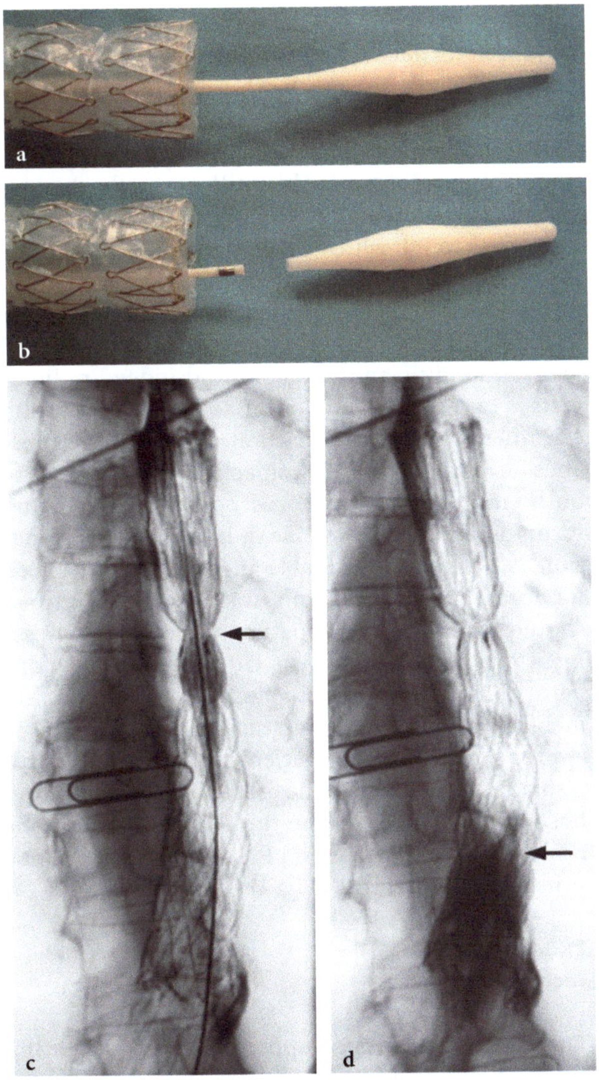

Fig. 11.5. **a,b** Detachable introducer tip (Ella-CS stents / UK Medical, Sheffield UK). A bayonet mechanism allows the olive to be released in case of difficulties on removal. **c,d** The tip (*arrow*) will not pass back through the incompletely expanded stent and is released, allowing easy removal of the delivery system (Boubella stent)

11.2.4.2
Outcomes

The commonest complication of stent placement is chest pain which usually lasts 24–48 h and should be managed with an ascending scale of analgesic power. Other immediate complications such as perforation or bleeding are extremely rare (BSIR 2004).

Normally the patient can be allowed to drink clear fluids once recovered from sedation and a soft diet accompanied by free fluids can start within 4 hours of stent placement. The patient should be given dietary advice regarding the escalating nature of consistency of their diet and also clear advice as to what they should do if dysphagia recurs. Routine contrast swallows to check for stent expansion and position are not required in asymptomatic patients (Owen et al. 2003).

Recurrent dysphagia in the early stages following stent placement is usually due to stent displacement which occurs in around 5% of stents placed in the oesophagus proper and around 15% in stents placed across the cardia (BSIR 2004). It is generally wise to remove a displaced stent before re-stenting.

Late recurrent dysphagia may be due to stent migration or to tumour overgrowth below or, much more frequently, above the stent (Fig. 11.6). In situations where the overgrowth has occurred above the level of the stent, stent removal may prove impossible and over-stenting with a second stent will be necessary. Other techniques to deal with tumour overgrowth such as alcohol injection, laser photocoagulation or photodynamic therapy may also be appropriate.

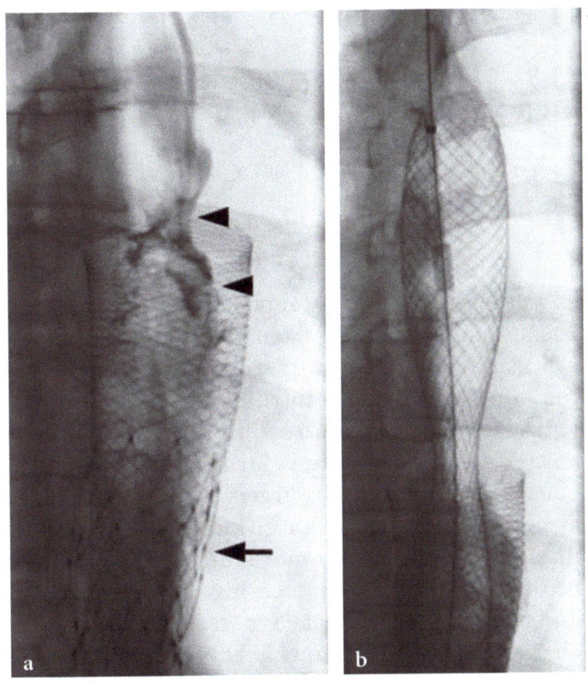

Fig. 11.6. **a** Recurrent overgrowth: A Flamingo Wallstent (Boston Scientific, St. Albans, UK) had been inserted for tumour overgrowing a previous Gianturco-Z stent (Cook, Letchworth, UK) (*arrow*). The lumen is now narrowed by tumour tissue growing over and into the top of the Flamingo stent (*arrowheads*). **b** A second Flamingo stent is inserted. Expansion is limited by tumour tissue at the top of the previous stent

11.2.5 Post-Operative Recurrence

Recurrence of tumour after gastro-oesophagectomy for distal oesophageal adenocarcinoma most often occurs at the level of the oesophago-gastric anastomosis and presents with recurrent dysphagia. Various non-interventional therapies such as chemotherapy or radiotherapy may be appropriate in this situation but the most effective method of rapid relief of dysphagia is placement of a stent. Generally the length of the stenotic lesion is quite short under these circumstances and a relatively short stent can be used. The technique for placement is exactly as described above for unoperated patients. Whilst the inevitable vagotomy which goes along with oesophagectomy will have reduced the gastric acid production, it is still best to place an anti-reflux stent in this situation. If pyloroplasty has not been performed, gastric emptying may be impaired and reflux of gastric contents can be expected if an open, non-valved stent is used.

11.3 Stomach

11.3.1 Gastric Tumours

The incidence of gastric carcinoma is reducing except at the gastro-oesophageal junction (ONS 2003). Tumours arising from the body of the stomach tend not to cause gastric outlet obstruction but tumours involving the antrum may do so. Patients with gastric outlet obstruction may present with a rapid feeling of fullness during meals, anorexia, nausea and vomiting. If surgery for resection is not an option because of advanced local stage, metastatic disease or because of co-morbidities then the choice of therapy lies between stenting the gastric outlet and performing a surgical bypass. Stent insertion is cheaper and results in quicker recovery than open gastro-jejunostomy (Maetani et al. 2004; Mittal et al. 2004) but patients with a good long-term prognosis might benefit from the lower re-intervention rate following surgery (Maosheng et al. 2001). First experience with laparoscopic gastro-enterostomy indicates this as a potential surgical alternative to stenting but definitive comparative information is awaited.

11.3.1.1 Patient Assessment

The best method of assessing a patient with lower gastric carcinoma who presents with vomiting is to undertake endoscopy. This will normally demonstrate a large circumferential tumour involving the antrum through which the endoscope will not pass into the pylorus. An inappropriately large fluid or food residue in the stomach is usually present under these circumstances. An important message to get across to physicians, surgeons and indeed radiologists is to resist the temptation to perform a barium examination of the stomach at all costs. The presence of barium in the stomach is a hindrance to both endoscopic and fluoroscopic procedures and it can take many days to clear. If contrast examination is considered valuable in assessing the need for intervention, non-ionic water soluble contrast should be used. For the patient undergoing assessment of operability for gastric cancer CT is mandatory. This will demonstrate the local, nodal and metastatic extent of the disease and determine the appropriateness of the patient for surgery. CT can also be used to evaluate the presence of gastric outlet obstruction caused by the tumour and therefore is probably the best method of assessing the patient's suitability for stenting (Fig. 11.7).

11.3.1.2 Technique

The basic principles of upper GI luminal stenting are the same wherever the lesion. It is however true to say, that the further the lesion from the mouth the greater the advantage of using an endoscope for guidance. The benefit is mainly that from the endoscope acting as an overtube rather than simply allowing direct visualisation of the stricture. Stenting the gastric outlet using catheter and guidewire alone is perfectly possible and specific catheters have been designed to avoid redundant loops forming in the capacious stomach. This happens easily and not only makes control of the catheter tip difficult, but even 100 cm long catheters may simply turn out to be too short to cross the stricture. It should be noted that the use of an endoscope does not obviate the need for fluoroscopy as it is imperative to assess the distal margin of the obstruction, which is usually impossible endoscopically. Most stent delivery systems are between 10 and 11 Fr in size necessitating the use of a therapeutic duodenoscope with a large ($\geq$ 3.8 mm) working channel.

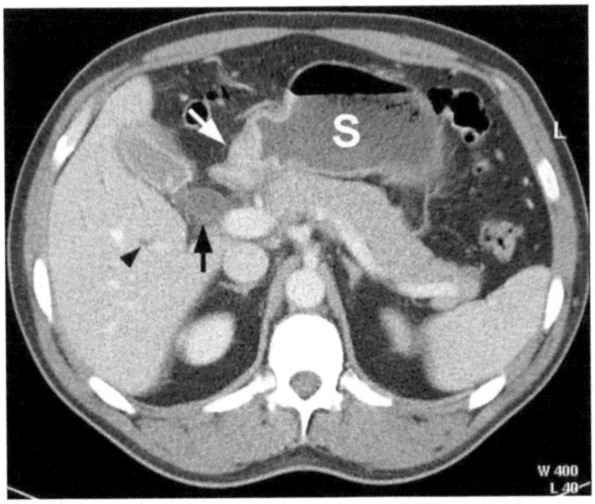

Fig. 11.7. CT of an obstructing pyloric tumour (*white arrow*). The stomach (*S*) is distended and there is dilatation of the common bile duct (*black arrow*) and some intrahepatic ducts (*arrowhead*)

Whether or not an endoscope is used, the principle of gastric outlet stenting is the same (LAASCH et al. 2005). The proximal margin of the lesion as assessed either endoscopically or fluoroscopically is marked with a marker on the patient's skin. A catheter and hydrophilic guidewire are negotiated through the tumour into the second or third part of the duodenum beyond. The guidewire is withdrawn and contrast injected to delineate the distal margin of the tumour and also to demonstrate the absence of further more distal obstructing lesions (Fig. 11.8). It is also helpful to inject air following contrast through the catheter to delineate and distend the small bowel adequately. Intravenous anti-peristaltic agents (e.g. 20 mg hyoscine butylbromide) can be used for better assessment. Once the proximal and distal margins of the tumour have been identified the catheter and hydrophilic guidewire are negotiated as far as possible along the duodenal loop. The hydrophilic guidewire is withdrawn and replaced with a guidewire suitable for stenting. The further the wire can be passed beyond the stricture, the better the guidance for the stent and the lower the risk of accidental displacement of the system. Depending upon the length of the stent delivery system a very long guidewire may be required. For endoscopic stenting a 400-cm long Teflon coated stainless steel wire as used for ERCP is adequate. Forming a J-tip on the end of the guidewire before insertion avoids inadvertent perforation. Nitinol wires are more kink-resistant, but at significantly increased cost. For fluoroscopic insertion a heavy duty wire provides better stabilisation through the distended stomach, but distorts the anatomy more.

Once the guidewire is in position the introducing catheter is withdrawn and the flushed and lubricated stent delivery system is mounted on the guidewire and advanced through the tumour. Occasionally it can be difficult to negotiate the stent through the tumour and on around the duodenal loop. It is particularly in these circumstances that the use of an endoscope with its additional options for directional control, stability and torque helps to guide the stent through the tumour and around the duodenum. When stenting around flexures, e.g. from the gastric antrum into the second part of the duodenum, it is important that the long axis of the deployed stent lies parallel to the long axis of the bowel lumen at either end. A stent placed with its end in the apex of a flexure may cause functional obstruction. Angulation of the stent end forcing it to impinge on the wall of either duodenum or stomach will impair stent function and may cause pressure necrosis of the wall and subsequent perforation. When stenting the gastric outlet it is therefore necessary to place the distal end of the stent well into the second part of the duodenum. This of course brings with it the possibility that the distal margin of the stent may cross the Papilla of Vater, possibly impairing biliary drainage but definitely making future biliary access more difficult, if not impossible. The role of preemptive biliary drainage will be considered below. Once the stent is in position deployment can begin. It is important to recognise that one of the common pitfalls of gastric outlet stenting is that the stent is placed too distally with the risk that the proximal margin of the tumour is not completely covered as the stent shortens following release (Fig. 11.9). This is best dealt with by deliberately placing the stent too far distally as deployment starts but by withdrawing the partly deployed stent slowly under constant fluoroscopic control until the distal part is seen to conform to the distal end of the stricture. In this way accurate stent position with regards to the flexures, the axis of the lumen as well as the extent of the tumour can be ensured. Woven stents can be recaptured if only partly deployed and repositioned. If after stent release there is doubt about the adequate coverage of the proximal margin of the tumour the guidewire should be left in position until this can be assessed either endoscopically or by the injection of contrast medium. A catheter should be introduced through the stent, the guidewire removed and contrast injected during steady withdrawal of the catheter until adequate stent function can be demonstrated. If there is any doubt that the proximal margin of the tumour has been properly cov-

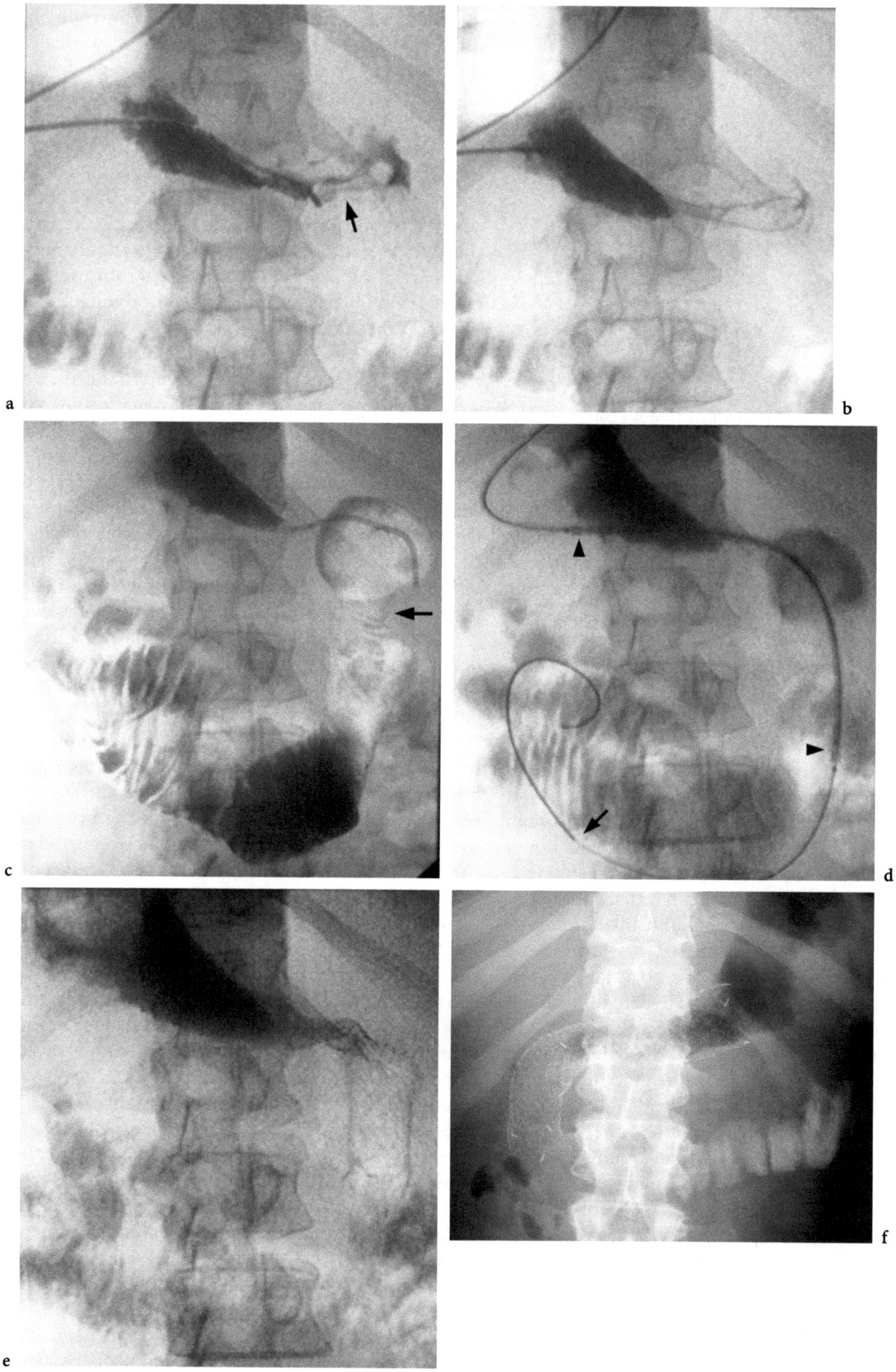
a
b
c
d
e
f

Fig. 11.8. a Obstructing pancreatic tumour: Fluoroscopic stent placement in prone position. Injection of contrast shows an irregular stricture at the pylorus (*arrow*). **b** The stricture is crossed with a looped, stiff hydrophilic wire (Aqualiner, UK Medical, Sheffield, UK). **c** Injection of air and contrast shows a possible further stricture in D2 (*arrow*). **d** The hydrophilic wire is exchanged for a heavy duty wire (Meier back-up wire, Boston Scientific, St. Albans, UK), note the junction of the flexible wire tip with the stiff shaft (*arrow*). The stent delivery system (*arrowheads*) is positioned, allowing for stent shortening on deployment. **e** A Niti-S stent (Pyramed, Sorbiton, UK) immediately after deployment. The stent is in excellent position, with an initially distorted appearance. **f** After 24 h the nitinol skeleton has regained its original configuration (patient supine)

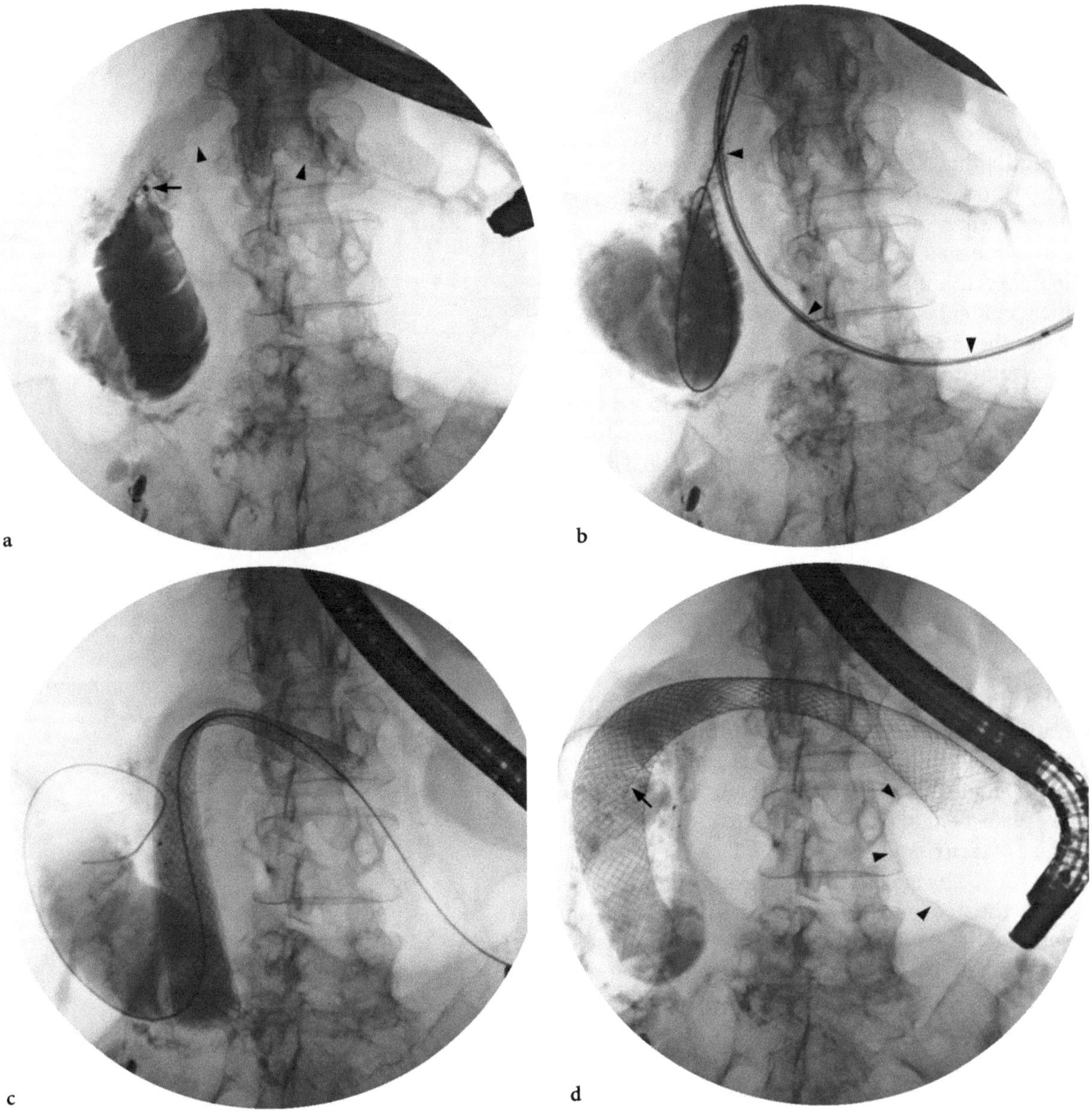

Fig. 11.9. a Injection of contrast shows a tight stricture at the gastric outlet (*arrowheads*). The radiopaque tip of the ERCP catheter (*arrow*) is seen at the distal end of the stricture in the second part of the duodenum (patient prone). **b** A wire has been passed across the stricture and a through-the-scope delivery system (*arrowheads*) is advanced over it (Enteral Wallstent, Boston Scientific, St. Albans, UK). **c** After stent release, marked waisting is seen at the level of the stricture. The stent has been placed too distally and the proximal end of the stricture is not covered. **d** A second Wallstent has been placed overlapping the first one and extending well into the gas-filled antrum (*arrowheads*). Note the position of the distal end of this (*arrow*) in the D1/D2 flexure, which may have caused impaction without the first stent

ered the guidewire can be reinserted, via the catheter through the lumen of the existing stent and a further stent placed more proximally.

It is rare for stents to expand to their full diameter immediately. At the end of the procedure most stents will have opened to about 50% of their nominal diameter at the site of the lesion and will continue to expand for 2–3 days after delivery. This particularly applies to nitinol stents, which only develop their full radial force after warming to body temperature. If considered appropriate, balloon dilatation can be used to open the stent further but this carries with it the risks of stent displacement and perforation and is generally not necessary. Stents constructed from individual segments rather than woven from a single strand of wire shorten less, but may look very distorted when released. Again these will reconfigure over the space of 24–48 h (Fig. 11.8e,f) and further intervention should be resisted unless there is clinical evidence of poor function.

After the procedure the patient can be allowed to drink immediately following recovery from sedation with a very soft light diet being introduced after 6 h. Dietary advice should be given to the patient regarding the escalating nature of the consistency of their diet but they should be warned that return to a normal diet is unlikely to be achievable.

11.3.1.3 Outcome

The majority of patients manage to return to a reasonable diet, which allows them to maintain nutrition although some dietary limitation such as the avoidance of meat is to be expected. Approximately 30% of patients who have undergone gastric outlet stent placement will need further intervention because of recurrence of vomiting. This is most commonly caused by stent occlusion from tumour overgrowing the stent ends, tumour growing through the skeleton of the stent or mucosal hypertrophy. Just as a patent gastro-enterostomy does not guarantee adequate gastric emptying some patients with a properly placed, adequately patent gastric stent will not empty their stomach adequately and will continue to vomit. This is presumably because of inadequate gastric peristalsis in the diseased stomach.

11.3.1.3.1 Restenting

If a stent should occlude, either because of overgrowth or through-growth, a new stent can be inserted using exactly the same technique. The crucial point to note is that it is easy when inserting a guidewire through the existing stent, to inadvertently pass the wire through the interstices of the stent without realising this until discovering the stent itself will not pass. This is best avoided by accessing the initial stent lumen using a J-wire or doubled-up wire, which passes through the stent lumen without making an exit through the mesh (Fig. 11.10). Passage of a catheter over the wire and contrast medium injection confirms its proper position.

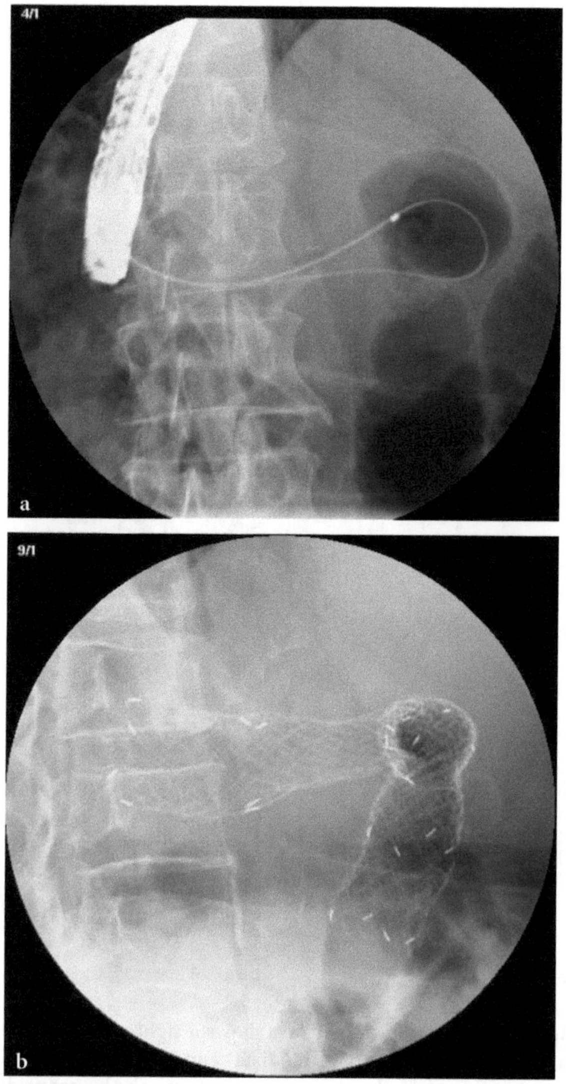

Fig. 11.10a,b. Obstruction of the gastric outlet: using a doubled-up wire is the safest way to traverse a stricture, avoiding perforation as well as exiting through the sides of an existing stent. (Hanaro stent, Diagmed, Thirsk, UK)

The second stent can snag on the proximal end of the first. It is best not simply to push as this can distort the first stent and damage the delivery system of the second. It is best to use the endoscope to alter the angle of approach of the new stent, slowly persuading it into the first stent lumen.

11.3.2 The Post-Operative Stomach

The procedure for stenting anastomotic tumour recurrence after Billroth I gastrectomy is exactly as described in the native stomach. Similarly tumour recurrence after Polya (Billroth II) gastrectomy can be treated with stenting of the gastro-enterostomy (Fig. 11.11). However, it is absolutely crucial to ensure that the stent is placed within the draining efferent and not the afferent loop. Whether the procedure is performed endoscopically with fluoroscopic assistance or under fluoroscopy alone, it is important to confirm the position of catheter and guidewire in the efferent loop by injecting contrast and air until the anatomy is unequivocally outlined. Once this has been achieved the stent can be placed as described above.

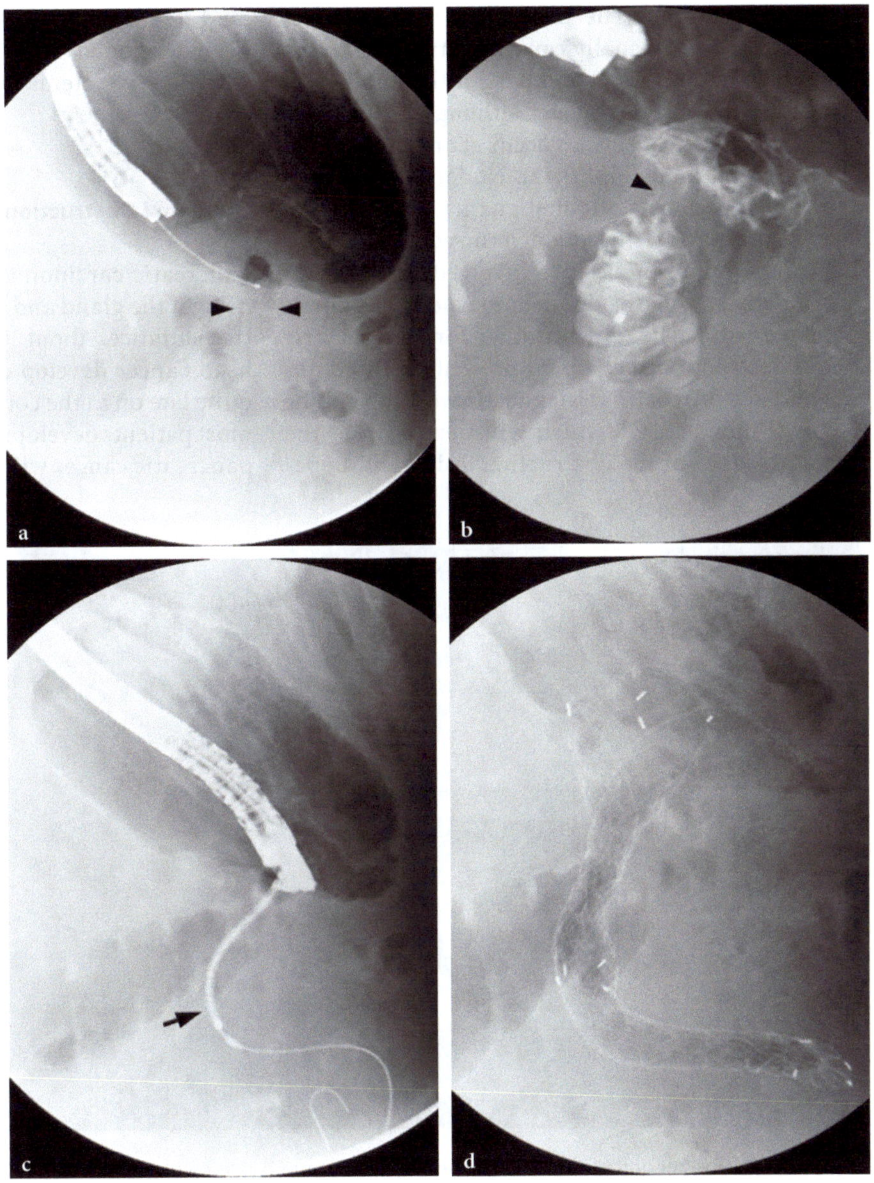

Fig. 11.11a–d. Recurrent tumour obstructing the efferent loop of a Polya (Billroth 2) gastro-jejunostomy. The stricture (*arrowheads*) is easily identified, a through-the-scope delivery system passed (*arrow*) and an uncovered Hanaro nitinol stent (Diagmed, Thirsk, UK) deployed. Initial limited expansion will increase over the space of several days

11.4 Duodenum

11.4.1 Duodenal Stents

The first part of the duodenum is an intra-peritoneal structure and obstructive lesions very rarely if ever occur at this site. However the second, third and fourth parts of the duodenum lie within the anterior para-renal space of the retroperitoneum and as such are relatively fixed in position. Mural lesions within the duodenum, for example duodenal carcinoma and tumours of the Papilla of Vater, can cause obstruction, but extrinsic lesions are far more common. The most frequent is pancreatic cancer which usually causes obstruction to the proximal part of the second part of the duodenum just above the Papilla of Vater although obstruction from pancreatic cancer can occur at any point along the duodenal loop (Fig. 11.12). Nodal masses from lymphoma or metastatic malignancy can obstruct the second part of the duodenum when the peri-pancreatic lymph nodes are involved or the third and fourth parts of the duodenum when para-aortic nodes are affected. As with other forms of gastric outlet obstruction the patient presents with vomiting and a fear of eating. Diagnostic work-up can be largely limited to CT which will demonstrate the site and extent of the obstructing lesion and hopefully give a clue to the presence of further pathology more distally within the small bowel which may lead to failure. Again it is important to understand that barium examination should be avoided as it contributes little to the assessment of the patient and creates significant problems for the interventionalist.

Historically, first attempts at duodenal stenting were performed with oesophageal stents inserted through a gastrostomy (Razzaq et al. 2001). On the whole the use of softer uncovered stents has become standard practice in the stomach and particularly in the duodenum. Covered stents have proved to have an unacceptably high migration rate and flexibility is of increased importance in order for the stent to conform to the flexures of the small bowel.

A range of dedicated partially covered and uncovered stents, as well as specialised double stents, have been developed (Song et al. 2004b) and are available on delivery systems for either fluoroscopic or endoscopic placement.

11.4.1.1 Duodenal Obstruction and the Bile Duct

Pancreatic carcinoma most frequently involves the head of the gland and usually presents with obstructive jaundice. About 10% of patients with pancreatic head cancer develop duodenal obstruction, usually quite late on in the course of their disease. Therefore most patients developing duodenal obstruction from pancreatic cancer will already have a biliary stent in

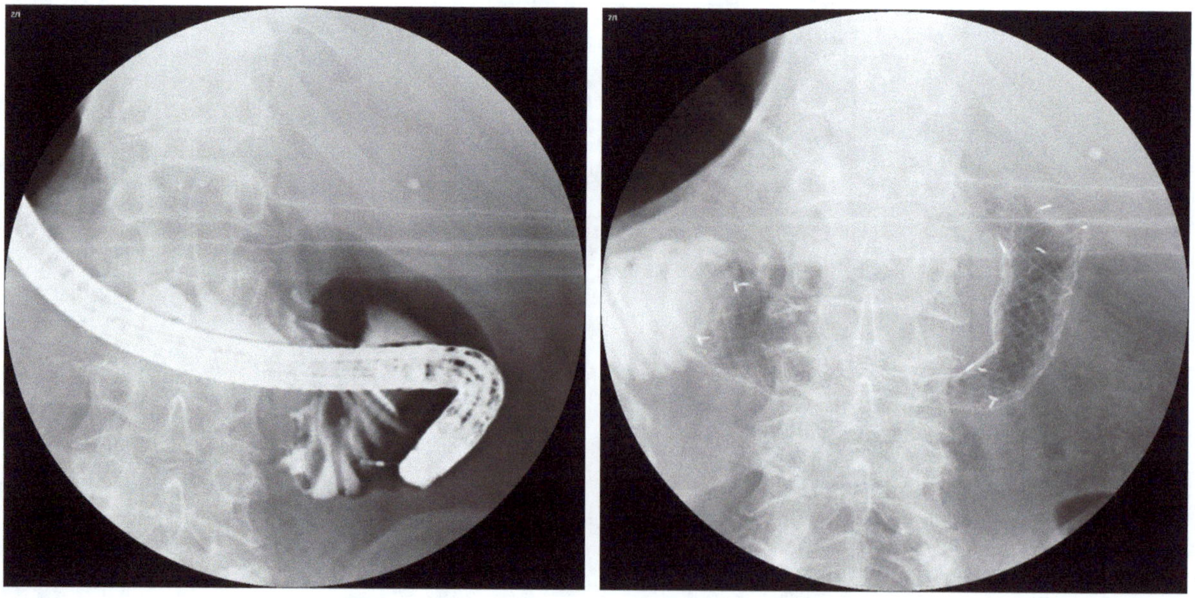

a b

Fig. 11.12a,b. Obstruction of the third part of the duodenum treated with a Hanaro stent (Diagmed, Thirsk, UK) situ, either a plastic stent, (usually 10-Fr/3.2-mm) or a self-expanding metal stent (usually 8–10 mm). If a metal stent was used and at the onset of duodenal obstruction this is still patent, then it is safe to simply go ahead and stent the duodenum. However, if the bile duct was previously stented with a plastic stent, it is desirable to remove this and replace it with a metal biliary stent prior to duodenal stenting (Fig. 11.13). This is generally a fairly easy task if endoscopic access to the plastic stent is still possible. However, more often than not endoscopic access is made impossible by the duodenal obstruction and the situation becomes more complicated:

If the plastic stent is draining, the best course of action is to leave it alone and stent the duodenum. Depending on the level of duodenal obstruction, endoscopic access may be regained through the duodenal stent, if this can be placed with the distal end short of the papilla. Otherwise one has to accept that a transhepatic approach will be necessary for any future biliary intervention.

If the duodenal stent is placed proximal to the plastic biliary stent, it may be possible to displace this into the duodenum percutaneously, should it occlude (Fotheringham et al. 2002). This is difficult, but gives better results than simply placing a metal stent alongside, as the plastic stent reduces expansion of the metal stent.

When duodenal obstruction occurs without jaundice and a biliary stent is not in situ, subclinical biliary obstruction must be excluded before duodenal stent placement. Careful assessment of the biliary system is important so that impending bile duct obstruction can be treated. Where ERCP is precluded by the duodenal tumour, information from CT may be complemented by ultrasound or magnetic resonance cholangio-pancreatography (MRCP). If the patient's liver function tests are abnormal in the absence of hepatic metastases, this should be assumed to reflect biliary obstruction and a biliary stent placed. It is wise to place a metal biliary stent first, either endoscopically or transhepatically before placing a duodenal stent.

If there is no biliary obstruction at the time of duodenal stenting there is no evidence to suggest that pre-emptive biliary drainage is of advantage to the patient. Naturally biliary obstruction may well develop after duodenal stenting, in which case a transhepatic approach is required. When placing a transhepatic biliary stent in a patient with a duodenal stent across the papilla, it is best to place the distal end of the biliary stent alongside the duodenal stent rather than through the interstices of the stent mesh (Fig. 11.14). Better drainage is provided this way and the route is still open for further transhepatic access in the future should this become necessary.

11.4.1.1.1
Duodenal Stenting: Technique

The principle outlined earlier that the further the lesion from the mouth the more useful is an endoscope certainly applies in the duodenum. Whilst lesions in the second part of the duodenum can be stented without an endoscope, particularly if dedicated catheters are available (Song et al. 2004a), those in the third and fourth parts of the duodenum become extremely difficult. Without the endoscope to straighten out the tortuous route through stomach and the duodenal 'C', the catheter and even stiff wires tend to form loops in the distended stomach.

Nonetheless the principle of stent placement is exactly as outlined for gastric outlet obstruction. A 100-cm long catheter and hydrophilic wire are negotiated to the proximal margin of the lesion where contrast is injected to outline its position. Very few lesions cannot be crossed using an angled catheter (e.g. Headhunter 1) and a straight hydrophilic wire. In case of difficulties an angled hydrophilic wire or a catheter of a different shape (e.g. Sidewinder) should be considered. After negotiating the hydrophilic wire and catheter through the tumour, contrast and air are injected to outline the distal end of the stricture and its relation to the duodenal flexures and to ensure that the bowel distal to the stenosis is not obstructed. A guidewire appropriate for the length of the delivery system is placed (minimum 260 cm) and the stent is positioned. As with gastric outlet obstruction it is very easy to place the stent too far into the bowel with the effect that the proximal margin of the tumour is not adequately stented. This is particularly important with shorter (< 10 cm) stents. Slow, careful deployment with correction of the position of the expanding stent during release is the key to success.

If an endoscope is used, a sphincterotome (a device used by endoscopists for performing endoscopic sphincterotomy) can be very helpful. The sphincterotome has a bow wire which deflects the tip of the device. This can be used with various levels of flexion to try and steer the tip of the catheter into the lumen of the obstruction. Once the guidewire has passed through the stricture, the sphincterotome is straightened, passed over the wire and then a standard wire placed for stenting.

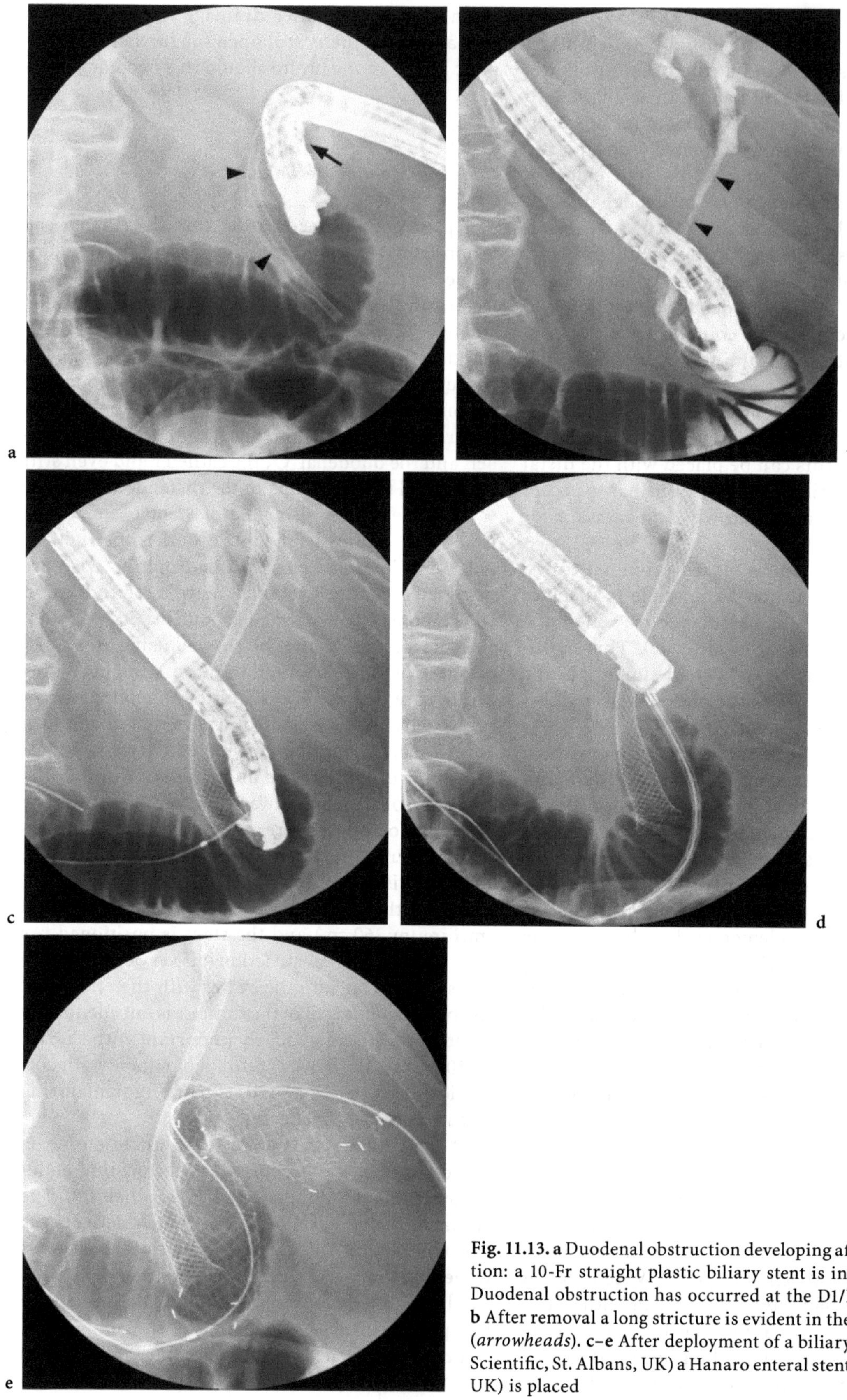

Fig. 11.13. a Duodenal obstruction developing after biliary obstruction: a 10-Fr straight plastic biliary stent is in situ (*arrowheads*). Duodenal obstruction has occurred at the D1/D2 flexure (*arrow*). **b** After removal a long stricture is evident in the common bile duct (*arrowheads*). **c–e** After deployment of a biliary Wallstent (Boston Scientific, St. Albans, UK) a Hanaro enteral stent (Diagmed, Thirsk, UK) is placed

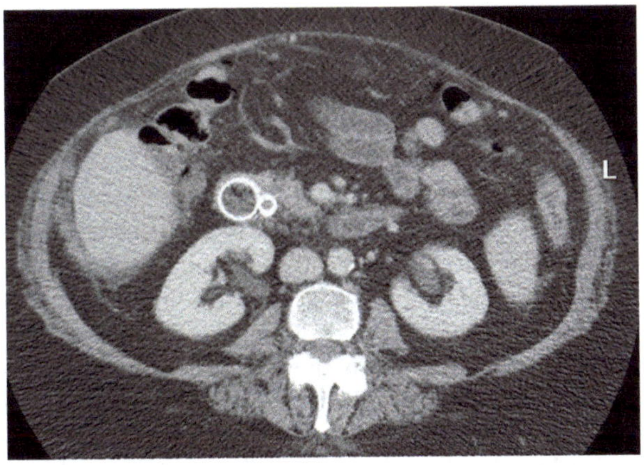

Fig. 11.14. Biliary stent placed alongside a duodenal stent. The stents lie parallel rather than crossing into each other

11.4.1.1.2
Outcomes

Duodenal stenting has a high technical success rate ranging from 80%–90% (Dormann et al. 2004). It is rare not to be able to cross the lesion and it is uncommon not to be able to place a stent. However, clinical outcome is slightly less good. Tough rubbery lesions, particularly those caused by lymph node metastases, may prevent full expansion of the stent. Balloon dilatation is not particularly effective in this context, as permanent dilatation is difficult to achieve. Mucosal hypertrophy or prolapse of oedematous duodenal mucosa through the interstices of the stent can also cause significant narrowing of the lumen. A second or even a third stent may narrow these interstices and allow effective widening of the stent lumen. For stent occlusion by ingrowth of tumour or mucosal hypertrophy, covered stents can be used as the risk of migration is reduced by the presence of the initial stent.

Most patients find relief from vomiting but do not return to a normal diet, although a soft diet will normally be tolerated in the majority of cases. A significant number of patients remain anorexic and cannot face food. It is important to differentiate this from the inability to eat because of stent failure.

As with gastric outlet obstruction up to 30% of patients will require further intervention before death for stent dysfunction.

11.5
Gastrostomy

Percutaneous gastrostomy for feeding support is a procedure for which there has been enormous demand since it was first described in children in 1980 (Gauderer et al. 1980). Before this, gastrostomy was a surgical procedure, which required opening the abdomen and stomach in order to place the feeding tube. The advent of percutaneous endoscopic gastrostomy (PEG) avoided the need for surgery and general anaesthesia and it has now become the mainstay for feeding support in a variety of clinical situations. The commonest indications in children are cerebral palsy and cystic fibrosis, and in adults, neurological or neuromuscular conditions, particularly those caused by cerebrovascular disease.

11.5.1
Percutaneous Endoscopic Gastrostomy (PEG)

Undoubtedly the quickest and simplest way to place a gastrostomy is with endoscopic support. The endoscope is passed into the stomach, which is inflated with air and a point in the body or antrum is chosen for entry. Localisation is either achieved using trans-illumination of the abdominal wall by the endoscope or by indenting the anterior abdominal and gastric wall with a finger and visualising this endoscopically. The stomach is easily punctured under local anaesthesia and a loop of string introduced through the puncture needle into the stomach. The string is grasped with a snare passed through the endoscope channel. The scope is then removed, withdrawing the string through the mouth. A pull-type gastrostomy tube is attached to the string and pulled down through the oesophagus and out through the abdominal wall to lie with its bumper up against the gastric mucosa. Alternatively a longer push-gastrostomy can be used over a guidewire instead of the string.

The tube is cut, the external fixator and feeding connectors are attached and the job is complete. Some endoscopists recommend checking by endoscopy to ensure the position of the bumper before feeding is commenced. However, if the procedure has gone smoothly, and the tube position indicates a bumper to skin exit distance of approximately 2–4 cm, check endoscopy is unnecessary (Sartori et al. 1996).

Percutaneous endoscopic gastrostomy has a high rate of success (90%–95%) (Wollman et al. 1995), but occasionally fails because of unsuccessful endoscopic access or inability to determine a safe point of puncture (Wollman and D'Agostino 1997; Laasch et al. 2003). This latter occurs most commonly in overweight patients or when the left lobe of the liver lies low in the epigastrium covering access to the stomach. Inadvertent puncture of the liver and particularly of the transverse colon are recognised complications of endoscopic gastrostomy and the possibility of this should call for the procedure to be abandoned (Fig. 11.15). Endoscopic access may also be precluded by the presence of a pharyngeal pouch, oesophageal stricture, oesophageal tumour or large hiatus hernia. Rather than attempting some of the more adventurous endoscopic approaches described (Taller et al. 2001; Vitale et al. 2005), radiological placement should be performed in these cases.

For patients with curable head and neck tumours there is an increasing tendency to establish a route of nutritional support prior to neck dissection or radical radiotherapy. The majority of these patients require feeding support at some stage, frequently for 2 months or longer, making feeding through a gastrostomy more appropriate than through a nasogastric tube. Elective gastrostomy insertion 1 week prior to surgery pre-empts nutritional failure and allows the stoma to heal before it needs to be used. Taking the gamble whether the patient can manage long enough with post-treatment dysphagia runs the risk of malnutrition compromising surgical recovery and wound healing. It also requires the procedure to be performed as a semi-emergency in a patient with increased procedural risk (Tyldesley et al. 1996).

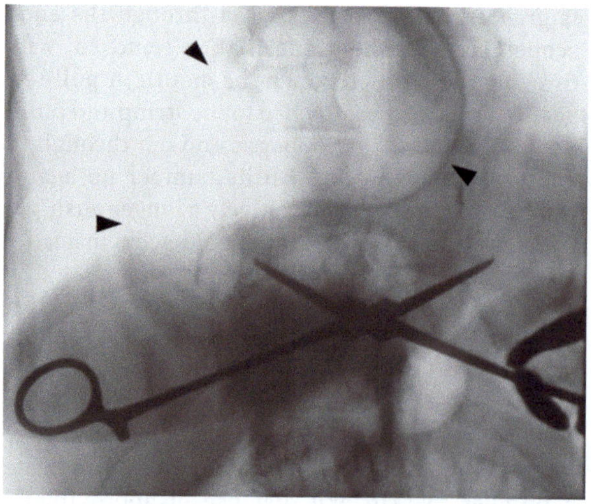

Fig. 11.15. The stomach (*arrowheads*) is completely contained in the chest. The forceps indicate the costal margin

For pre-operative gastrostomy insertion in patients with *curable* upper GI cancer, passing the tube through the mouth should be avoided. This carries a low, but definite risk of seeding of malignant disease to the gastrostomy track by the gastrostomy tube passing through the tumour (Potochny et al. 1998; Douglas et al. 2000; Sinclair et al. 2001; Wacke et al. 2004). In these circumstances insertion of the tube from the outside through the skin is advisable. This is traditionally performed radiologically, but the first endoscopic alternatives are being developed.

11.5.2 Fluoroscopic Gastrostomy

There are a variety of options for the radiological placement of a gastrostomy tube. The main difference is whether the tube is inserted directly through the skin into the stomach or – as in PEG – advanced through the mouth, oesophagus and stomach and brought out through the abdominal wall. An essential requirement is an inflation catheter in the stomach as the single most important factor for success is adequate gastric distension. A pre-existing nasogastric tube is ideal as it also allows the administration of barium sulphate for opacification of the transverse colon (e.g. 100 ml of 100% w/v $BaSO_4$ on the evening before the procedure). This is not strictly required as the colon is usually adequately outlined by gas, but removes any doubt as to possible colonic transgression. If the patient can swallow, this can of course be administered orally. If the patient cannot tolerate a nasogastric tube, a catheter is inserted through the mouth after the patient has been sedated, using a hydrophilic guidewire as for oesophageal stenting. This is much kinder to the patient, but adds a non-sterile part to the procedure and increases cost and room time.

11.5.2.1 Radiologically Inserted Gastrostomy (RIG)

Radiologically inserted gastrostomy (RIG), also termed percutaneous radiologic gastrostomy (PRG), allows a tube to be placed directly percutaneously into the stomach (Preshaw 1981; Wills and Oglesby 1983). A variety of tubes can be used for this purpose. The advantages are a reduced infection rate as the tube is not contaminated by oral flora, avoiding the risk of stoma metastasis from upper GI tumour seeding and provides the option to perform this under local anaesthesia in high-risk patients (e.g. motor neurone disease). The technique also allows the primary placement of low-profile devices ("button gastrostomy") (Lyon et al. 2003). Disadvantages include the use of balloon-retained devices with their high requirements for maintenance and risk of balloon rupture, the necessity for gastropexy and the need for track dilatation.

11.5.2.1.1 Technique

If a nasogastric tube is not in situ, a 5- to 6-Fr angled torque catheter of any type (we use Headhunter 1) together with a hydrophilic guidewire is placed into the stomach under fluoroscopic control and light sedation as described above prior to oesophageal stenting. Approximately 800–1000 ml of room air is insufflated through the gastric catheter under fluoroscopic control until the stomach extends well below the costal margin (Fig. 11.16). This displaces the colon into the mid-abdomen, which is then readily avoided. The use of a barium enema inflation device and intravenous smooth muscle relaxant (e.g. 20 mg hyoscine butylbromide) greatly enhances gastric distension and a puncture site on the anterior abdominal wall is usually picked with ease. If there is anxiety about the position of the left lobe of the liver ultrasound examination will demonstrate a safe route for entry.

The patient's abdomen is prepared with a skin cleansing agent and draped. The point of access chosen for the gastrostomy is marked on the skin. Gastropexy sutures need to be placed around the tube site in order to anchor the stomach to the anterior abdominal wall. These are short metal T-fasteners on a surgical suture, which fix the stomach during track dilatation and tube insertion and prevent gastric retraction while the stoma is healing (Fig. 11.17). Radiologists vary on the number of T-fasteners that are placed but three in a triangle with the chosen point of gastrostomy access at the centre of the triangle is usually simple and straightforward. At the anticipated position of the T-fasteners and the gastrostomy track the anterior abdominal wall is liberally infiltrated with lidocaine down to the peritoneum. T-fasteners are inserted into the stomach in the tip of a slotted needle, pushed into the gastric lumen with a metal rod, pulled back and

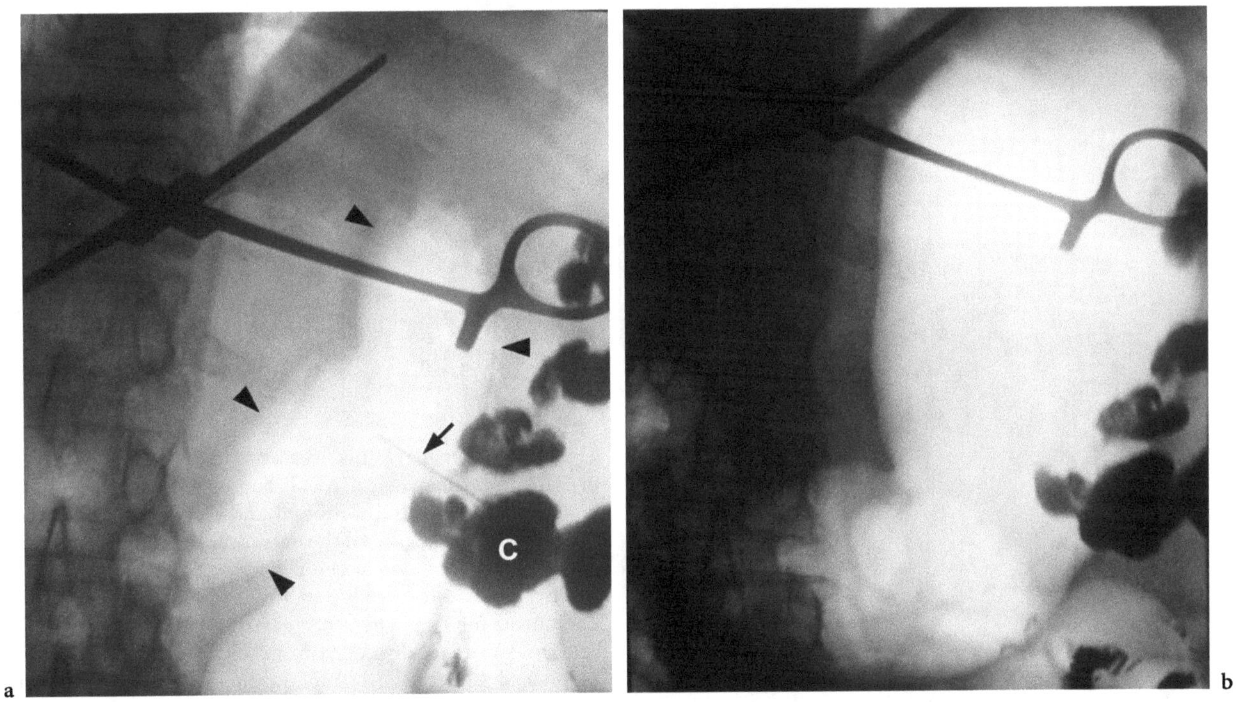

Fig. 11.16. **a** Undistended stomach: the air-filled contour is seen below the costal margin (*forceps*) and the colon outlined by barium given the night before (*C*). *Arrow:* Needle from local anaesthetic injection. **b** After administration of hyoscine bromide and insufflation of 1000 ml air the stomach is well distended, displacing the colon and approximating the anterior abdominal wall

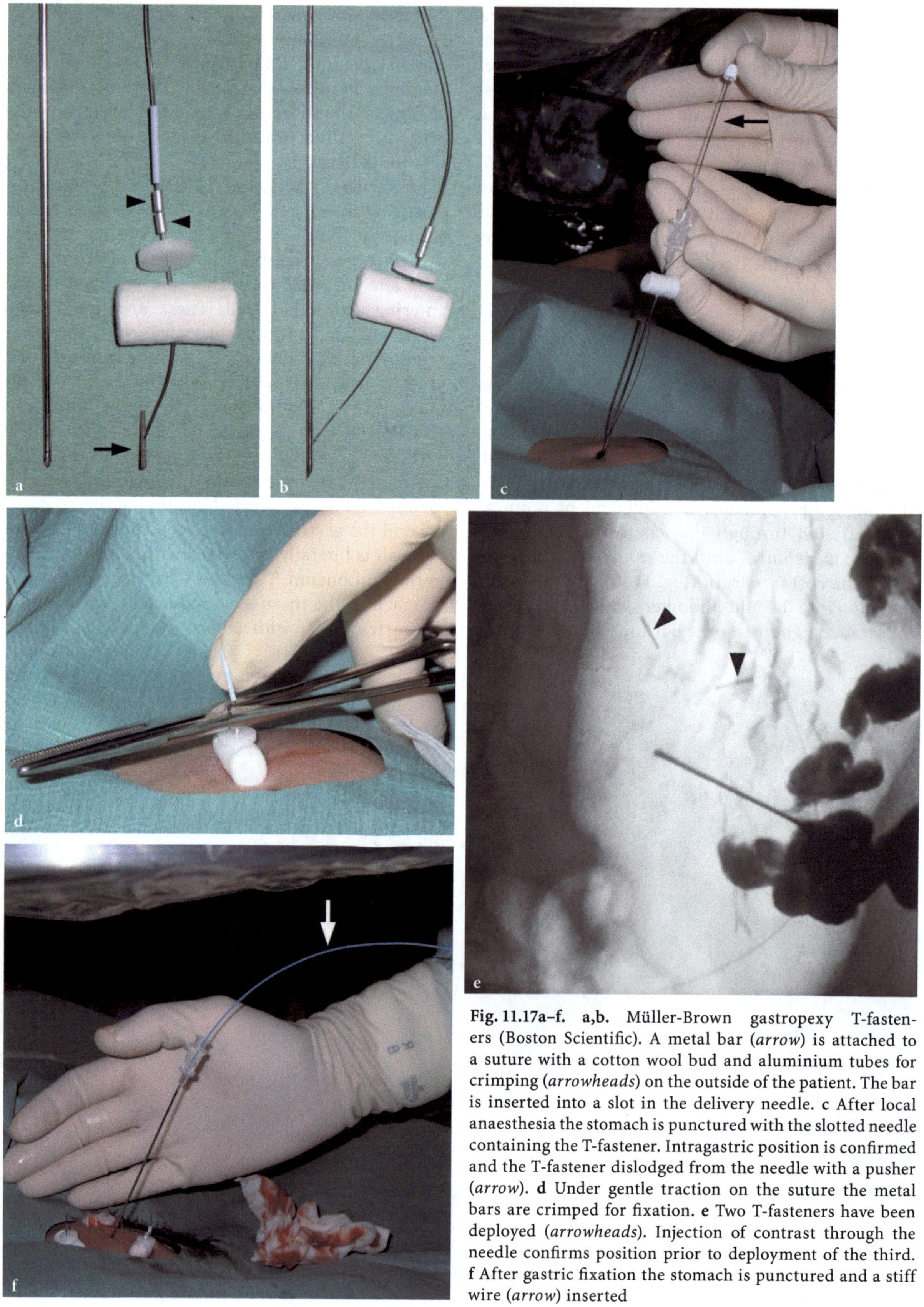

Fig. 11.17a–f. **a,b.** Müller-Brown gastropexy T-fasteners (Boston Scientific). A metal bar (*arrow*) is attached to a suture with a cotton wool bud and aluminium tubes for crimping (*arrowheads*) on the outside of the patient. The bar is inserted into a slot in the delivery needle. **c** After local anaesthesia the stomach is punctured with the slotted needle containing the T-fastener. Intragastric position is confirmed and the T-fastener dislodged from the needle with a pusher (*arrow*). **d** Under gentle traction on the suture the metal bars are crimped for fixation. **e** Two T-fasteners have been deployed (*arrowheads*). Injection of contrast through the needle confirms position prior to deployment of the third. **f** After gastric fixation the stomach is punctured and a stiff wire (*arrow*) inserted

the suture secured on the skin, either by crimping a retaining tube or with a surgical stitch. The stomach is punctured with a needle capable of carrying a 0.035-in. guidewire (the gastropexy needle can be used) and a stiff wire inserted into the stomach. The track is dilated, a peel-away sheath inserted and the gastrostomy tube is placed through this. The traditional tube for this is a 10- to 11-Fr catheter with a retaining loop and multiple side holes distal to this. The end of the tube can be placed in the duodenum if necessary. The tube is secured in position by a locking pigtail at its centre point (Fig. 11.18). After the procedure the position of the RIG is checked by injection of contrast medium. Some radiologists prefer to avoid the use of gastropexy sutures because their placement lengthens the duration of the procedure, creates further sites for haemorrhage or infection and also increases the radiation dose to the operator's hands. However, the risk of displacement of the stomach from the abdominal wall and the inadvertent entry of the guidewire or the gastrostomy tube into the peritoneal cavity is definitely increased without the use of gastropexy sutures. Furthermore, small, flexible or inflatable retaining devices may allow displacement of the tube out of the stomach into the peritoneum, if the gastrostomy track is not supported by gastropexy while fresh.

After the procedure the patient can start to feed with water via the gastrostomy tube at about six hours progressing to half strength and later full strength feeds over the course of the next 48 hours.

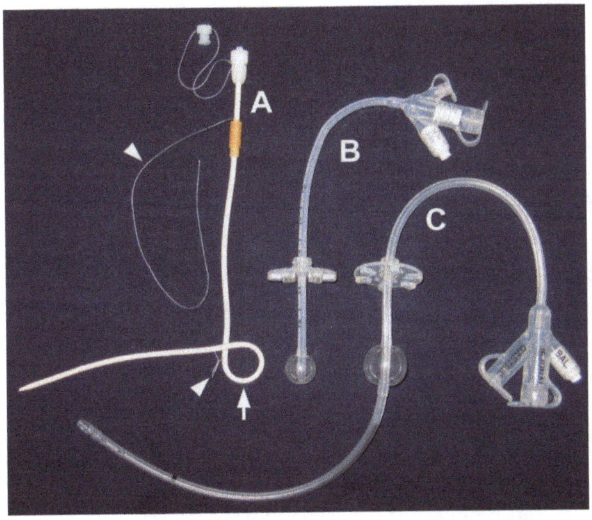

Fig. 11.18. RIG-tubes: *A*, 10.5-Fr Tilma gastrostomy tube with pigtail retaining loop (*arrow*). *Arrowhead*: locking string (Cook, Letchworth, UK). *B*, A 14-Fr MicKey balloon replacement gastrostomy tube (Vygon, Cirencester, UK). *C*, A 16-Fr MicKey balloon-retained transgastric jejunostomy tube

11.5.2.1.2
Problems

Infection at the skin site is common, which previously occurred in up to 20% of patients with endoscopic gastrostomy. This is because organisms from the patient's mouth are inevitably transferred with the gastrostomy tube to the skin wound and prophylactic antibiotics are now considered mandatory for patients having endoscopic gastrostomy. However with RIG the risk of skin site sepsis is much lower, between 2% and 5% and antibiotic prophylaxis is not considered compulsory (Funaki et al. 2000; Laasch et al. 2003).

The main problem with the relatively small diameter loop-retained tubes described above is dislodgement. The locking pigtail is not a particularly effective retention device. Displacement of the tube within a month of placement can pose significant difficulties because a transperitoneal track may not have formed adequately to allow replacement of the tube.

Recently, different types of tubes have been used more widely in order to try to avoid the problem of displacement (Fig. 11.18). Balloon replacement tubes which are designed like a short Foley urinary bladder catheter can be inserted using a similar technique as described above. It is also possible to place a low-profile gastrostomy ("button gastrostomy") directly during the initial procedure (Given et al. 2004).

11.5.2.1.3
Technique for Placing Balloon-Retained Gastrostomy Tubes

The procedure is as described above for RIG placement but once guidewire access to the lumen of the stomach has been gained, a larger track needs to be created. In order to accommodate the deflated gastrostomy tube balloon, the track needs to be oversized by 4 Fr above the gastrostomy tube (e.g. 16 Fr for a 12-Fr balloon-retained tube). Dilatation can either be performed using increments of rigid dilators (e.g. 11 and 14 Fr), which is cheaper or with a 5- to 6-mm/4-cm long angioplasty balloon, which is less traumatic. Dilatation is completed by inserting a 16-Fr peel-away sheath over the wire into the stomach, the sheath dilator is removed and the lubricated tube passed through the sheath into the stomach (Fig. 11.19). The sheath is peeled away and the retaining balloon inflated with 5 ml of water. Saline should be avoided as crystallisation can occur, blocking the valve. After removal of the guidewire the balloon

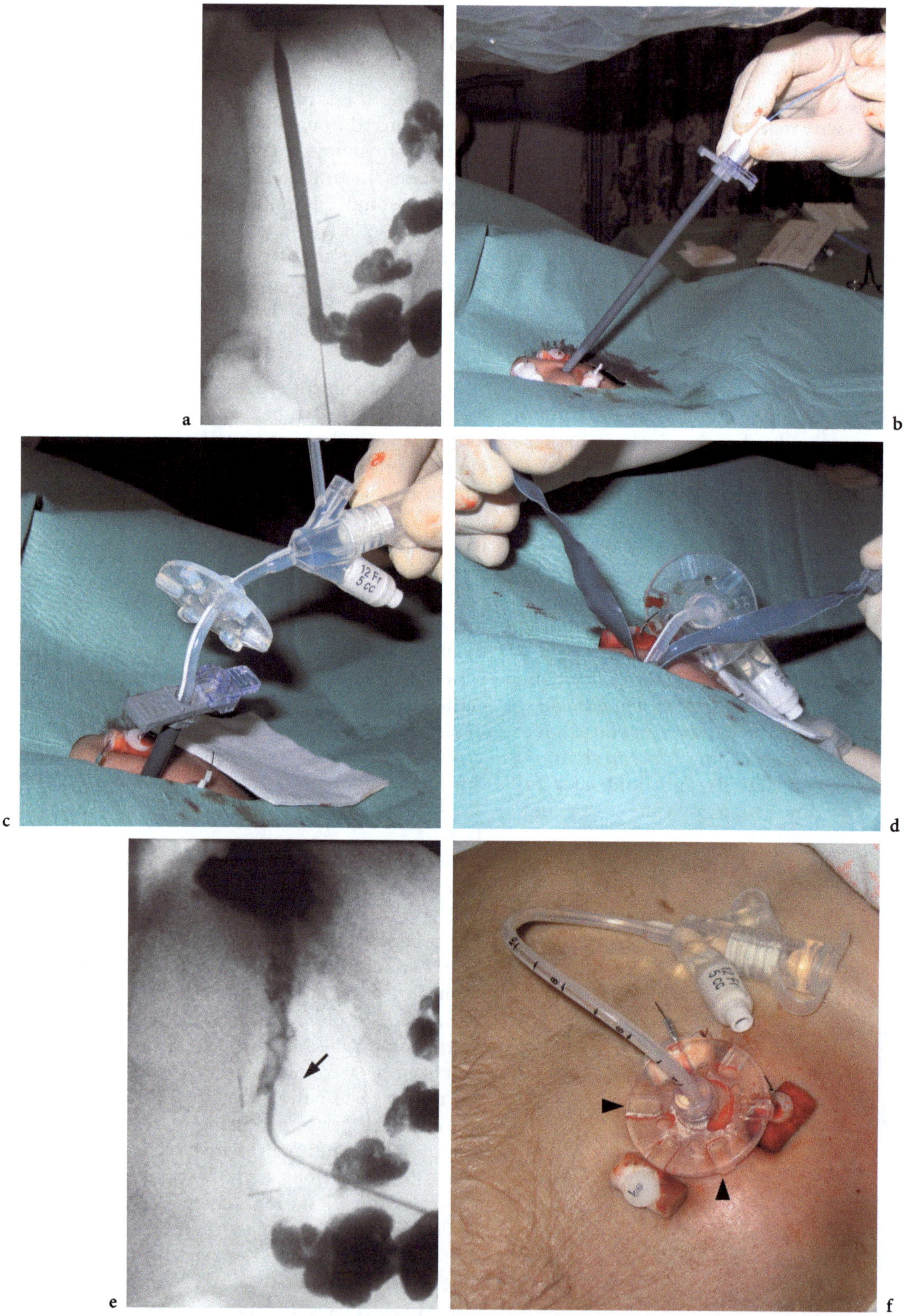

Fig. 11.19a–f. After dilatation of the track, a peel-away sheath is inserted and the lubricated tube inserted through this. The sheath is split, peeled away and removed and the balloon (*arrow*) inflated. The outer retention disc (*arrowheads*) needs re-adjusting after removal of the gastropexy sutures

is gently withdrawn to lie snug against the gastric mucosa and an external bumper placed against the skin to anchor the tube. This should be snug enough to seal the track from the inside, but not so tight as to prevent free rotation of the tube and to cause pain. Post-procedural instructions for feeding are as for loop-retained tubes.

Alternatively a button gastrostomy can be placed at the initial procedure if the patient prefers and has the required manual dexterity or the care support to handle the extension tubes. The outer connector of a button gastrostomy lies flush against the patient's skin and it is therefore necessary to determine the length of the tube shaft prior to its insertion (Fig. 11.20). Button gastrostomies are available in a variety of lengths with quarter centimetre increments. Once access to the stomach has been achieved and the guidewire placed the 6 mm balloon used for dilatation is first passed into the stomach and inflated. It is then pulled back against the gastric mucosa and the skin level marked on the catheter. The balloon is deflated and withdrawn and the distance between the catheter mark and the proximal margin of the balloon measured which represents the required shaft length of the button gastrostomy. If in doubt the next longer size should be chosen, as traction on the tube increases when the stomach deflates at the end of the procedure and again after cutting the gastropexy sutures. Dedicated stoma measuring devices are available; however, these require an established track for insertion and at present none is available for use over a guidewire. If dilatation is performed with rigid dilators only, the stoma length can also be estimated prior to insertion of the peel-away sheath using an 8-Fr Foley bladder catheter instead of the dilatation balloon.

Once the required tube length has been determined, dilatation of the track is completed, the peel-away sheath inserted and the button gastrostomy tube placed through this over the guidewire. Passing the wire retrogradely up the tube will damage the one-way valve in the hub of the gastrostomy.

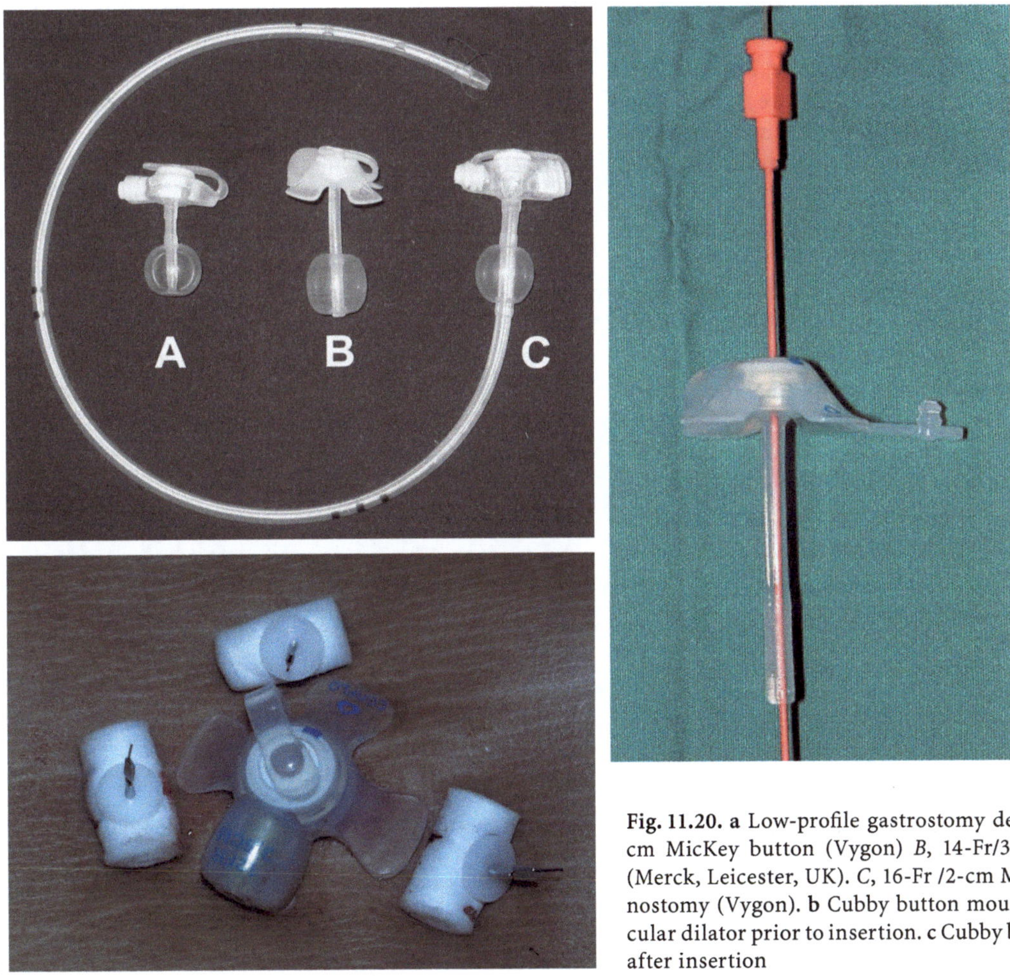

a

b

c

Fig. 11.20. **a** Low-profile gastrostomy devices: *A*, 12-Fr/1.7-cm MicKey button (Vygon) *B*, 14-Fr/3-cm Cubby button (Merck, Leicester, UK). *C*, 16-Fr /2-cm MicKey Button-jejunostomy (Vygon). **b** Cubby button mounted on a 6-Fr vascular dilator prior to insertion. **c** Cubby button immediately after insertion

To open the valve a 6-Fr vascular dilator should be inserted through the hub of the tube, and the wire fed through this. This also stiffens the button tube making it easier to pass into the stomach. Again feeding instructions are as above. Button gastrostomies are also available with retaining devices constructed from folding struts removing the anxieties about balloon failure, but are more difficult to insert and remove and also require a larger track (Rio et al. 2005).

There is little benefit in using a tube larger than 12 Fr if the device is conscientiously flushed after every use and liquid medicine preparations are used instead of crushed tablets. A growing number of drugs are specifically manufactured for use through feeding tubes.

11.5.2.1.4
Removal of Gastropexy Sutures

The normal recommendation is that gastropexy sutures should be removed after 10–14 days. However their presence is uncomfortable for the patient and makes nursing care of the stoma difficult. Recently some authors have brought this time down to 3–4 days and some are now removing them immediately after the placement of the tube at the end of the procedure (Griffiths 1996; Given et al. 2005). Naturally this will bring with it some risk of tube displacement and peritonitis but insufficient data exist to determine the frequency of this problem. Manufacturers recommend a change of water in the retention balloon every week, in order to avoid the inevitable small losses of volume which add up. However, it is prudent to change the water immediately prior to removal of the gastropexy sutures and then leave it for a fortnight, particularly if the sutures are removed early. Balloon replacement tubes have the great advantage of being able to be pushed far into the stomach during deflation of the balloon which avoids displacement even if the stomach retracts. Accidental feeding outside the stomach usually causes instant severe abdominal pain and peritonism. Feeding must be stopped immediately and the stoma careful evaluated.

11.5.2.2
Per-oral Image-Guided Gastrostomy (PIG)

Wire-guided placement of push-PEG tubes, also termed radiological per-oral gastrostomy (RPG) has been described by a number of authors since 1994 (Rosenzweig et al. 1994; Clark et al. 1999; Yip et al. 2004), but has had a surprisingly low take-up. As a hybrid of PEG and RIG it combines the success rate of radiological placement and the robustness of a bumper-retained PEG tube (Fig. 11.21) with outcomes superior to both methods (Laasch et al. 2003). It can be used as a routine alternative to PEG, and is also appropriate for use where endoscopic gastrostomy has failed but RIG is not necessarily indicated. The procedure is simple and does not require the use of gastropexy sutures or the use of an endoscope. In keeping with guidelines for per-oral endoscopic tube placement antibiotic prophylaxis is required (ESGE 1998; BSG 2001). The technique should be avoided in patients with treatable upper GI cancer to avoid the risk of tumour seeding to the stoma.

11.5.2.2.1
Technique

A nasogastric tube or a vascular catheter and guidewire are passed into the stomach, which is inflated after i.v. administration of a smooth muscle relaxant (20 mg hyoscine butylbromide). The puncture site is prepared and draped and local anaesthetic instilled down to the peritoneum. Gastropexy sutures are not required. The aim of the procedure is to pass a catheter and guidewire from the stomach into the oesophagus so that ultimately it exits through the patient's mouth. The gastric puncture site must therefore allow straight access to the gastro-oesophageal junction. Normally it is best to puncture in the mid-body of the stomach. Low access through the gastric antrum requires negotiating the gastric incisura in order to intubate the oesophagus.

Once the puncture site has been anaesthetised a needle capable of carrying a 0.035-in. guidewire is

Fig. 11.21a–g. **a** Over-the-wire push gastrostomy tubes: *A*, assembled 20-Fr Corflo gastrostomy (Merck). *B*, 14-Fr MicKey gastrostomy (Vygon). The tube itself is joined (*arrow*) to a long tapered dilator shaft (*arrowheads*). **b** The stomach is inflated through a naso-gastric tube (*arrow*). **c** The puncture needle (*arrow*) is inserted in a straight line below the cardia. **d** Over a wire the needle is exchanged for a valved vascular sheath (*arrow*). **e** A Headhunter 1 catheter (*arrow*) is advanced onto the cardia. In this case cannulation is made easy by the presence of an axial hiatus hernia (*arrowheads*). **f** Catheter and wire (*arrow*) are manipulated up the oesophagus following the line of the nasogastric tube (*arrowhead*). **g** Push-gastrostomy in situ

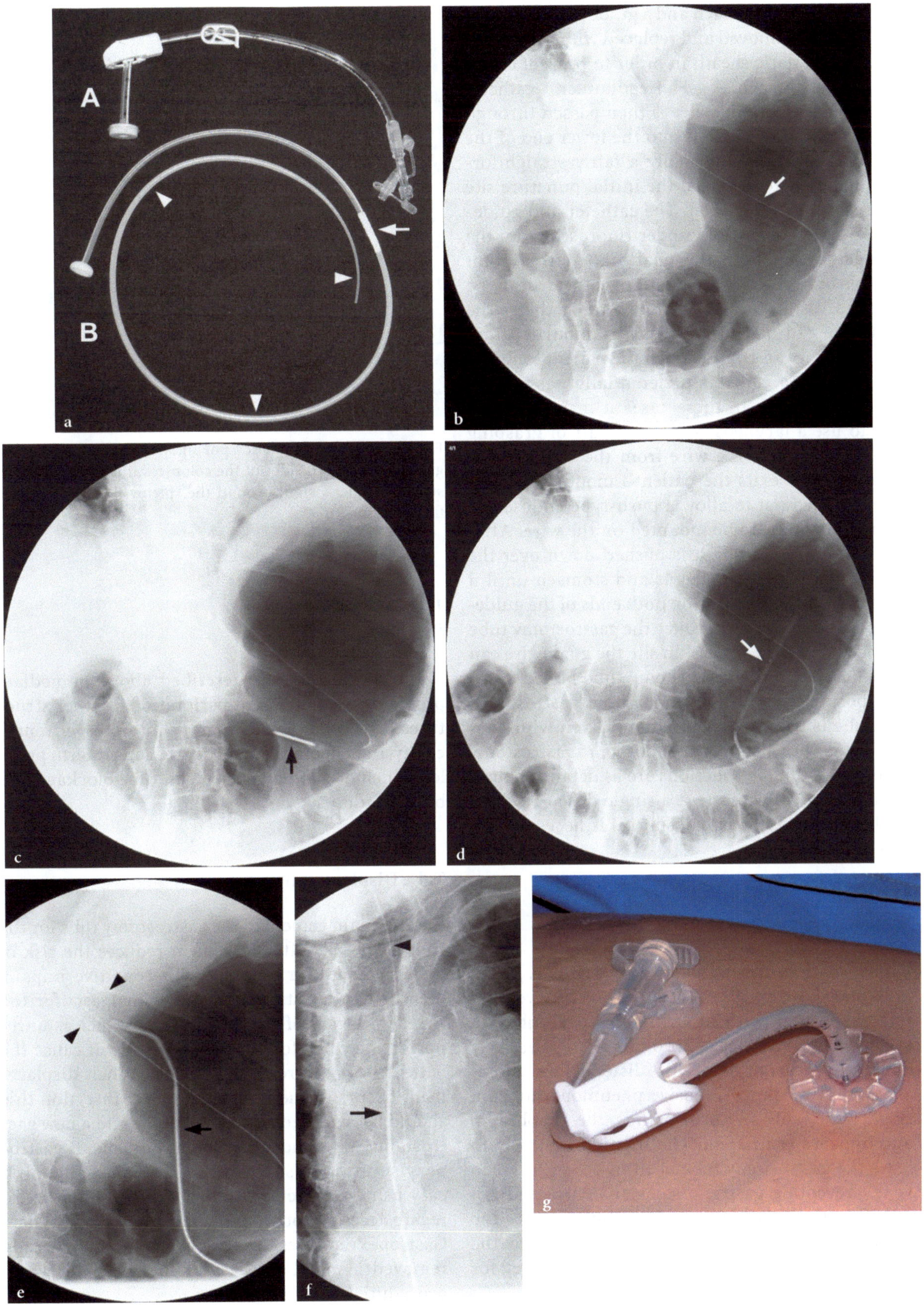
A
B
a
b
c
d
e
f
g

inserted into the stomach and a guidewire is passed. The needle is removed and replaced with a 4-Fr vascular haemostatic sheath in order to prevent deflation of the stomach. A 4-Fr Headhunter 1 catheter preloaded with a guidewire is then passed through the sheath and negotiated into the lower end of the oesophagus. This is normally a fairly straightforward manoeuvre provided the initial puncture site has been properly chosen. The catheter and guidewire are then negotiated under fluoroscopy up the oesophagus and into the pharynx. At this point the per-oral gastric insufflation catheter can be removed. Using torque control of the catheter the guidewire can usually be easily manipulated into the oral cavity and out through the patient's mouth. Sometimes the catheter preferentially passes into the nasopharynx. In these cases it may be necessary to use a laryngoscope and a pair of grasping forceps to retrieve the wire from the oropharynx. Once the wire exits the patient's mouth sufficient wire is pulled out to allow a push-type endoscopic gastrostomy tube to be mounted on the wire. After lubrication of the tube it is pushed down over the wire through the oesophagus and stomach until it exits at the skin. Traction on both ends of the guidewire assists this process. Once the gastrostomy tube has been retrieved at the skin site the guidewire can be removed and the gastrostomy tube pulled down into position just as for endoscopic gastrostomy. The tube is trimmed, secured and fixed with connectors as with a standard endoscopic gastrostomy tube and feeding instructions are as detailed above. Antibiotic prophylaxis (e.g. a single dose of second or third generation cephalosporin) is necessary for this procedure.

11.5.2.2.2 *Ventilatory Support*

Patients with neuro-muscular disorders (e.g. MND, muscular dystrophies) on positive pressure ventilatory support but without an endotracheal tube can swallow large volumes of air or air passes passively down the oesophagus. This distends the stomach and can lead to extensive pneumoperitoneum (Fig. 11.22). This in turn, splints the diaphragm and impedes ventilation. The solution is simply to leave the gastrostomy tube open in order for air to vent, preventing gastric distension. This need not significantly impair long-term feeding as, once the track forms and the risk of gas leakage into the peritoneum subsides, venting is only necessary for comfort.

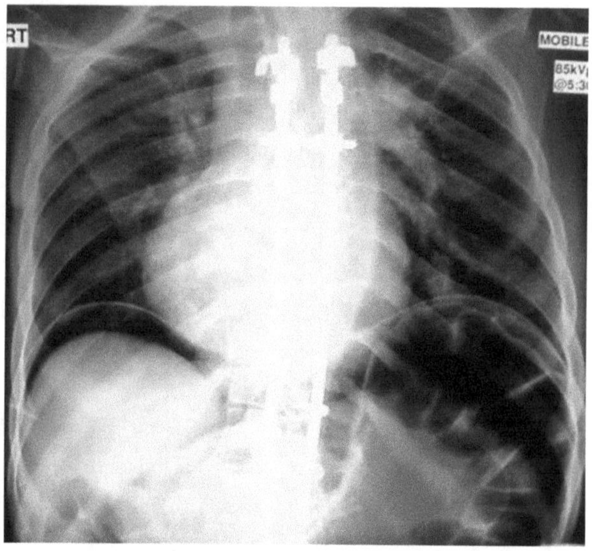

Fig. 11.22. Asymptomatic pneumoperitoneum following gastrostomy. Both sides of the colonic wall are well demonstrated (Rigler's sign) around the splenic flexure. A spinal fixator is in situ

11.5.2.2.3 *Problems*

Using the techniques described above immediate problems of inadvertent perforation of other structures, loss of access with entry into the peritoneal cavity and haemorrhage are rare. Longer term problems include tube displacement, tube blockage and buried bumper.

Tube Displacement

Careful management of the gastrostomy tube for the first few weeks after placement reduces the risk of displacement. For patients with cognitive impairment (e.g. after stroke) adequate analgesia for the first few days is of paramount importance as unreported and therefore untreated pain will cause the patient to try to remove the tube. When displacement occurs in the first month after insertion this should be regarded as an emergency and a new gastrostomy tube placed as soon as possible. If gastropexy sutures are still in place this is usually fairly easy using a catheter and hydrophilic guidewire to regain access through the gastrostomy track. Where Gastropexy sutures have not been placed or already removed it may be necessary to repeat the whole procedure from *de novo*.

When the tube displaces after a mature track has formed it is important to make certain that the patient and those looking after the patient realise that the gastrostomy track will close down and seal very quickly. We give our patients a spare replacement balloon tube so they can insert this themselves in the event of tube dislodgement. The longer it takes for the patient to seek advice following displacement the more difficult it is to regain access through the old gastrostomy track and the more likely it is that a completely new procedure will become necessary. If a standard replacement gastrostomy tube cannot be passed into the track at the time the patient arrives, it is usually possible to gain access using a straight or short tipped angled catheter (e.g. biliary manipulation catheter) together with a hydrophilic guidewire. Under fluoroscopic control these can be fairly easily manipulated down the closing gastrostomy track into the stomach. The track can be dilated over a stiff guidewire and a fresh balloon replacement gastrostomy tube inserted.

Tube Blockage

Patients and their carers insert all sorts of items down gastrostomy tubes including crushed medication. Some materials can set like concrete within the tube and it is important to give careful advice to patients and their attendants regarding the care of the tube. A growing number of medications are available in liquid form for tube feeding from specialist manufacturers (e.g. Rosemont Pharmaceuticals, Leeds, UK) and instillation of crushed tablets can and should be avoided. When tube blockage occurs, forceful flushing using water or saline may clear the tube. Wrapping the tube in a hot towel to soften the consistency of the blockage may allow flushing to succeed. Various dispersing agents are available and these occasionally work. Anecdotally good results have been achieved with warm lubricating jelly, but this is not licensed for this purpose. Alternatively passing a guidewire (e.g. a stiff hydrophilic wire) through the tube under fluoroscopic control may break up the debris and re-establish patency. In case of a loop- or balloon-retained gastrostomy with a mature track the easiest option is usually to replace the tube.

Buried Bumper

Some endoscopic gastrostomy tubes can migrate into the wall of the stomach so that gastric mucosa grows over the internal bumper leaving only a small central orifice through which feed can still enter the stomach (Fig. 11.23). This occurs usually because the outer bumper securing the tube in position has been fixed too tightly against the skin. This happens easily because the bumper is usually fixed with the patient lying supine but when the patient sits up the length of tube within the gastrostomy track becomes inappropriately short and the bumper of the tube is pulled into the gastric wall.

The clinical hallmarks of buried bumper are that feeding becomes slow and increasingly more difficult. Automated pumps used for slow overnight feeding may alarm because of increased pressure due to the closing gastric orifice. The patient may also experience pain because of accumulation of

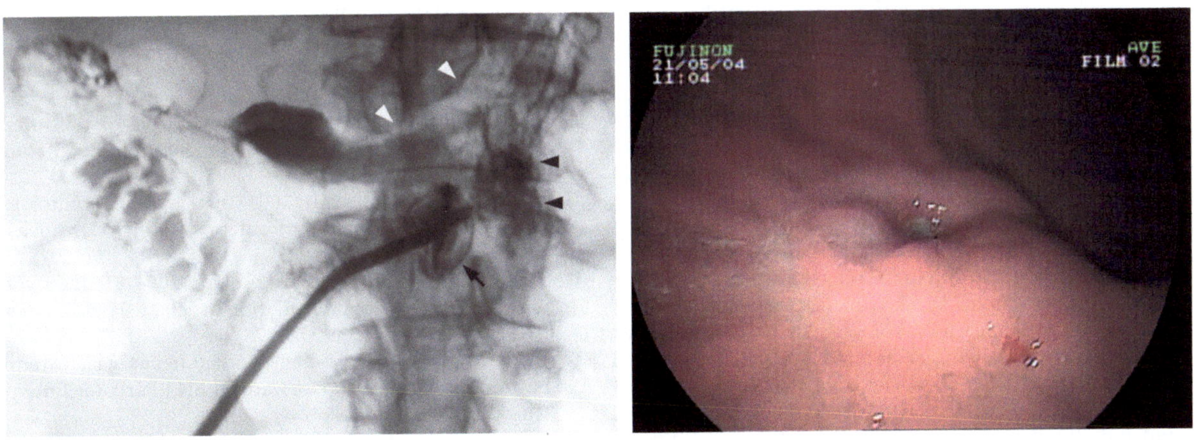

a b

Fig. 11.23. a The internal bumper (*arrow*) is seen deformed outside the line of the stomach (*white arrowheads*). Injection of contrast fills a cavity below the greater curve (*black arrowheads*). **b** Endoscopic view of a buried bumper feed between the gastric mucosa and the main gastric wall. Also an abscess may develop. The tube will still rotate within the track, but the diagnostic warning sign is the inability to push the tube into the stomach.

A wide variety of endoscopic techniques have been described for the management of the patient with a buried bumper. These include a diathermy incision of the mucosa over the bumper or the passage of a balloon to dilate the gastric mucosa followed by pushing the gastrostomy tube back into the stomach (Braden et al. 2003; Strock and Weber 2005).

As long as the gastrostomy tube is traction removable the solution to the problem is normally simple. After local anaesthesia to the track, a guidewire is placed through the gastrostomy tube into the stomach under fluoroscopic control. The gastrostomy tube is then pulled out leaving the guidewire in position. A balloon replacement gastrostomy tube is then placed, dilating the gastrostomy track beforehand if necessary. If the internal bumper consists of a rigid disk, removal other than by surgery may be impossible.

Prevention

Proper care of a gastrostomy tube is necessary to reduce the risk of a buried bumper. The simplest manoeuvre is to loosen the external bumper device 2–3 times a week and push the gastrostomy tube into the stomach by about 3 cm at the same time rotating the tube. This is a painless manoeuvre and will guarantee no buried bumper. Obviously this is not possible with a low-profile gastrostomy, which emphasises the need for accurate measuring of the track length and over-sizing in case of uncertainty.

References

Bell JK, Laasch HU, Wilbraham L et al. (2004) Bispectral index monitoring for conscious sedation in intervention: better, safer, faster. Clin Radiol 59:1106–1113

Bollschweiler E, Wolfgarten E, Gutschow C et al. (2001) Demographic variations in the rising incidence of esophageal adenocarcinoma in white males. Cancer 92:549–555

Botterweck AA, Schouten LJ, Volovics A et al. (2000) Trends in incidence of adenocarcinoma of the oesophagus and gastric cardia in ten European countries. Int J Epidemiol 29:645–654

Braden B, Brandstaetter M, Caspary WF et al. (2003) Buried bumper syndrome: treatment guided by catheter probe US. Gastrointest Endosc 57:747–751

BSIR, British Society of Interventional Radiology (2004) ROST – registry of oesophageal stenting, first report 2004. Dendrite Clinical Systems, Henley-on-Thames

BSG, British Society of Gastroenterology (2001) Antibiotic prophylaxis in gastrointestinal endoscopy. http://www.bsg.org.uk/pdf_word_docs/prophylaxis2001.pdf

Cappell MS (2005) Clinical presentation, diagnosis, and management of gastroesophageal reflux disease. Med Clin North Am 89:243–291

Chan KC, Wong SK, Lee DW et al. (2004) Short-term and long-term results of endoscopic balloon dilation for achalasia: 12 years' experience. Endoscopy 36:690–694

Clark JA, Pugash RA and Pantalone RR (1999) Radiologic peroral gastrostomy. J Vasc Interv Radiol 10:927–932

Demeester SR (2006) Adenocarcinoma of the esophagus and cardia: a review of the disease and its treatment. Ann Surg Oncol 13:12–30

Dobrucali A, Erzin Y, Tuncer M et al. (2004) Long-term results of graded pneumatic dilatation under endoscopic guidance in patients with primary esophageal achalasia. World J Gastroenterol 10:3322–3327

Dormann A, Meisner S, Verin N et al. (2004) Self-expanding metal stents for gastroduodenal malignancies: systematic review of their clinical effectiveness. Endoscopy 36:543–550

Douglas JG, Koh W and Laramore GE (2000) Metastasis to a percutaneous gastrostomy site from head and neck cancer: radiobiologic considerations. Head Neck 22:826–830

ESGE, European Society of Gastroenterology (1998) Antibiotic prophylaxis for gastrointestinal endoscopy. http://www.esge.com/guideantib2.html

Evrard S, Le Moine O, Lazaraki G et al. (2004) Self-expanding plastic stents for benign esophageal lesions. Gastrointest Endosc 60:894–900

Falk GW (2001) Gastroesophageal reflux disease and Barrett's esophagus. Endoscopy 33:109–118

Fotheringham T, Abbass S, Varghese JC et al. (2002) Displacement of occluded plastic endoprostheses into the duodenum during percutaneous biliary drainage: description of an under-reported technique. Clin Radiol 57:1113–1117

Funaki B, Zaleski GX, Lorenz J et al. (2000) Radiologic gastrostomy placement: pigtail- versus mushroom-retained catheters. AJR Am J Roentgenol 175:375–379

Gauderer MW, Ponsky JL, Izant RJ, Jr. (1980) Gastrostomy without laparotomy: a percutaneous endoscopic technique. J Pediatr Surg 15:872–875

Given MF, Lyon SM, Lee MJ (2004) The role of the interventional radiologist in enteral alimentation. Eur Radiol 14:38–47

Given MF, Hanson JJ, Lee MJ (2005) Interventional radiology techniques for provision of enteral feeding. Cardiovasc Intervent Radiol 28:692–703

Gockel I, Junginger T, Bernhard G et al. (2004) Heller myotomy for failed pneumatic dilation in achalasia: how effective is it? Ann Surg 239:371–377

Griffiths M (1996) Single-stage percutaneous gastrostomy button insertion: a leap forward. JPEN J Parenter Enteral Nutr 20:237–239

Ho HS, Ong HS (2004) A rare life-threatening complication of migrated nitinol self-expanding metallic stent (Ultraflex). Surg Endosc 18:347

Homs MY, Steyerberg EW, Eijkenboom WM et al. (2004a) Single-dose brachytherapy versus metal stent placement for the palliation of dysphagia from oesophageal cancer: multicentre randomised trial. Lancet 364:1497–1504
Homs MY, Wahab PJ, Kuipers EJ et al. (2004b) Esophageal stents with antireflux valve for tumors of the distal esophagus and gastric cardia: a randomized trial. Gastrointest Endosc 60:695–702
Kim HC, Han JK, Kim TK et al. (2000) Duodenal perforation as a delayed complication of placement of an esophageal stent. J Vasc Interv Radiol 11:902–904
Kocher M, Dlouhy M, Neoral C et al. (1998) Esophageal stent with antireflux valve for tumors involving the cardia: work in progress. J Vasc Interv Radiol 9:1007–1010
Laasch HU, Marriott A, Wilbraham L et al. (2002) Effectiveness of open versus antireflux stents for palliation of distal esophageal carcinoma and prevention of symptomatic gastroesophageal reflux. Radiology 225:359–365
Laasch HU, Wilbraham L, Bullen K et al. (2003) Gastrostomy insertion: comparing the options – PEG, RIG or PIG? Clin Radiol 58:398–405
Laasch HU, Martin DF, Maetani I (2005) Enteral stents in the gastric outlet and duodenum. Endoscopy 37:74–81
Lee S, Osugi H, Tokuhara T et al. (2005) Self-expandable metallic stent for unresectable malignant strictures in the esophagus and cardia. Jpn J Thorac Cardiovasc Surg 53:470–476
Lees NP, Reid F, Lee SH et al. (2003) Distal small bowel obstruction caused by a migrated self expanding metal oesophageal stent. Eur J Surg [Suppl]:66–68
Lyon SM, Haslam PJ, Duke DM et al. (2003) De novo placement of button gastrostomy catheters in an adult population: experience in 53 patients. J Vasc Interv Radiol 14:1283–1289
Maetani I, Tada T, Ukita T et al. (2004) Comparison of duodenal stent placement with surgical gastrojejunostomy for palliation in patients with duodenal obstructions caused by pancreaticobiliary malignancies. Endoscopy 36:73–78
Maosheng D, Ohtsuka T, Ohuchida J et al. (2001) Surgical bypass versus metallic stent for unresectable pancreatic cancer. J Hepatobiliary Pancreat Surg 8:367–373
Marsman WA, Tytgat GN, ten Kate FJ et al. (2005) Differences and similarities of adenocarcinomas of the esophagus and esophagogastric junction. J Surg Oncol 92:160–168
Mayberry JF (2001) Epidemiology and demographics of achalasia. Gastrointest Endosc Clin N Am 11:235–248
Mikaeli J, Yaghoobi M, Montazeri G et al. (2004) Efficacy of botulinum toxin injection before pneumatic dilatation in patients with idiopathic achalasia. Dis Esophagus 17:213–217
Mittal A, Windsor J, Woodfield J et al. (2004) Matched study of three methods for palliation of malignant pyloroduodenal obstruction. Br J Surg 91:205–209
NCEPOD, National Confidential Enquiry into Patient Outcome and Death (2004) Scoping our practice. http://www.ncepod.org.uk/2004.htm
ONS, Office for National Statistics (2003) Cancer Statistics. http://www.statistics.gov.uk/downloads/theme_health/MB1_34/MB1_34.pdf
Owen A, Laasch H-U, Marriott A et al. (2003) Oesophageal stent follow-up: Routine contrast swallow does not add to the management. (Abstract). CardioVasc Intervent Radiol 26:197
Park W, Vaezi MF (2005) Etiology and pathogenesis of achalasia: the current understanding. Am J Gastroenterol 100:1404–1414
Potochny JD, Sataloff DM, Spiegel JR et al. (1998) Head and neck cancer implantation at the percutaneous endoscopic gastrostomy exit site. A case report and a review. Surg Endosc 12:1361–1365
Preshaw RM (1981) A percutaneous method for inserting a feeding gastrostomy tube. Surg Gynecol Obstet 152:658–660
Razzaq R, Laasch HU, England R et al. (2001) Expandable metal stents for the palliation of malignant gastroduodenal obstruction. Cardiovasc Intervent Radiol 24:313–318
RCR, Royal College of Radiologists (2003) Safe sedation, analgesia and anaesthesia within the radiology department. http://www.rcr.ac.uk/pubtop.asp?PublikationID=186
Riley SA, Attwood SE (2004) Guidelines on the use of oesophageal dilatation in clinical practice. Gut 53[Suppl 1]:i1–6
Rio A, Ampong MA, Turner MR et al. (2005) Comparison of two percutaneous radiological gastrostomy tubes in the nutritional management of ALS patients. Amyotroph Lateral Scler Other Motor Neuron Disord 6:177–181
Rosenzweig TB, Palestrant AM, Esplin CA et al. (1994) A method for radiologic-assisted gastrostomy when percutaneous endoscopic gastrostomy is contraindicated. Am J Surg 168:587–590; discussion 590–581
Sartori S, Trevisani L, Nielsen I et al. (1996) Percutaneous endoscopic gastrostomy placement using the pull-through or push-through techniques: is the second pass of the gastroscope necessary? Endoscopy 28:686–688
Sharma P, Sidorenko EI (2005) Are screening and surveillance for Barrett's oesophagus really worthwhile? Gut 54[Suppl 1]:i27–32
Shim CS, Jung IS, Cheon YK et al. (2005) Management of malignant stricture of the esophagogastric junction with a newly designed self-expanding metal stent with an antireflux mechanism. Endoscopy 37:335–339
Siersema PD, Homs MY, Haringsma J et al. (2003) Use of large-diameter metallic stents to seal traumatic nonmalignant perforations of the esophagus. Gastrointest Endosc 58:356–361
Sinclair JJ, Scolapio JS, Stark ME et al. (2001) Metastasis of head and neck carcinoma to the site of percutaneous endoscopic gastrostomy: case report and literature review. J Parenter Enteral Nutr 25:282–285
Song HY, Park SI, Do YS et al. (1997) Expandable metallic stent placement in patients with benign esophageal strictures: results of long-term follow-up. Radiology 203:131–136
Song HY, Shin JH, Lim JO et al. (2004a) Use of a newly designed multifunctional coil catheter for stent placement in the upper gastrointestinal tract. J Vasc Interv Radiol 15:369–373
Song HY, Shin JH, Yoon CJ et al. (2004b) A dual expandable nitinol stent: experience in 102 patients with malignant gastroduodenal strictures. J Vasc Interv Radiol 15:1443–1449
Strock P, Weber J (2005) Buried bumper syndrome: endoscopic management using a balloon dilator. Endoscopy 37:279
Taller A, Horvath E, Ilias L et al. (2001) Technical modifications for improving the success rate of PEG tube place-

ment in patients with head and neck cancer. Gastrointest Endosc 54:633–636

Tyldesley S, Sheehan F, Munk P et al. (1996) The use of radiologically placed gastrostomy tubes in head and neck cancer patients receiving radiotherapy. Int J Radiat Oncol Biol Phys 36:1205–1209

Vitale MA, Villotti G, D'Alba L et al. (2005) Unsedated transnasal percutaneous endoscopic gastrostomy placement in selected patients. Endoscopy 37:48–51

Wacke W, Hecker U, Woenckhaus C et al. (2004) Percutaneous endoscopic gastrostomy site metastasis in a patient with esophageal cancer. Endoscopy 36:472

Wadhwa RP, Kozarek RA, France RE et al. (2003) Use of self-expandable metallic stents in benign GI diseases. Gastrointest Endosc 58:207–212

Wills JS, Oglesby JT (1983) Percutaneous gastrostomy. Radiology 149:449–453

Wollman B, D'Agostino HB (1997) Percutaneous radiologic and endoscopic gastrostomy: a 3-year institutional analysis of procedure performance. AJR Am J Roentgenol 169:1551–1553

Wollman B, D'Agostino HB, Walus-Wigle JR et al. (1995) Radiologic, endoscopic, and surgical gastrostomy: an institutional evaluation and meta-analysis of the literature. Radiology 197:699–704

Yip D, Vanasco M, Funaki B (2004) Complication rates and patency of radiologically guided mushroom gastrostomy, balloon gastrostomy, and gastrojejunostomy: a review of 250 procedures. Cardiovasc Intervent Radiol 27:3–8

The Acute Stomach and Duodenum

12

Evis Sala and Alan H. Freeman

CONTENTS

12.1 Perforation of Peptic Ulcer

Perforation of peptic ulcer is the most common cause of pneumoperitoneum. Anterior wall ulcers of the stomach and duodenal bulb usually perforate freely into the intraperitoneal space, whereas posterior wall gastric ulcers perforate into the lesser sac. However, a significant proportion of perforated gastric and duodenal ulcers seal off immediately, and free intraperitoneal air can be detected on plain radiography in only 70% of the patients (Rubesin and Levine 2003). An erect chest radiograph and a supine abdominal radiograph are usually obtained if perforation is suspected. Both are very sensitive, and as little as 1 ml of free air can be detected on the horizontal beam examination, which may be aided by the use of a decubitus abdominal radiograph (Fig. 12.1a,b) (Levine et al. 1991). On the erect chest radiograph, air may be shown under one or other diaphragmatic surfaces but rarely both are outlined by air, hence the "continuous diaphragm" sign (Fig. 12.2). Signs of free intraperitoneal air on a supine abdominal radiograph include the "lucent liver" sign, which is air overlying the liver (Fig. 12.3), the "Doges' cap" sign due to a triangle of air in Morrison's pouch (Fig. 12.4), and the "falciform ligament" sign. Note that these are all found in the right upper quadrant, an area that is often not fully included on the supine abdominal film. "Rigler's sign" is the demonstration of both sides of the bowel wall and usually requires the presence of a substantial quantity of intra-abdominal air (Fig. 12.5). Posterior wall duodenal ulcers usually perforate into the retroperitoneal space. A plain abdominal radiograph may reveal a small amount of free retroperitoneal air that sometimes outlines the kidneys or psoas muscles.

A perforation may be confirmed by the administration of water-soluble contrast medium either orally or via a nasogastric tube. Extravasation of

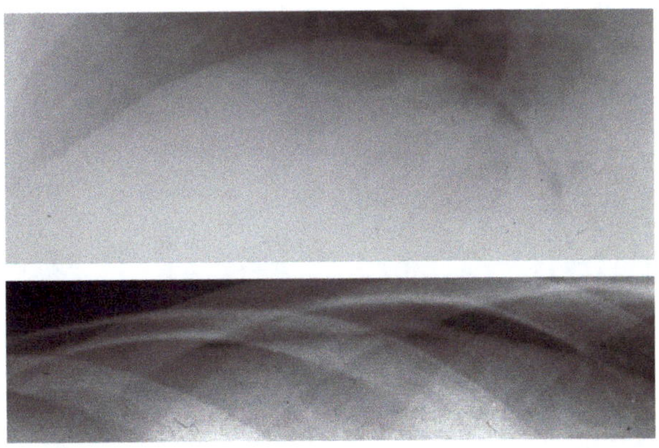

a

b

Fig. 12.1a,b. Perforation of peptic ulcer. **a** Erect abdominal film showing tiny sliver of air under the medial aspect of the right hemidiaphragm. This minimal amount of air was confirmed on a decubitus film (**b**)

E. Sala, MD, PhD, FRCR
Univerity Lecturer/Honorary Consultant Radiologist, Department of Radiology, Addenbrooke's Hospital, Box 219, Hills Road, Cambridge, CB2 2QQ, UK
A. H. Freeman, MB, BS, FRCR
Consultant Radiologist, Department of Radiology, Addenbrooke's Hospital, Box 219, Hills Road, Cambridge, CB2 2QQ, UK

contrast medium from the stomach or duodenal lumen into the peritoneal cavity is only seen in 50% of patients with perforated peptic ulcer (Jacobson et al. 1961). However, CT is the most sensitive imaging technique for diagnosis of free intra-peritoneal air (Jeffrey et al. 1983; Madrazo et al. 1984; Fultz et al. 1992; Rubesin and Levine 2003). Fine bubbles of air or pockets of fluid are usually seen around the wall of stomach and duodenum or adjacent to gastrohepatic and hepatoduodenal ligaments. Small amounts of free intra-abdominal air can be seen in the greater or lesser peritoneal sac, anterior to the liver, in the midline abdomen, and in the peritoneal recesses or retroperitoneal spaces (Fig. 12.6). CT may also demonstrate associated complications such as peritonitis, abscess, pancreatitis, and presence of fistulas to adjacent hollow viscera (Rubesin and Levine 2003).

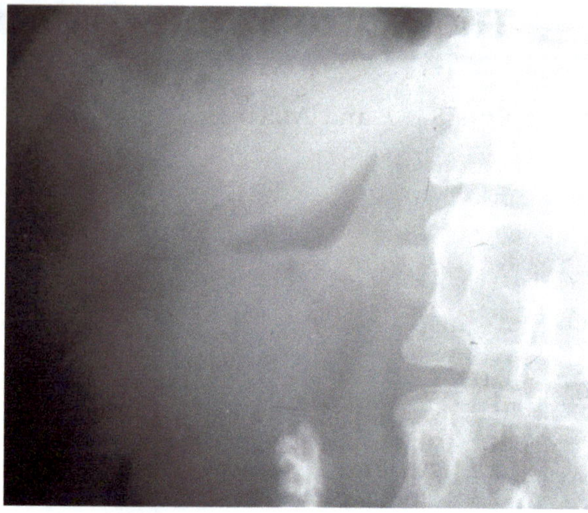

Fig. 12.4. Pneumoperitoneum. "Doges cap" sign due to air in Morrison's pouch

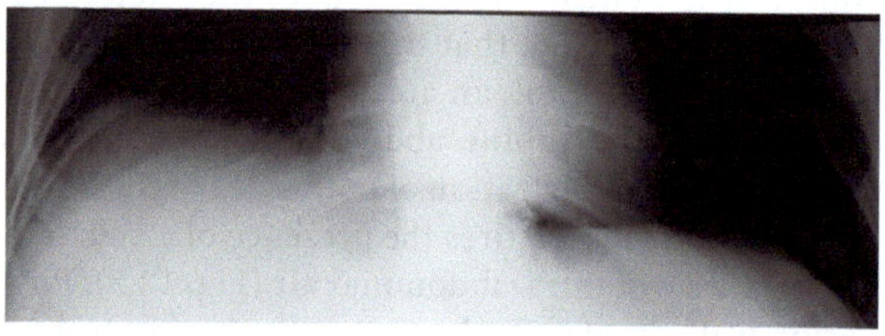

Fig. 12.2. Pneumoperitoneum. Supine abdominal film showing the "continuous diaphragm" sign

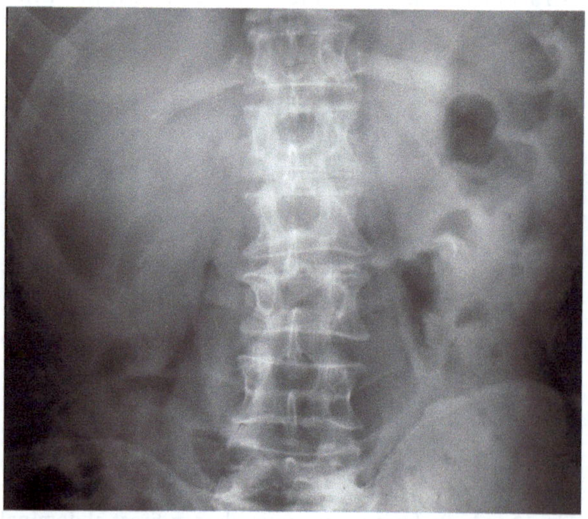

Fig. 12.3. Pneumoperitoneum. Supine abdominal film showing the "lucent liver" sign. Note the opaque left renal calculus

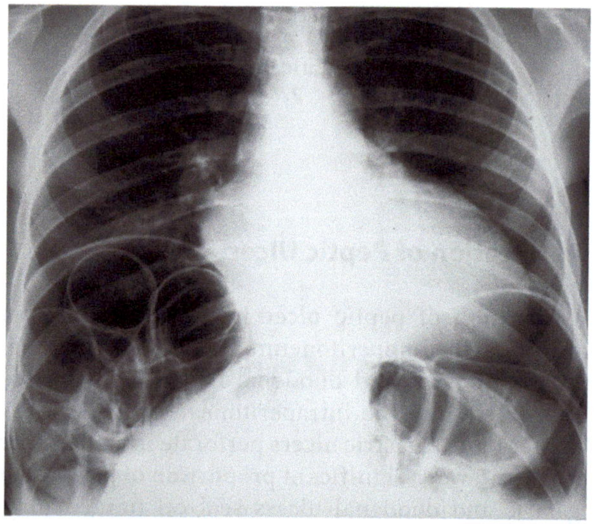

Fig. 12.5. Pneumoperitoneum. Demonstration of Rigler's sign with air outlining both sides of the bowel wall

12.2 Acute Gastric Volvulus

Gastric volvulus occurs when there is abnormal rotation of one part of the stomach around another centred on its normal anatomical fixation. It is a surgical emergency, because a more than 180° of twisting will produce complete obstruction that may lead to vascular compromise. An understanding of the varied clinical features, including both thoracic

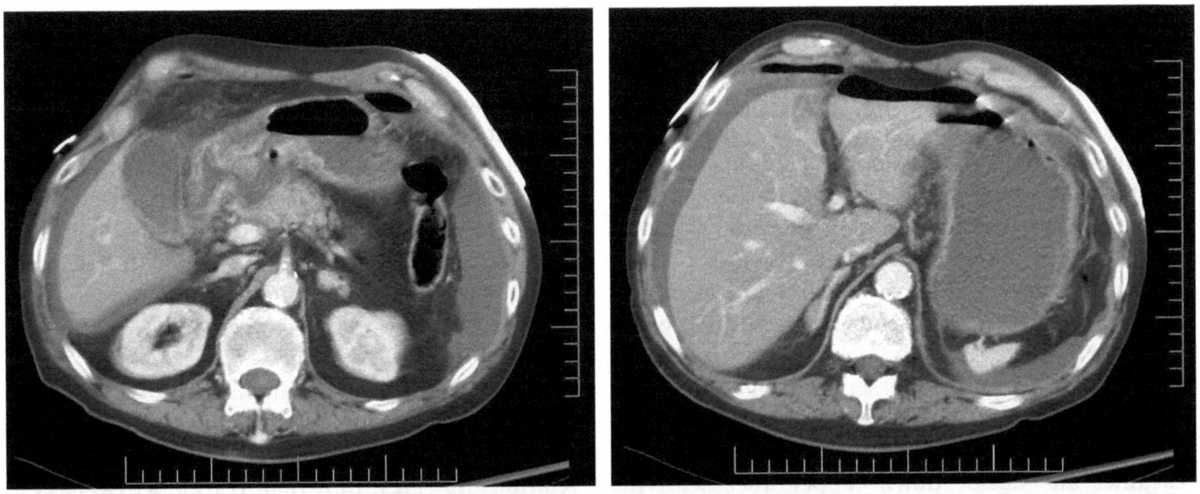
a b

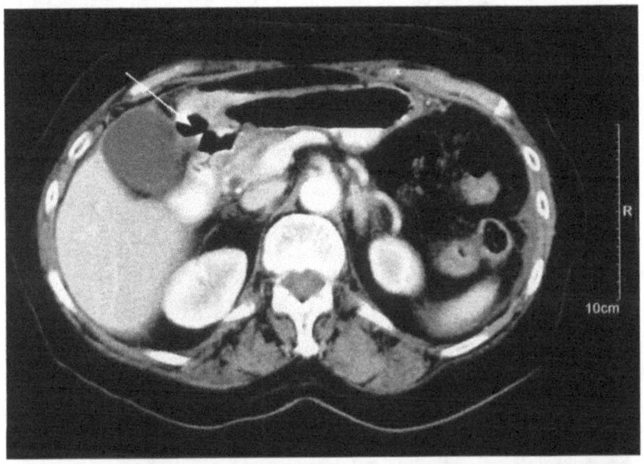

c

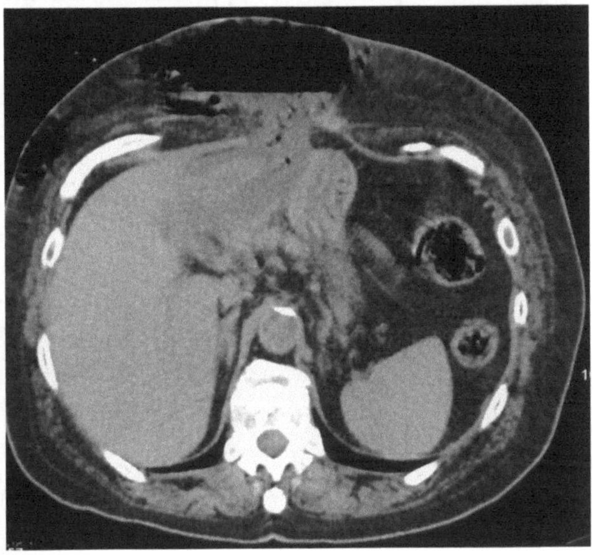
d

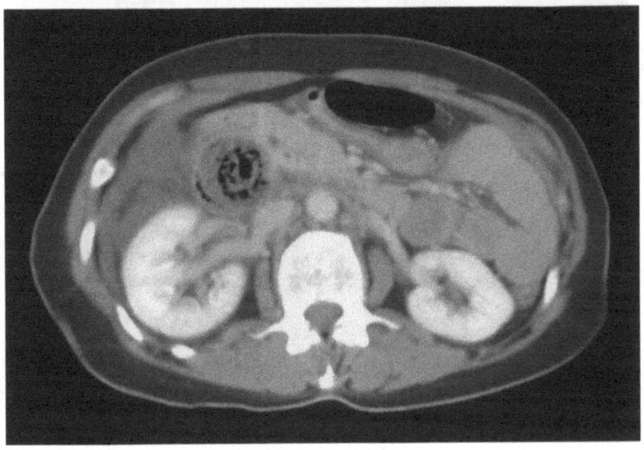
e

Fig. 12.6a–e. Perforation of peptic ulcer. Contrast enhanced CT (CECT) images in five different cases demonstrating: **a** free air anterior to the stomach and free air and fluid in the lesser sac due to perforation of posterior gastric wall ulcer; **b** free intraabdominal air and fluid due to perforation of anterior duodenal bulb ulcer; **c** free air due to duodenal ulcer perforation (*arrow*); **d** free air extending into the anterior abdominal wall due to perforation of a duodenal ulcer; **e** retroperitoneal abscess complicating perforation of a posterior duodenal ulcer

and abdominal manifestations, is essential to early recognition and prompt treatment. Gastric volvulus is most commonly seen in elderly patients with large pre-existing paraoesophageal hiatus hernia (Carter et al. 1980). There is a high incidence of strangulation (up to 28%), which attests to the urgency of this condition and is a compelling reason for the elective repair of paraesophageal hiatus hernias whenever possible (Carter et al. 1980). Other predisposing factors include abnormalities of the suspensory ligaments of the stomach, long gastrohepatic and gastrocolic mesenteries, and eventration of the diaphragm. Diaphragmatic hernia may be complicated by gastric volvulus (Shivanand et al. 2003).

There are two types of gastric volvulus depending on the plane of torsion, organo-axial and mesentero-axial. Organo-axial volvulus is the most common and occurs when the stomach rotates around its long axis, being the line extending from cardia to pylorus. The appearance of the twisted stomach depends on its original position: i.e. if the stomach was in the vertical position, the volvulus causes a right to left twist of the greater curve, whereas if the stomach was in the horizontal position the volvulus flips the greater curve superior to the lesser curve. In the mesentero-axial volvulus, rotation occurs along the plane of the mesenteric attachments of the stomach to the lesser and greater omentum, i.e. the line extending from mid-lesser to mid-greater curve and perpendicular to the long axis of the stomach (Gerson and Lewicki 1976). The twisted stomach assumes an "upside down" appearance with the pylorus and antrum being cranial to the fundus. Mesentero-axial volvulus is often associated with a wide diaphragmatic hiatus and is more likely to have significant clinical consequences due to mesenteric ischaemia (Shivanand et al. 2003).

Plain chest radiograph shows a gas-filled viscus in the lower chest or upper abdomen with an air-fluid level on erect projection. Obstruction at the site of volvulus and abnormal position to different parts of the stomach are best demonstrated by an emergency upper gastrointestinal contrast series (Menuck 1976; Carter et al. 1980; Wasselle and Norman 1993; Shivanand et al. 2003). CT is very useful as it provides a quick diagnosis with very good anatomical details, although the appearances can be confusing because of the changed spatial relationship (Figs. 12.7, 12.8) (Cherukupalli et al. 2003).

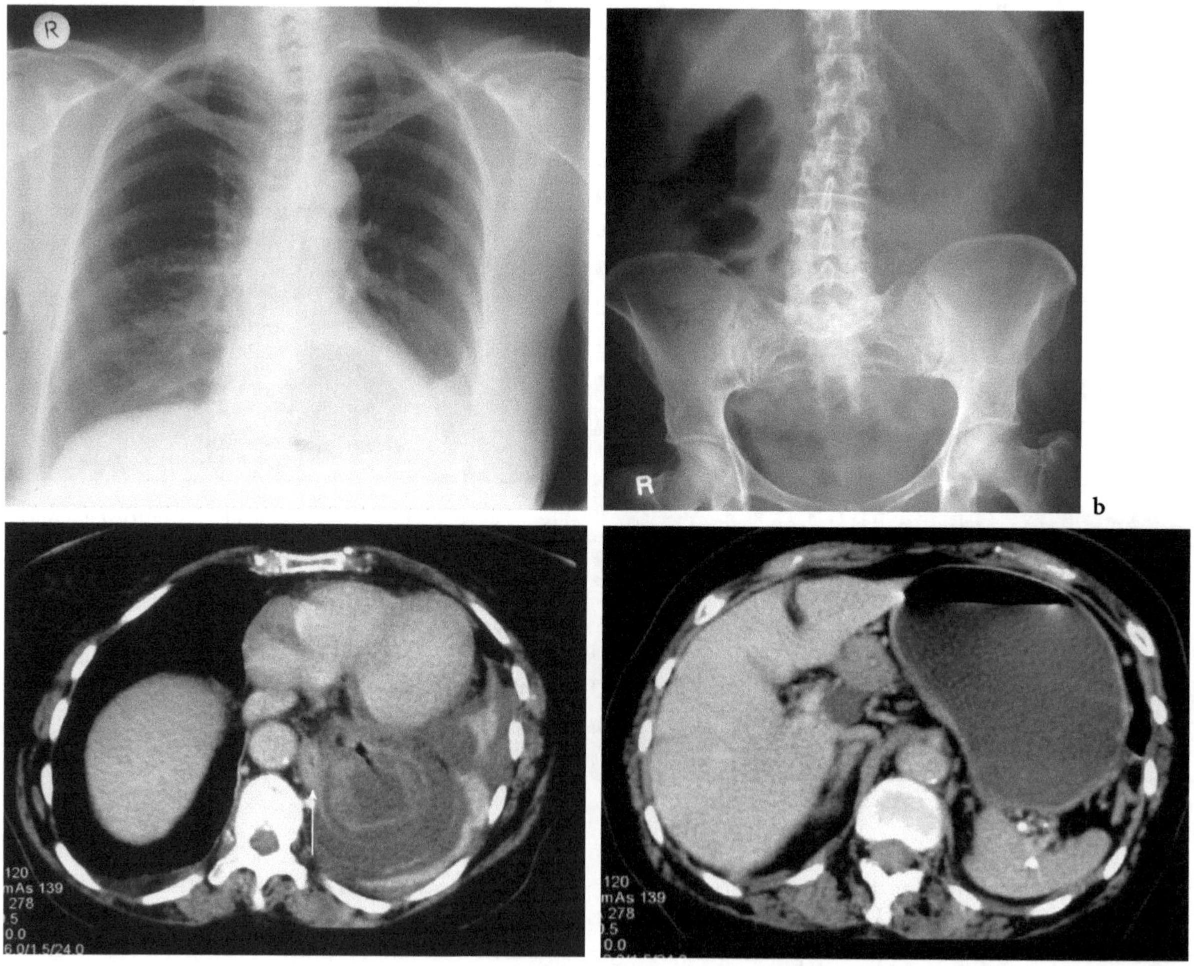

a b c d

Fig. 12.7a–d. Mesentero-axial gastric volvulus: **a** CXR demonstrating an air-filled viscus in the central lower chest that represents the antrum of the volved stomach; **b** AXR showing a gas-filled dilated centrally placed viscus which represents the distended fundus and body; **c** CECT image through the lower chest demonstrates the twisted antrum of the stomach compressing the oesophagus (*arrow*); **d** Images through the upper abdomen demonstrating the dilated fluid filled fundus and body of stomach

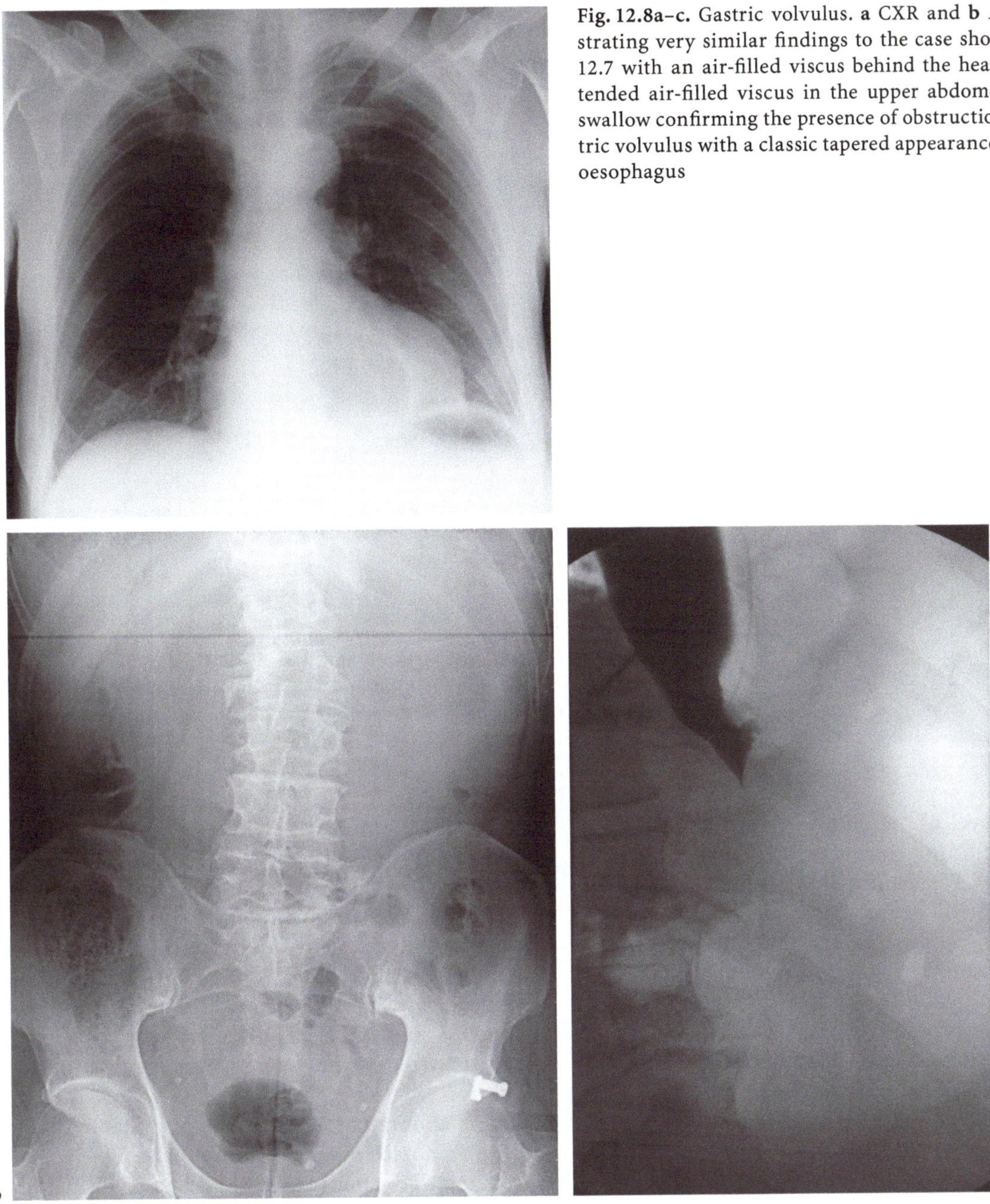

Fig. 12.8a–c. Gastric volvulus. **a** CXR and **b** AXR demonstrating very similar findings to the case shown in Figure 12.7 with an air-filled viscus behind the heart and a distended air-filled viscus in the upper abdomen; **c** barium swallow confirming the presence of obstruction due to gastric volvulus with a classic tapered appearance to the distal oesophagus

12.3 Proximal Small Bowel Volvulus

Midgut volvulus usually occurs in neonates and young children and is due to an abnormal rotation or fixation of both the duodenum and colon, resulting in narrowing of the mesenteric base with potential for mid-gut volvulus (Long et al. 1996). In adults, congenital anomalies of intestinal rotation are usually incidental findings. Any symptoms present may be the result of intermittent volvulus of the small bowel (Bernstein and Russ 1998). In children, plain abdominal X-ray (AXR) may show a distended stomach and proximal duodenum. The diagnosis of the malrotation is confirmed on a contrast study, which may also show the abnormally placed caecum (Fig. 12.9). In adults, plain AXR may show a paucity of small bowel loops on one side of the abdomen. Barium studies demonstrate a malpositioned duodenal-jejunal junction that is sited

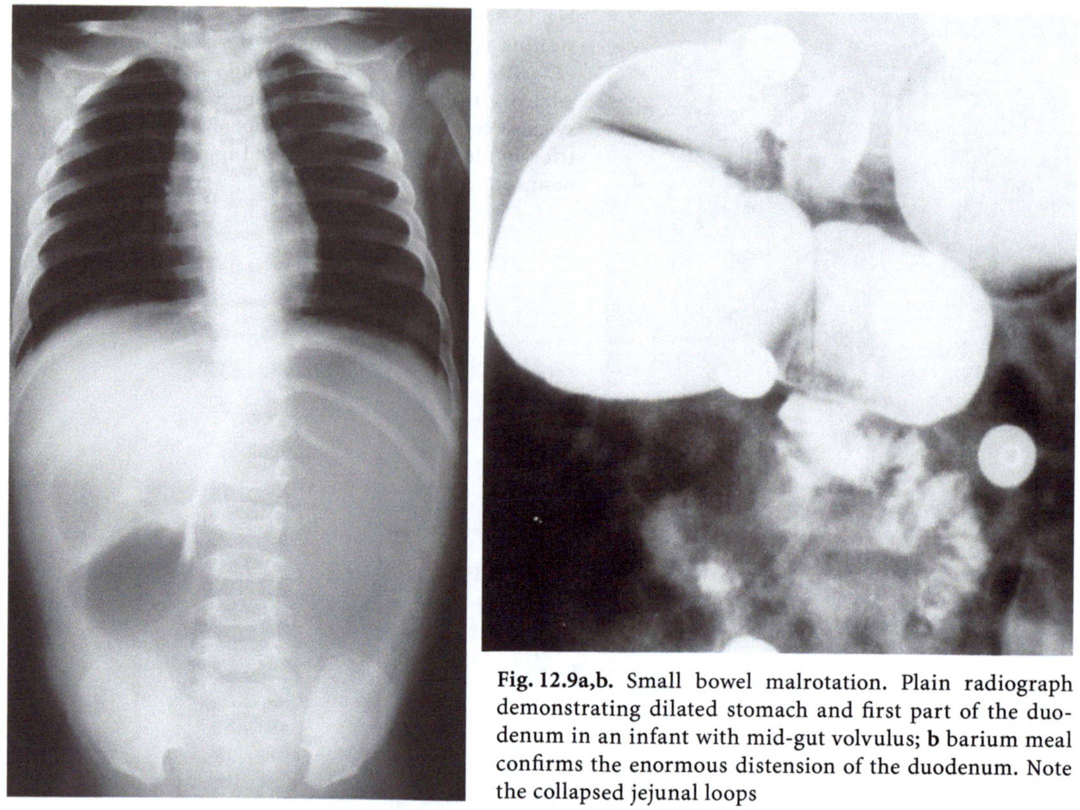

a

b

Fig. 12.9a,b. Small bowel malrotation. Plain radiograph demonstrating dilated stomach and first part of the duodenum in an infant with mid-gut volvulus; **b** barium meal confirms the enormous distension of the duodenum. Note the collapsed jejunal loops

below the level of the duodenal bulb on the right. Additional findings include thickening of the duodenal folds. CT elegantly demonstrates a whirl-like pattern of small bowel loops and mesenteric vessels with adjacent mesenteric fat converging to the point of torsion. The superior mesenteric vein may also be seen to the left of the superior mesenteric artery (SMA), i.e. reverse vessel position (Figs. 12.10, 12.11) (Paul and Dean 1990). Complications include intestinal ischaemia and necrosis in the SMA supply territory.

12.4 Emphysematous Gastritis

Emphysematous gastritis is caused by an infection of an already disrupted mucosa by gas-forming organisms, most commonly *Escherichia coli* and *Clostridium welchii* (Fishman et al. 1996). Predisposing factors that lead to disruption of gastric mucosa include ingestion of toxic or corrosive substances, alcohol abuse, trauma, peptic ulcer disease, gastric infarction, and recent gastro-duodenal surgery. There is no age or sex predilection and no association with diabetes mellitus (Meyers and Parker 1967; Grayson et al. 2002). Gas in the stomach wall is thought to be a combination of nitrogen and carbon dioxide secondary to the fermentation of glucose by bacteria (Grayson et al. 2002). Emphysematous gastritis carries a bad prognosis with up to 80% mortality, hence appropriate imaging and accurate interpretation play an important role in the prompt management of this condition.

Plain abdominal radiograph may demonstrate multiple bubbles of air outlining the stomach causing a mottled appearance (Meyers and Parker 1967). Water-soluble contrast meal may demonstrate thickened gastric folds due to mucosal oedema and confirm the intramural presence of gas (Meyers and Parker 1967). However, conventional studies are superseded by CT, which is currently the imaging modality of choice for detection of gas within the grossly thickened gastric wall (de Lange et al. 1986; Fishman et al. 1996; Grayson et al. 2002; Horton and Fishman 2003). CT is also valuable in demonstrating additional features such as pneumoperitoneum or gas in the portal vein, and late complications such as strictures and fistulas if present (Grayson et al. 2002).

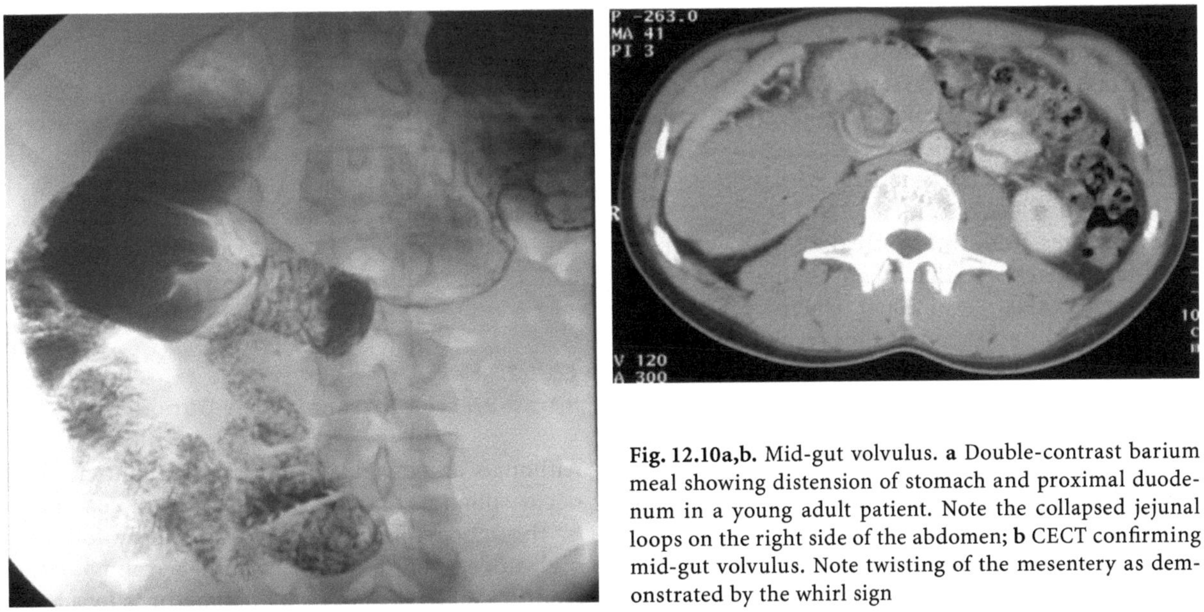

a b

Fig. 12.10a,b. Mid-gut volvulus. **a** Double-contrast barium meal showing distension of stomach and proximal duodenum in a young adult patient. Note the collapsed jejunal loops on the right side of the abdomen; **b** CECT confirming mid-gut volvulus. Note twisting of the mesentery as demonstrated by the whirl sign

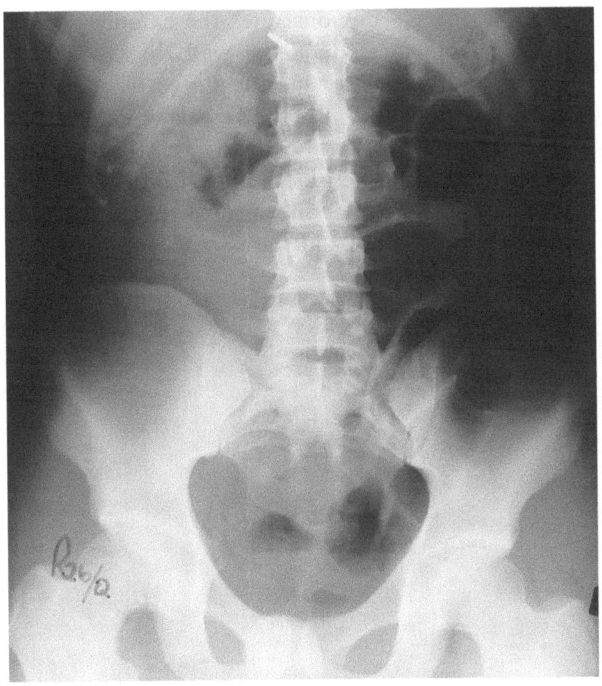

a

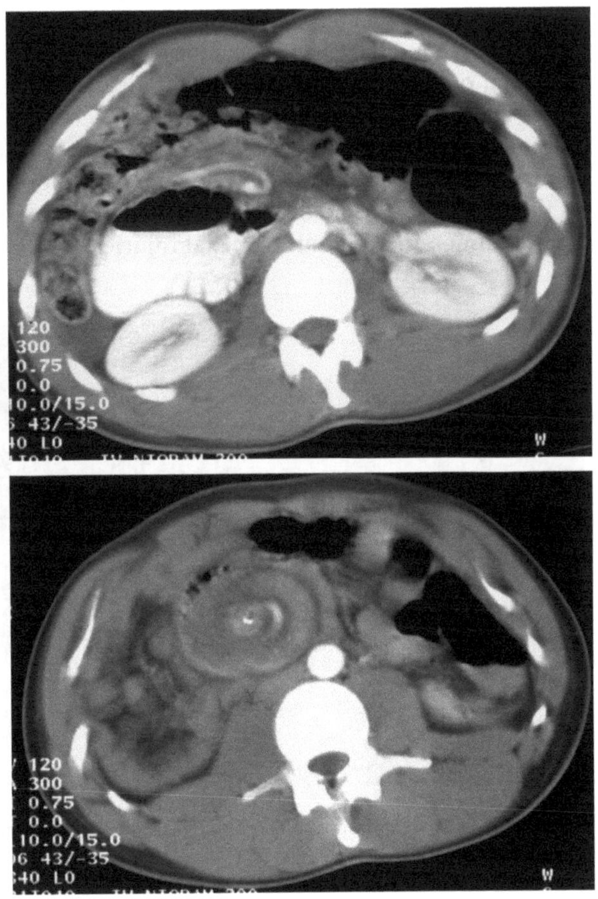

b c

Fig. 12.11a-c. Mid-gut volvulus. **a** AXR showing paucity of bowel gas in the right abdomen in a young adult patient; **b** CECT showing the dilated descending duodenum and the superior mesenteric artery curving towards the right. **c** A more caudal image demonstrating the “whirl” sign through the mesentery. Note all the collapsed jejunal loops in the right abdomen

Air in the stomach wall can also be seen in gastric emphysema, which is a benign condition and thus is important to differentiate from emphysematous gastritis. It is usually associated with severe obstructive pulmonary disease, violent coughing or vomiting, instrumentation, gastric outlet obstruction, and gastric volvulus (Fig. 12.12) (Grayson et al. 2002). CT demonstrates thin, linear streaks of air within the normal stomach wall that do not change with patient position (Grayson et al. 2002). The patient is usually asymptomatic, and spontaneous resolution occurs.

12.5 Injuries to the Stomach and Duodenum

Gastric or duodenal injuries are frequently part of multi-organ trauma that can be classified as penetrating or blunt. The major causes of blunt injuries are road traffic accidents (mainly due to steering wheel impact) or direct blows to the mid-abdomen. Serious blunt trauma to the abdomen can lead to the rupture of the stomach or duodenum, the former being very rare. Blunt injuries to the duodenum (typically associated with seat-belt injuries) usually affect the second part, resulting in intra-mural haematoma; or they cause rupture of the third/fourth parts due to a shearing effect against the vertebral bodies. Very occasionally, blunt trauma can cause avulsion of the pancreatic and bile duct at the level of the papilla. Associated trauma of the pancreas is very common in all blunt duodenal injuries.

12.5.1 Rupture of the Stomach

This is a rare event, the stomach being more susceptible if distended with food or fluid. Direct blows may produce partial or full thickness tear, with the latter allowing spillage of gastric content into the general peritoneal cavity well demonstrated by CECT (Fig. 12.13).

12.5.2 Intramural Haematoma of the Duodenum

Although duodenal intramural haematoma may occur spontaneously, particularly in anticoagulated or thrombocytopenic patients, it usually follows a high-impact blunt mid-abdominal trauma either from a road traffic accident or sometimes by a horse kick. Plain abdominal radiograph is often unhelpful. Contrast studies show a concentric intraluminal filling defect, usually in the second part of the duodenum (Fig. 12.14a). A "coil spring" appearance is produced by thickening of valvulae conniventes due to blood infiltration and oedema (Felson and Levin 1954). CT demonstrates the extent of injury ranging from focal duodenal wall thickening to a large mixed attenuation mass typical of a haematoma together with stranding of the peri-pancreatic fat, etc. (Darrah and Nolan 1999; Jayaraman et al. 2001). Sometimes extensive blood clot within the duodenum may give a similar appearance, though its intraluminal position is usually apparent (Fig. 12.14b).

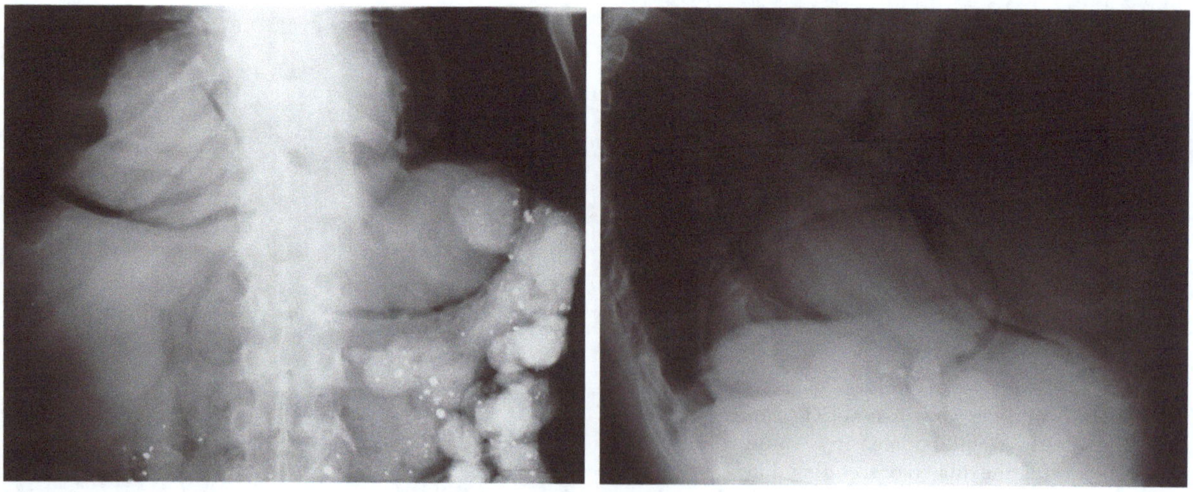

a b

Fig. 12.12a,b. Gastric emphysema complicating gastric volvulus. **a** Upper AXR and **b** lateral CXR showing the presence of the intramural air in a patient with a volvulus of an intrathoracic stomach. Residual barium is present from a contrast study performed a few days before

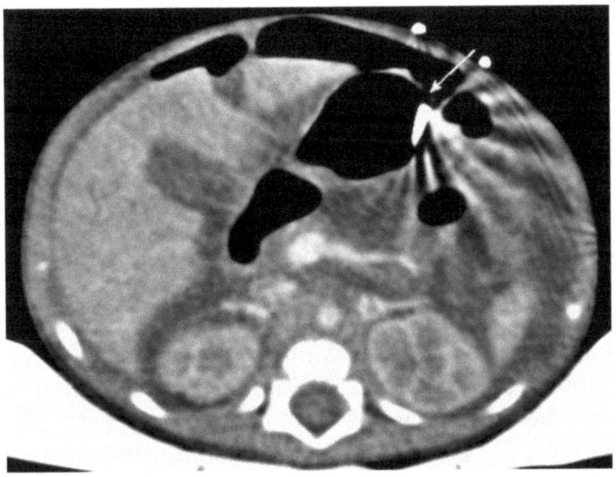

a

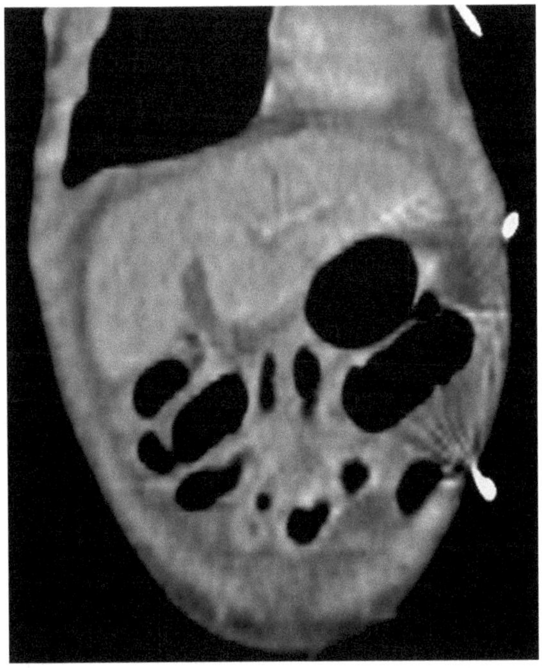

b

Fig. 12.13a,b. Traumatic gastric tear. CECT axial **a** and coronal **b** images demonstrating free intraperitoneal air and fluid due to a 3-cm tear (*arrow*) of the greater curve of the stomach in a 6-week-old baby who suffered blunt trauma to his abdomen. Note the tip of the nasogastric tube at the site of the tear

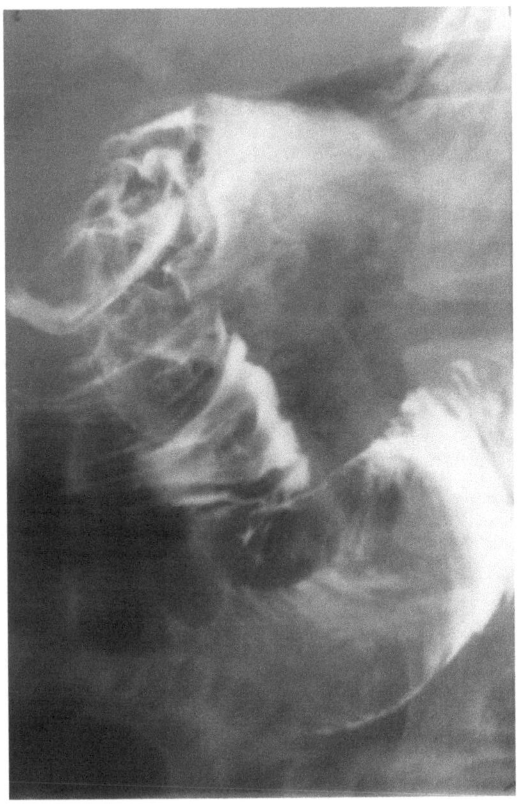

a

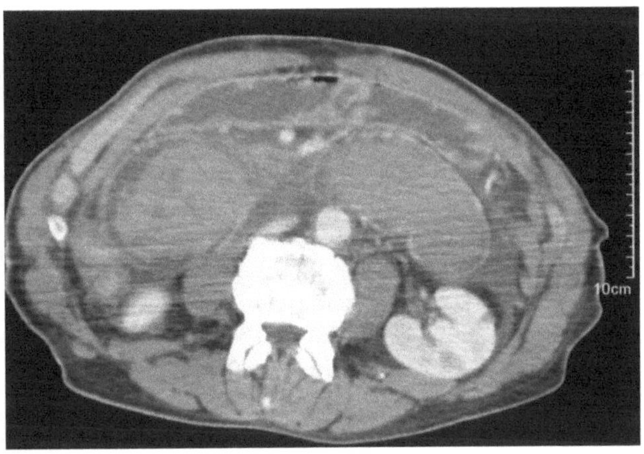

b

Fig. 12.14a,b. Duodenal haematomas. **a** A barium study showing an intramural haematoma in an anticoagulated patient; **b** CECT demonstrating massive intraluminal clot arising from a bleeding duodenal ulcer also in an anticoagulated patient

12.5.3
Retroperitoneal Rupture of the Duodenum

At CT the diagnosis of duodenal rupture should be suspected in the presence of free air or contrast medium in the retroperitoneum (adjacent to the duodenum, kidneys, and psoas muscles), free retroperitoneal fluid, mesenteric haematoma, and pancreatic transection (Hofer and Cohen 1989; Brody et al. 2000; Maniatis et al. 2000; Jayaraman et al. 2001). Focal discontinuity of the duodenal wall can be seen occasionally (see Fig. 12.25).

Imaging plays a crucial role in the diagnosis and management of patients with blunt duodenal trauma, as the choice of treatment is dependent on whether there is just a haematoma present or a perforation. Intramural haematoma is usually managed conservatively, whereas duodenal rupture represents a genuine surgical emergency (Weigelt 1990; Darrah and Nolan 1999). CT is the investigation of choice (Hofer and Cohen 1989; Brody et al. 2000; Maniatis et al. 2000), particularly with the multiplanar reconstruction abilities of multi-slice CT.

12.6
Diaphragmatic Rupture

Diaphragmatic rupture can occur due to both significant penetrating and blunt thoraco-abdominal trauma. It occurs in up to 8% of patients after blunt trauma, 90% of which are due to road traffic accidents (Iochum et al. 2002). There is a high incidence of associated injuries (52–100%), with pelvic fractures, liver, splenic, and renal injuries being the most common. Thoracic injuries such as rib fractures and pneumohaemothorax are very common (Iochum et al. 2002). Most tears are at least 10 cm long, radially oriented and usually occur at the weakest part of the diaphragm in the postero-lateral aspect (Kuhlman et al. 1998). Left- and right-sided tears occur with equal frequencies, but left-sided ones are diagnosed more easily than the right-sided tears, the majority of which are missed. This is due to the fact that liver herniation through a right-sided tear retains the smooth contour of the hemidiaphragm, which is taken to be of normal appearance on a chest radiograph (Killeen et al. 1999). Herniated organs in order of frequency include stomach, colon, small bowel, omentum, spleen, etc. Extension of tears into the central tendon and bilateral tears are uncommon (2%–6%) (Shanmuganathan et al. 2000). Penetrating injuries are more common than blunt ones, and the tear is usually less then 1 cm in diameter and more likely to be overlooked (Shackleton et al. 1998).

Prompt diagnosis of diaphragmatic rupture is very important since surgical repair of tears is mandatory, as they do not heal spontaneously. The chest radiograph is not very sensitive in the diagnosis of diaphragmatic rupture, being abnormal in under 60% of left-sided injuries and only 17% of right-sided injuries (Shanmuganathan and Mirvis 1999). Radiographic findings include elevation of the hemidiaphragm, loss of the diaphragmatic contour, contralateral mediastinal shift, and presence of hollow viscera within the thorax (Figs. 12.15, 12.16a). Sometimes, a coiled nasogastric tube may be seen within the left hemithorax (Gelman et al. 1991; Dee 1992; Shackleton et al. 1998). Ultrasound (US) is very good in visualising the diaphragm, especially if outlined by fluid and can reliably diagnose tears. However, this examination is difficult if the patient is very tender or if there are complications such as extensive surgical emphysema, pneumothorax, etc. which will impair visualisation of the diaphragm.

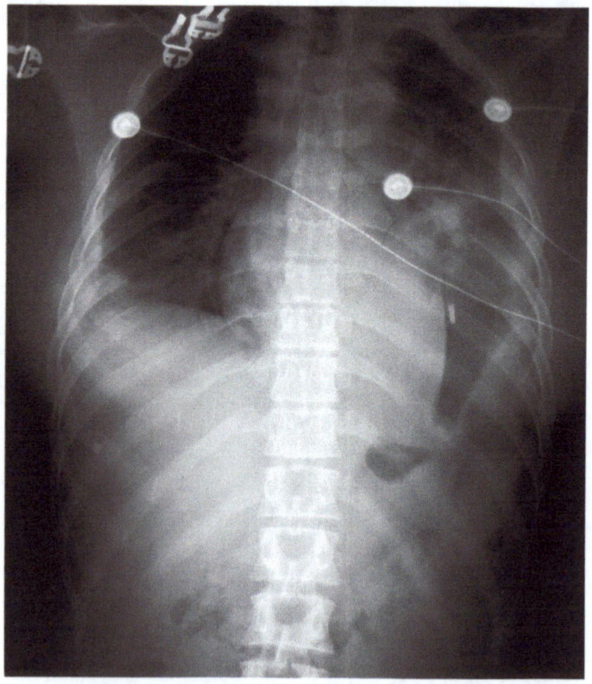

Fig. 12.15. Traumatic diaphragmatic hernia. Plain radiograph in a patient with left-sided traumatic diaphragmatic hernia showing loss of diaphragmatic contour and presence of a hollow viscus within the left hemithorax. Note the position of the nasogastric tube confirming the viscus as being stomach. Image courtesy of Dr. Robin Gibney

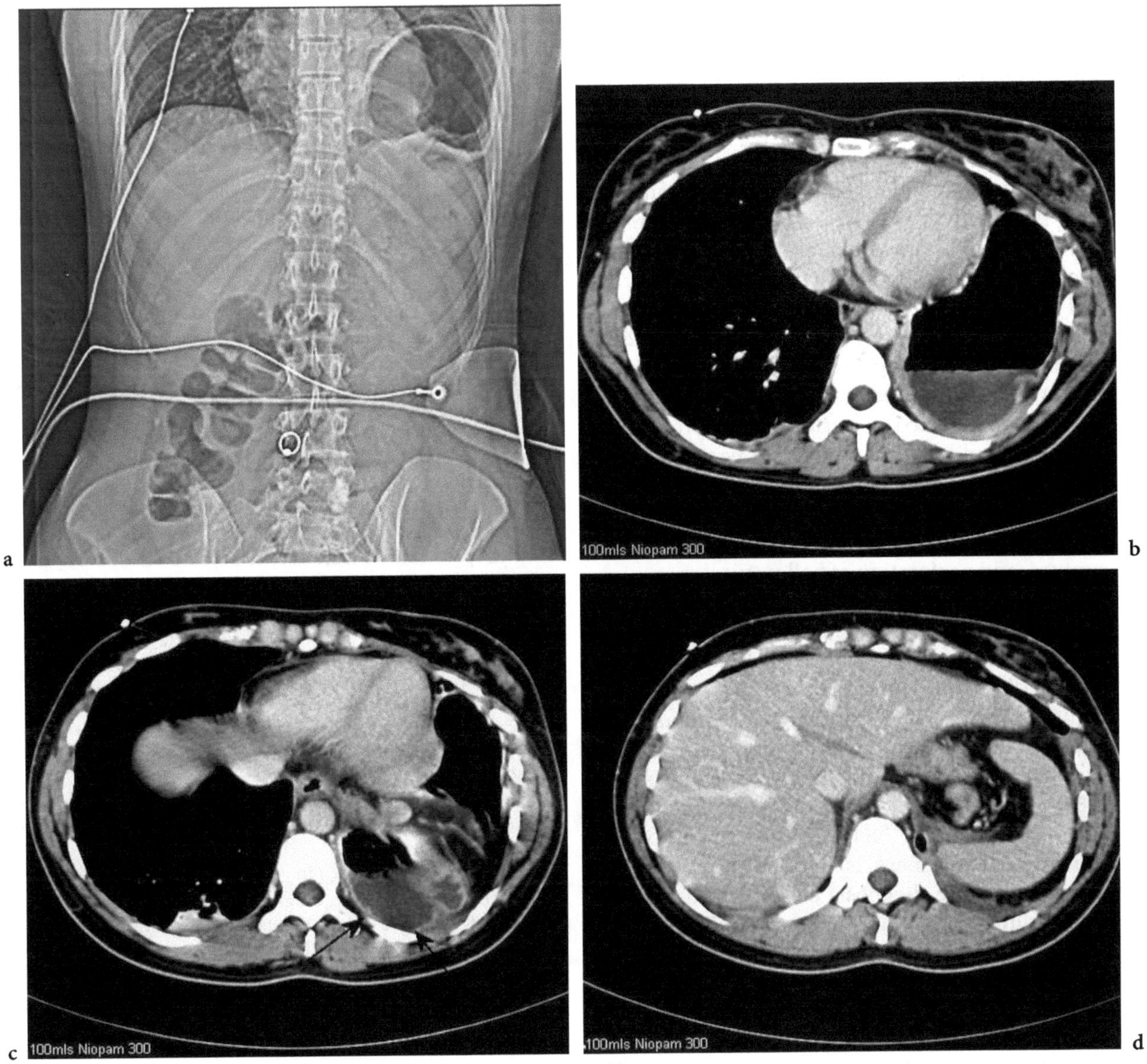

Fig. 12.16a–d. Traumatic diaphragmatic rupture. **a** Scanogram and **b–d** CECT images of a young female patient with a traumatic diaphragmatic rupture following a road traffic accident. Note the "dependent viscera" sign (*black arrows*)

These factors together with its operator dependence limit the role of US in routine imaging of the diaphragmatic rupture (Shackleton et al. 1998).

CT is the best available technique, though it is sometimes difficult to visualise the dome of the diaphragm, as it usually lies tangential to the axial plane. Multi-slice CT with its ability to produce coronal and sagittal reformatted images has significantly improved the sensitivity and specificity of CT in this role (Shanmuganathan et al. 2000; Killeen et al. 2002). The sensitivity of CT approaches 70% (78% for left-sided and 50% for right-sided tears), with a specificity of 100%. It has an accuracy of over 85% for left-sided tears and 70% for right-sided tears (Killeen et al. 1999; Shanmuganathan et al. 2000). Features of diaphragmatic rupture on CT include interruption of normal diaphragmatic contour, which is the most sensitive sign of rupture (Worthy et al. 1995; Murray et al. 1996). It should be noted that the presence of a diaphragmatic defect is not specific for a rupture, as postero-lateral defects, thought to represent congenital asymptomatic Bochdalek hernias, are detected in 6% of asymptomatic adults attending for routine CT examination (Caskey et al. 1989).

Herniation of abdominal contents into the chest such as omentum, stomach, and colon on the left and liver in the right are very helpful signs (Murray et al. 1996). The most frequently encountered sign is the "collar sign", i.e. constriction of the stomach as it passes through the tear into the chest on the left side. In right-sided tears, an indentation of the liver is caused as it passes through the tear. This can be very subtle and often overlooked if only axial images are reviewed, making reformats in coronal and sagittal plane mandatory (Murray et al. 1996; Shackleton et al. 1998; Killeen et al. 1999, 2002). A very useful early sign is the "dependent viscera" sign, which is produced by herniated viscera that are no longer supported posteriorly by the torn hemidiaphragm and fall to a dependent position against the posterior ribs (Fig. 12.16b–d) (Bergin et al. 2001; Iochum et al. 2002). CT can also diagnose any associated injuries such as fractures of lower ribs, splenic rupture, and perforation of hollow viscera.

Magnetic resonance imaging (MRI) is excellent in diagnosis of diaphragmatic injuries, as direct multiplanar imaging is very helpful in detecting small tears. These are best shown on T1W sequence, where the diaphragm appears as a low-intensity line outlined on either side by high-intensity mediastinal and abdominal fat (Mirvis et al. 1988; Shanmuganathan et al. 1996; Mirvis and Shanmuganathan 2000). The use of intravenous contrast enhancement is optional but is usually indicated for the diagnosis of associated intrathoracic injuries. MRI findings are similar to those seen in CT and include abrupt disruption of normal diaphragmatic contour and intrathoracic herniation of omentum or various intra-abdominal viscera (Mirvis et al. 1988; Shanmuganathan et al. 1996; Mirvis and Shanmuganathan 2000). The use of MRI in acute settings is limited due to MRI incompatibility of some life support devices used in trauma patients. However, it can be effectively used in patients with a doubtful CT diagnosis and in subacute or chronic tears (Iochum et al. 2002).

References

Bergin D, Ennis R et al (2001) The "dependent viscera" sign in CT diagnosis of blunt traumatic diaphragmatic rupture. AJR Am J Roentgenol 177:1137–1140

Bernstein SM, Russ PD (1998) Midgut volvulus: a rare cause of acute abdomen in an adult patient. AJR Am J Roentgenol 171:639–641

Brody JM, Leighton DB et al (2000) CT of blunt trauma bowel and mesenteric injury: typical findings and pitfalls in diagnosis. Radiographics 20:1525–1536; discussion 1536–1537

Carter R, Brewer LA 3rd et al (1980) Acute gastric volvulus. A study of 25 cases. Am J Surg 140:99–106

Caskey CI, Zerhouni EA et al (1989) Aging of the diaphragm: a CT study. Radiology 171:385–389

Cherukupalli C, Khaneja S et al (2003) CT diagnosis of acute gastric volvulus." Dig Surg 20:497–499

Darrah ER, Nolan DJ (1999) Radiology of the duodenum. Hosp Med 60:10–18

De Lange EE, Slutsky VS et al (1986) Computed tomography of emphysematous gastritis. J Comput Assist Tomogr 10:139–141

Dee PM (1992) The radiology of chest trauma. Radiol Clin North Am 30:291–306

Felson B, Levin EJ (1954) Intramural hematoma of the duodenum: a diagnostic roentgen sign. Radiology 63:823–831

Fishman EK, Urban BA et al (1996) CT of the stomach: spectrum of disease. Radiographics 16:1035–1054

Fultz PJ, Skucas J et al (1992) CT in upper gastrointestinal tract perforations secondary to peptic ulcer disease. Gastrointest Radiol 17:5–8

Gelman R, Mirvis SE et al (1991) Diaphragmatic rupture due to blunt trauma: sensitivity of plain chest radiographs. AJR Am J Roentgenol 156:51–57

Gerson DE, Lewicki AM (1976) Intrathoracic stomach: when does it obstruct? Radiology 119:257–264

Grayson DE, Abbott RM et al (2002) Emphysematous infections of the abdomen and pelvis: a pictorial review. Radiographics 22:543–561

Hofer GA, Cohen AJ (1989) CT signs of duodenal perforation secondary to blunt abdominal trauma. J Comput Assist Tomogr 13:430–432

Horton KM, Fishman EK (2003) Current role of CT in imaging of the stomach. Radiographics 23:75–87

Iochum S, Ludig T et al (2002) Imaging of diaphragmatic injury: a diagnostic challenge? Radiographics 22 Spec No: S103–S116; discussion S116–118

Jacobson G, Berne CJ et al (1961) The examination of patients with suspected perforated ulcer using a water-soluble contrast medium. Am J Roentgenol Radium Ther Nucl Med 86:37–49

Jayaraman MV, Mayo-Smith WW et al (2001) CT of the duodenum: an overlooked segment gets its due. Radiographics 21 (Spec No):S147–S160

Jeffrey RB, Federle MP et al (1983) Value of computed tomography in detecting occult gastrointestinal perforation. J Comput Assist Tomogr 7:825–827

Killeen KL, Mirvis SE et al (1999) Helical CT of diaphragmatic rupture caused by blunt trauma. AJR Am J Roentgenol 173:1611–1616

Killeen KL, Shanmuganathan K et al (2002) Imaging of traumatic diaphragmatic injuries. Semin Ultrasound CT MR 23:184–192

Kuhlman JE, Pozniak MA et al (1998) Radiographic and CT findings of blunt chest trauma: aortic injuries and looking beyond them. Radiographics 18:1085–1106; discussion 1107–1108; quiz 1

Levine MS, Scheiner JD et al (1991) Diagnosis of pneumoperitoneum on supine abdominal radiographs. AJR Am J Roentgenol 156:731–735

Long FR, Kramer SS et al (1996) Radiographic patterns of intestinal malrotation in children. Radiographics 16:547–556; discussion 556–560
Madrazo BL, Halpert RD et al (1984) Computed tomographic findings in penetrating peptic ulcer. Radiology 153:751–754
Maniatis V, Chryssikopoulos H et al (2000) Perforation of the alimentary tract: evaluation with computed tomography. Abdom Imaging 25:373–379
Menuck L (1976) Plain film findings of gastric volvulus herniating into the chest. Am J Roentgenol 126:1169–1174
Meyers HI, Parker JJ (1967) Emphysematous gastritis. Radiology 89:426–431
Mirvis SE, Shanmuganathan K (2000) MR imaging of thoracic trauma." Magn Reson Imaging Clin North Am 8:91–104
Mirvis SE, Keramati B et al (1988) MR imaging of traumatic diaphragmatic rupture. J Comput Assist Tomogr 12:147–149
Murray JG, Caoili E et al (1996) Acute rupture of the diaphragm due to blunt trauma: diagnostic sensitivity and specificity of CT. AJR Am J Roentgenol 166:1035–1039
Paul AB, Dean DM (1990) Computed tomography in volvulus of the midgut. Br J Radiol 63:893–894
Rubesin SE, Levine MS (2003) Radiologic diagnosis of gastrointestinal perforation. Radiol Clin North Am 41:1095–1115, v
Shackleton KL, Stewart ET et al (1998) Traumatic diaphragmatic injuries: spectrum of radiographic findings. Radiographics 18:49–59
Shanmuganathan K, Killeen K et al (2000) Imaging of diaphragmatic injuries." J Thorac Imaging 15:104–111
Shanmuganathan K, Mirvis SE (1999) Imaging diagnosis of nonaortic thoracic injury. Radiol Clin North Am 37:533–551, vi
Shanmuganathan K, Mirvis SE et al (1996) MR imaging evaluation of hemidiaphragms in acute blunt trauma: experience with 16 patients. AJR Am J Roentgenol 167:397–402
Shivanand G, Seema S et al (2003) Gastric volvulus: acute and chronic presentation. Clin Imaging 27:265–268
Wasselle JA, Norman J (1993) Acute gastric volvulus: pathogenesis, diagnosis, and treatment. Am J Gastroenterol 88:1780–1784
Weigelt JA (1990) Duodenal injuries. Surg Clin North Am 70:529–539
Worthy SA, Kang EY et al (1995) Diaphragmatic rupture: CT findings in 11 patients. Radiology 194:885–888

The Postoperative Stomach and Duodenum

13

Peter Pokieser, Ahmed Ba-Ssalamah, and Mazda Memarsadeghi

CONTENTS

13.1 Introduction

The goal of imaging, when investigating the postoperative stomach and duodenum, is to rule out or to detect early and late postoperative complications. Clinical and laboratory findings, as well as endoscopy and imaging have to be considered in an interdisciplinary setting. Fluoroscopy and CT represent the basic imaging modalities which provide specific information on the evaluation of the normal postoperative state, as well as the detection of leaks, fistulas, haematomas, abcesses, obstruction, malignant disease and functional disorders.

Fluoroscopy, best combined with video recording, is ideal to follow directly the course of contrast material and the movements of the bowel wall. However, CT is the best modality to depict morphologic details, abnormalities of the bowel wall and of extraintestinal structures.

This chapter concentrates on the numerous surgical procedures in groups, and reviews the specific radiologic findings pertinent to the clinical background and the therapeutic intentions.

13.1.1 General Considerations

Immediate complications are managed during or just after the procedure and usually do not require imaging, although it may be necessary in some cases such as hematoma or cardio pulmonary problems. For many later postoperative complications, radiologic imaging plays the key role for diagnosis.

P. Pokieser, MD
Medical Media Services of the Core Unit of Medical Education and Department of Radiology, University of Vienna, Waehringer Gürtel 18–20, 1090 Vienna, Austria

A. Ba-Ssalamah, MD
M. Memarsadeghi, MD
Department of Radiology, University of Vienna, Waehringer Gürtel 18–20, 1090 Vienna, Austria

13.1.2 Postoperative Complications after Gastric Surgery

13.1.2.1 Early Complications

Common
- Anastomotic or staple-line leak
- Leak after dilatation
- Anastomotic oedema
- Anastomotic narrowing
- Hypotony or atony of the gut

Uncommon
- Haematoma, abscess
- Ischemia
- Intestinal injury

13.1.2.2 Late Complications

Common
- Stricture of anastomosis or leak after dilatation
- Gastroesophageal reflux and its sequelae
- Gastrointestinal obstruction
- Recurrent carcinoma

Uncommon
- Fistula or leaks
- Malnutrition
- Functional disorders

13.2 Imaging Techniques

Precontrast images are very useful, since calcifications, drains, clips and contrast material from previous investigations can mimic leaks (Fig. 13.1).

Leak or staple line dehiscences are the most likely cause of postoperative problems (Woodfield and Levine 2005). Leaks may appear as small tracks or collections near the anastomosis or suture line (Fig. 13.2). Iodinated water soluble contrast material is recommended for the early postoperative phase as it does not have any damaging effects on the surrounding structures in case of leakage (Woodfield and Levine 2005). Erect and horizontal positions

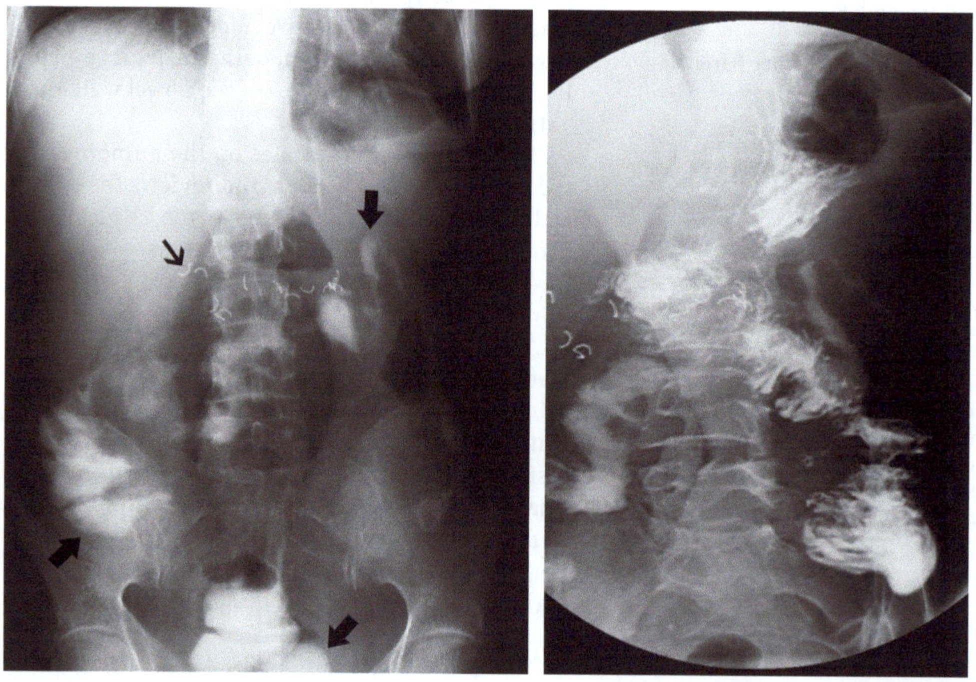

a b

Fig. 13.1a,b. A 47 year old woman after multiple abdominal operations, including a Bilroth II procedure and extensive resections of small bowel. A fistula at the level of the anastomosis of the gastric remnant was suspected at endoscopy. **a** Precontrast images show contrast in the colon from a previous study one week ago (*thick arrows*) and suture material (*thin arrow*). **b** Upper GI images show no sign of a fistula. No change in the appearance of the contrast of the colon also suggests a negative study based on information from the precontrast images

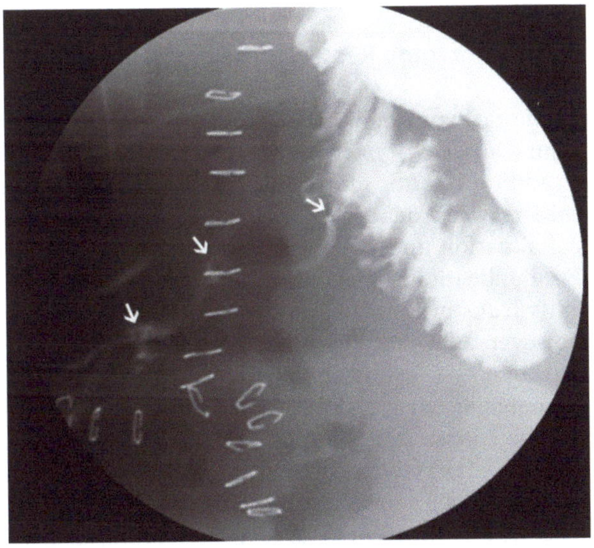

Fig. 13.2. A 25 year old man suffered a penetrating knife injury, with laceration of the duodenum. Fever, tachycardia and general condition of the patient suggested postoperative complications. *Arrows* indicate the persistent duodenal leak. This was followed by successful reoperation

allow coating of the anastomoses and the upper gastro-intestinal (GI) tract. Imaging and video recording should be obtained in two perpendicular planes for optimal projection of structures. Barium may be utilised when a leak has been ruled out by water soluble contrast material. The higher sensitivity of barium for small leaks is an argument for such a strategy. On the other hand, barium causes artifacts, which will affect a CT examination if performed shortly after an upper GI series. An alternative is to proceed directly to CT when the water soluble upper GI series is suspicious for a leak. If possible an interval of some hours is recommended to allow precontrast CT images to be acquired. Double contrast barium studies with effervescent powder are suitable for patients in the late period, 30 or more days after surgery. When general symptoms are present, CT is crucial to detect fluid collections, haematomas, recurrent tumour, metastases and wound complications. Finally, it is worth remembering that the stomach may undergo severe hypotonia after gastric surgery or other abdominal procedures (Fig. 13.3).

Close communication with the surgeon is of the utmost importance to achieve a successful outcome, and it is crucial that the radiologist has a clear understanding of the operative procedures; many of which are complex and varied. A good result is much more likely to be achieved if these principles are followed.

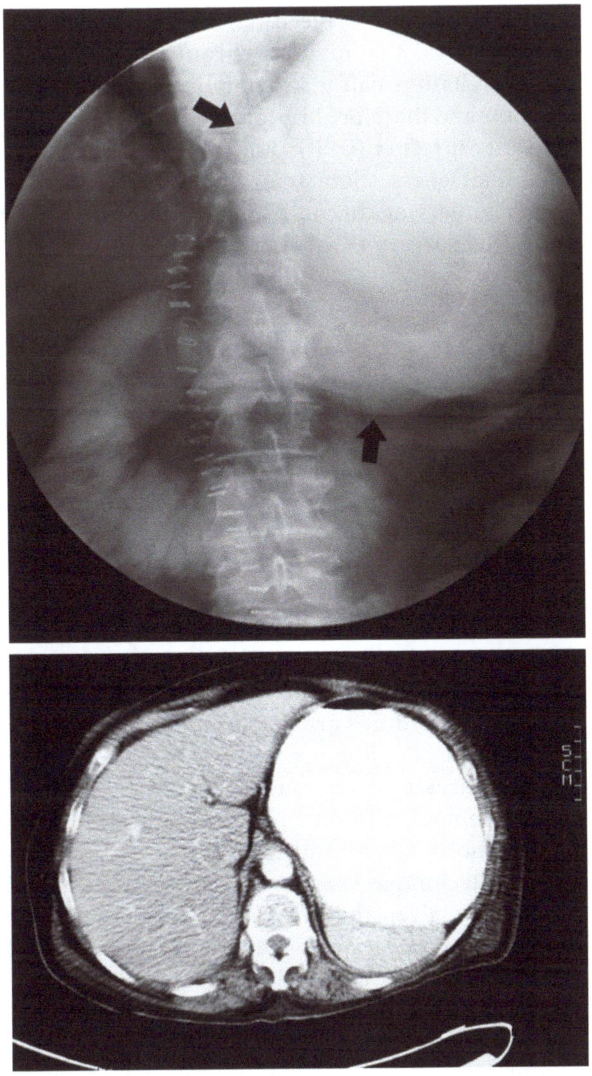

Fig. 13.3a,b. A 67 year old woman admitted to the intensive care unit for peritonitis after colon resection, demonstrated gas distension on chest X-ray. **a** Upper GI series showed a markedly distended stomach (*arrows*) with no sign of outlet obstruction and the duodenum rapidly filled with contrast material. **b** The degree of gastric dilatation is shown on CT images. Gastric function became normal during general improvement of the patient

13.3 Antireflux Surgery

13.3.1 Indication

Young healthy patients with chronic gastro-oesophageal reflux disease (GORD) who cannot contemplate lifelong medical therapy are candidates for a surgical antireflux procedure. Bleeding, recurrent strictures, failed medical therapy and chronic problems due to regurgitation can also complicate conservative attempts and therefore indicate surgery. Oesophago-pharyngeal reflux (OPR) can cause asthma, laryngitis, hoarseness, globus, laryngospasm and other ENT disorders, again contributing to indications for antireflux surgery (Kahrilas 2001).

13.3.2 Procedure

The rapid advances of surgical and endoscopic antireflux procedures have led to a wide variation of the number and types of invasive therapeutic approaches. Laparoscopic fundoplication is now established as a safe and effective procedure, and there are two main types. The Nissen or complete fundoplication (Fig. 13.4) creates an antireflux valve by wrapping the gastric fundus 360° around the intra- abdominal oesophagus. The Toupet procedure uses a 270° wrap and both procedures are performed either open or via the laparoscopic approach. The main advantage of the laparoscopic approach is the lower morbidity rate compared to the open fundoplication, with reduced hospital stay and recovery time. The laparoscopic technique is safer than open surgery and as effective, given that the rate of surgical failures leading to reoperation is 2%–17% with an overall mortality rate of 0%–3% (Waring 1999; Graziano et al. 2003).

As a general rule, total fundoplication is the best option. After the Nissen fundoplication, 8% of patients suffer from symptoms of recurrent GORD; after the Toupet procedure it is 20%.

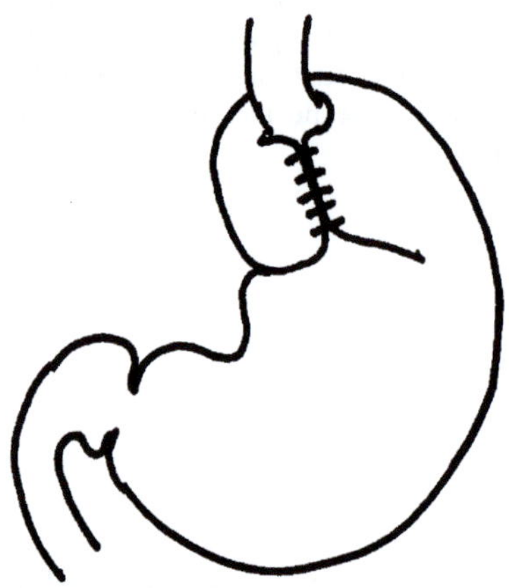

Fig. 13.4. Diagram of Nissen fundoplication with the typical "wrap" around the oesophagogastric junction

13.3.3 Normal Imaging Results and Complications

In the early postoperative period, suspected visceral injury, abscess or haematoma are evaluated with CT. In addition, routine fluoroscopy is performed within the first week, depending on the procedure, the clinical situation and patient's postoperative condition. Fundoplications have no anastomoses and therefore early leaks or fistulas are very rare. They can occur however as a late complication after dilatation of too tight or secondarily narrowed wraps. A narrow oesophagogastric junction during the early postoperative course is a common finding and represents oedema of the wrap. This finding is also typical after dilatation of a too tight fundoplication. The "wrap" after fundoplication (Fig. 13.4) appears as a mass with smooth contours at the level of the oesophagogastric junction, just below the diaphragm. The wrap can have an oval or more irregular shape with the oesophageal lumen passing through the centre. When postoperative oedema has disappeared contrast material should pass through the wrap without hindrance and there should not be a persistent level of contrast material above it. Retention of food or mucus, detected in the later postoperative phase indicates a narrowing of the wrap (Fig. 13.5). If solid food dysphagia has to be investigated in the later postoperative course, a 13-mm or 14-mm placebo tablet can be utilized to display the maximal diameter of the lumen. The sutures of the wrap may disrupt partially, leading to one or more small outpouchings of the fundus, or an incomplete encircling of the esophagus. A complete disruption of the sutures can present as a recurrent hiatal hernia with or without a broadening of the oesophagogastric junction (Fig. 13.6). Furthermore, complete disruption can be suggested when the expected "mass" of the wrap is not present, compared to earlier postoperative images. Comparison with earlier images is crucial in this setting, since some wraps present relatively little mass at the level of the oesophagogastric junction. This is because very experienced surgeons reconstruct the oesophagogastric junction in such a way that it resembles the appearance of the normal physiological state. Therefore, if wrap complication are suspected, it is extremely useful to have early post-operative studies in order to compare with later studies, which thus takes into account the variation of normal wraps. Another late complication is a slipped Nissen, when the wrap slips downward over the stomach, leading to an hour glass configuration of the stomach. Also without disrup-

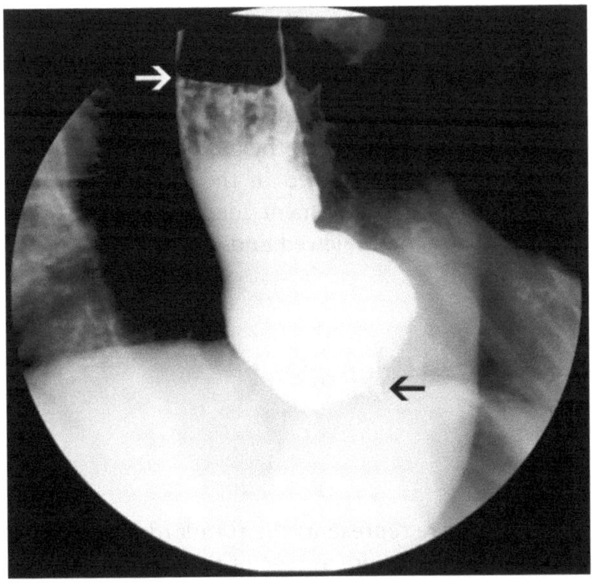

Fig. 13.5. An 80 year old lady, 3 years after fundoplication presented with severe solid food dysphagia, weight loss and heartburn. Endoscopy revealed severe esophagitis. Upper GI series showed a constant level of mucus and sedimented contrast material as a sign of delayed oesophageal clearance (*white arrow*). Small parts of the stomach are above the diaphragmatic hiatus (*black arrow*), indicating a partial migration of the fundoplication without disruption of the wrap itself. pH monitoring did not reveal reflux and the oesophagitis was suspected to be due to retention. Dilatation of the wrap was successful

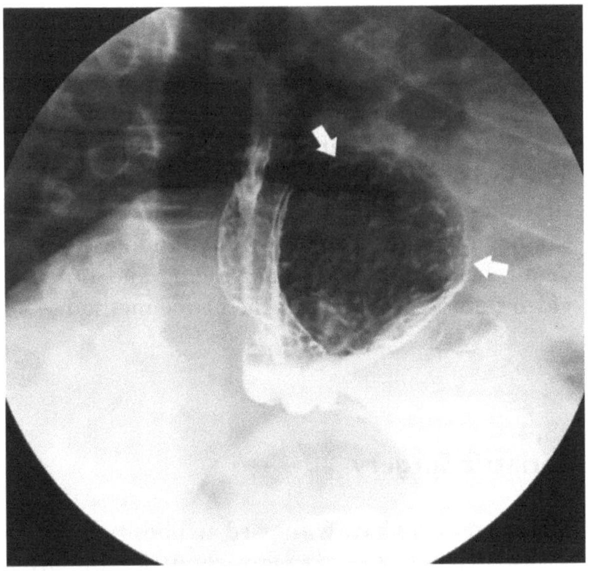

Fig. 13.7. A 36 year old male presents with symptoms of reflux and epigastric pain, 2 years after fundoplication. A recurrent paraesophageal hernia was present (*arrows*), parts of the wrap are visible under the level of the diaphragm. Reoperation was successful

a

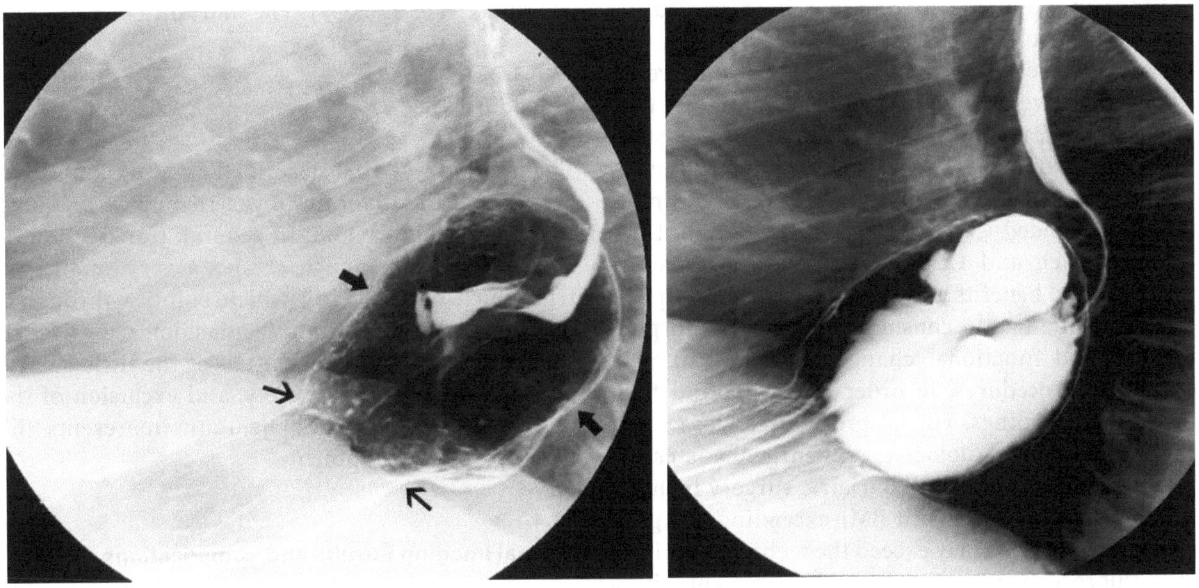

b

Fig. 13.6a,b. A 62 year old male, 13 months after laparoscopic fundoplication. **a** Hiatus hernia, measuring 8 cm is present (*thick arrows*), shown in the erect position with double contrast. Wide broadening of the region of the hiatus (*thin arrows*) is a sign of disruption of the hiatal closure. **b** Right lateral view in the horizontal position

tion, the intact wrap can migrate upward through a reopened hiatus. This is more common with parts of the wrap (Fig. 13.7), than herniation of the entire fundoplication. To study the morphology and function of these complications, video fluoroscopy combined with mono or double contrast images is the first choice. Multislice CT with reformatted images can depict the morphology of the fundoplication in detail, but for estimating narrowing and function, video fluoroscopy remains the prime method.

13.4 Bariatric Surgery

The last decades have witnessed an obesity epidemic with a high prevalence in many countries. In Europe the prevalence of obesity varies between 10% in Denmark to 28% in Switzerland and 32% in Romania. In the USA the incidence of overweight adults has tripled to 35% (Bohdjalian et al. 2004; Kluthe and Scubert 1985). Conservative treatment has yielded disappointing results. To obtain sustained substantial weight loss, bariatric surgery is an accepted option. This is considered when body mass index exceeds 35 kg/m^2 with attendant co morbidity, such as diabetes, obstructive sleep apnoea or cardiovascular disease. Without co morbidity 40 kg/m^2 is the recommended threshold (National Institutes of Health Consensus Development Conference Statement 1992). Different bariatric procedures are performed. Two basic principles of bariatric surgery have been developed within the last 50 years. The restrictive procedures limit the volume of food intake, whereas others create a malabsorption state. Gastric Banding (restrictive) and Roux-en-Y Gastric Bypass (restrictive and malabsorption) are common, Vertical Banded Gastroplasty, Gastric sleeve, Duodenal Switch and Gastric pacing are alternatives with several benefits and disadvantages. Postoperative imaging has to consider the specific morphological and functional changes of these different bariatric procedures, in order to understand their radiologic findings. For all procedures close interaction between radiologists and surgeons is essential (Toppino et al. 2001). Bariatric surgery includes super-obese patients with BMI exceeding 40 kg/m^2 and these patients may exceed the technical limits of the fluoroscopy unit. For example, a patient with a body weight of 180 kg may not be tilted up or down on the usual fluoroscopic equipment and requires the following strategy. For safety and to avoid damage to the equipment, the patient is investigated in the upright position and leaves the fluoroscopic equipment before it is moved. Only then is the table tilted to the horizontal position without the patient on it, who has to remount with the aid of a footstool. The table is then only moved in the horizontal plane. In addition, the equipment manufacturers' advice should always be reviewed and adhered to.

13.4.1 Roux-en-Y Gastric Bypass

13.4.1.1 Indication

The procedure represents the standard procedure in the USA. A major advantage of this approach is the positive influence on Type 2 diabetes as the majority of patients become euglycaemic, even insulin dependent patients. The mechanism for this is not completely understood but is thought to relate to the exclusion of passage of nutrients through the duodenum (Rubino and Marescaux 2004; Rubino et al. 2006). In addition, the early delivery of nutrients to the hindgut adds to weight loss by causing malabsorption. The results of this restrictive procedure combined with malabsorption results in better weight loss and a reduced number of failures compared with Gastric Banding, despite the longer operation time and life-threatening complications (Angrisani et al. 2007). The mortality rate is 0.4%.

13.4.1.2 Procedure

The method was first described by Mason and Ito (1969), and the diagram of gastric bypass anatomy is shown in Figure 13.8. In general, transsection or stapling of the stomach creates a very small gastric pouch of 15–35 m^3, which empties through a Rouxen-gastrojejunostomy, anastomosed side to side to the jejunum. Distention of the little gastric pouch results in early satiety, and exclusion of the duodenum and proximal jejunum represents the malabsorptive component.

13.4.1.3 Normal Imaging Results and Complications

An upper GI study is recommended within 24 h after surgery and is repeated if a leak is present. Plain films show the gastric pouch with a globu-

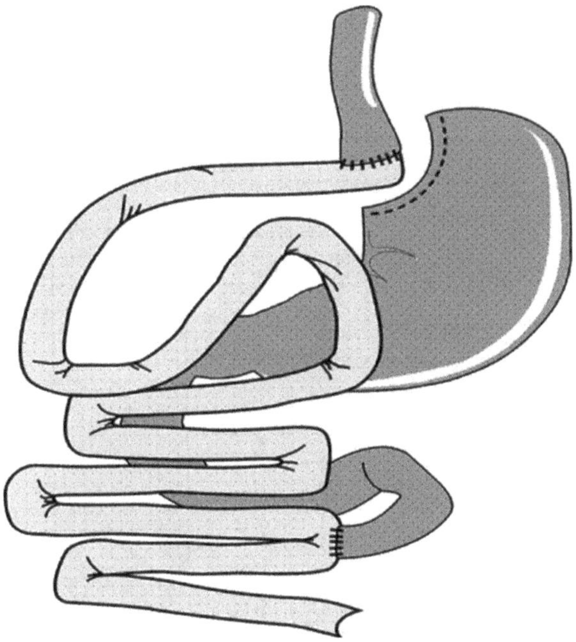

Fig. 13.8. Diagram of Roux-en-Y-gastric bypass. A small gastric pouch is created with stapling of the stomach, followed by an anastomosis of the pouch with a Roux-en-Y limb, 75–180 cm long

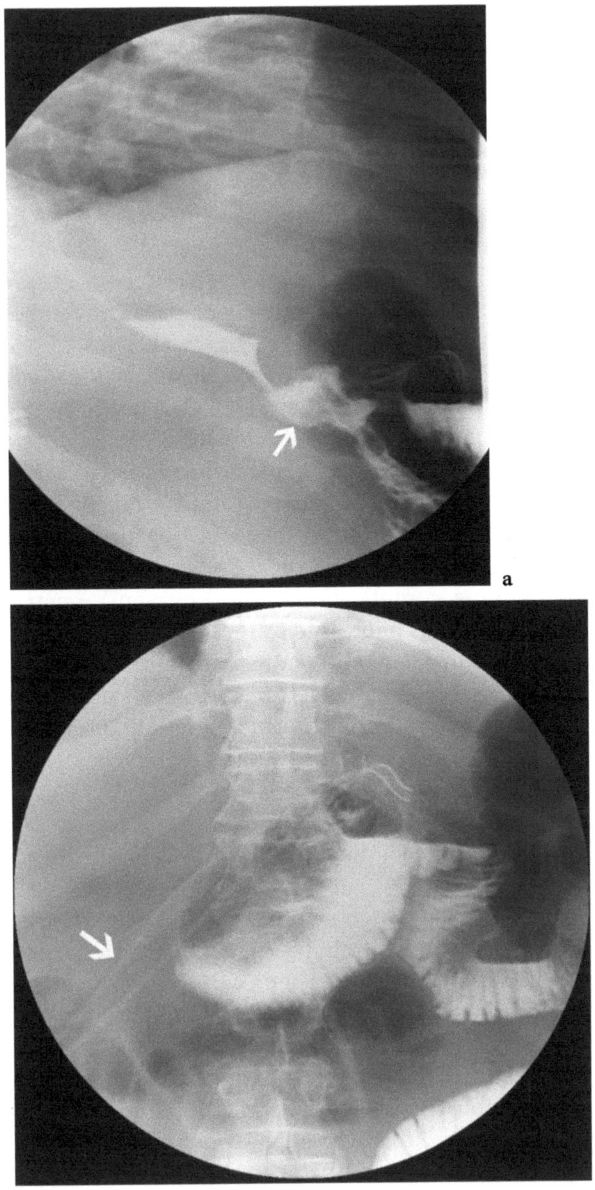

a

b

Fig. 13.9. **a** Normal postoperative upper GI study includes the tubular oesophagus and the little gastric pouch (*arrow*). **b** The jejunal limb is filled with constrast material demonstrating smooth mucosal folds. Surgical drains (*arrow*) are carefully inspected and should remain of similar density to precontrast images. Contrast within the drains would be an indirect sign of leakage

lar shape, emptying the contrast material into the jejunal limb (Fig. 13.9). Narrowing of the anastomosis in the early postoperative period is a typical sign of oedema and is a normal finding. Contrast in the jejunal limb should demonstrate normal mucosal folds and motility (Toppino et al. 2001). The excluded stomach can be outlined by refluxed contrast material. CT can add to the visualisation of the excluded stomach and also depict the proximal efferent Roux jejunal loop. In addition the blind oversewn loop and the distal jejunojejunal anastomosis are seen in more than 60% of patients (Yu et al. 2004). Anastomotic leaks (incidence of 1%–6%) occur most commonly at gastrojejunal anastomosis and within 10 days. Leaks are less frequent at the distal Roux anastomosis or stomach. Small bowel obstruction (incidence 4%–5%) may be due to internal hernias, adhesions, mesocolic tunnel stenosis or intussusceptions. Hypotonia of the excluded stomach must not be confused with an extra intestinal fluid collection. In case of bowel obstruction a transition zone between dilated bowel proximal to the obstruction and the collapsed bowel distal to the obstruction is observed. When a narrowing of the gastrojejunal anastomosis is present, the gastric pouch is dilated and has a spherical shape with delayed passage of contrast material. A stenosis of the jejunojejunal anastomosis is rare (Blachar et al. 2002). Phytobezoars occur when seeded fruits or other indigestible components of food impact in the proximal jejunum- which is the most common site (Sandrasegaran et al. 2005). In addition, CT is used when bowel obstruction or extra intestinal complications are suspected.

13.4.2 Gastric Banding and Other Bariatric Procedures

13.4.2.1 Indication

Whilst gastric banding and Roux-en-Y gastric bypass are the most common operations of laparoscopic obesity surgery, the selection criteria for these two procedures remain controversial. Many centres offer both methods and inform candidates of the risks and benefits of both procedures (Angrisani et al. 2007; Bohdjalian et al. 2004). At our centre (Bohdjalian et al. 2004), the Roux-en-Y gastric bypass is the method of choice whilst gastric banding is performed in selected patients. A recent study demonstrated that for gastric banding there was a weight loss after 5 years of 47.5% and without life-threatening complications. The Roux-en-Y gastric bypass also has a low rate of severe early complications, but an easier and better weight loss of 66.6%. The final choice will be strongly influenced by the patient's expectations (Angrisani et al. 2007; Kim et al. 2006).

13.4.2.2 Procedures and Findings

Adjustable laparoscopic gastric band is a restrictive method, limiting passage of ingested food (Fig. 13.10). Following the early postoperative period, the inner width of the band can be adjusted by injecting fluid (saline solution/water soluble contrast material) into the port (Fig. 13.11). An implantable silicon band is placed around the proximal stomach, forming a small neostomach – the "pouch". The width of the stoma can be adjusted with injection or suction through a catheter, which connects the silicon band and a subcutaneously implanted port. After surgery the width of the band's lumen can be adjusted at any time under fluoroscopic guidance by puncture of the port. Thus the restriction of food passage can be varied. A typical complication is slippage of the band with dilatation of the pouch (Fig. 13.12). This may occur as an early or late complication (Belachew et al. 1997; Szucs et al. 1998; Wiesner et al. 2001). The acute concentric pouch dilatation is mainly caused by a too narrow stoma and leads to a prestenotic dilatation of the pouch from normally 20 mL up to a size of 10 cm. Overfilling of the band, focal weakness of the band with mechanic obstruction from band herniation, overfilling of the oesoph-

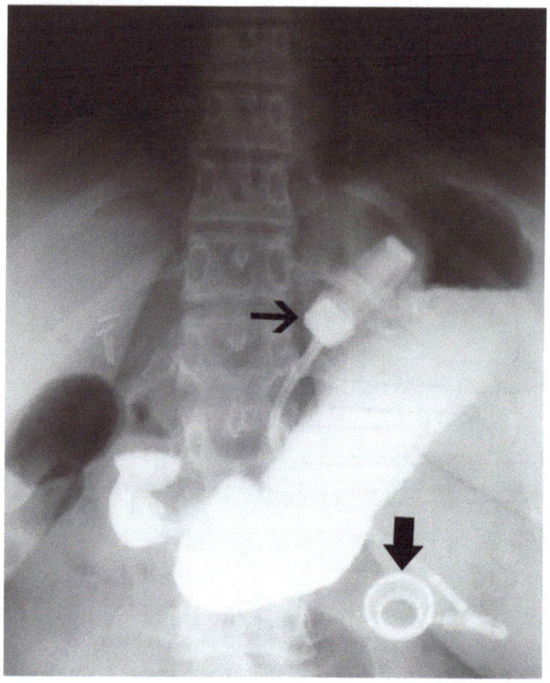

Fig. 13.10. A 29 year old man with a BMI of 42 kg/m². An adjustable laparoscopic gastric band has been inserted. Early postoperative images show the band in place (*thin arrow*), connected to a subcutaneous port (*thick arrow*). The lumen is adjusted from 3 to 8mm. Passage and filling of the stomach was normal

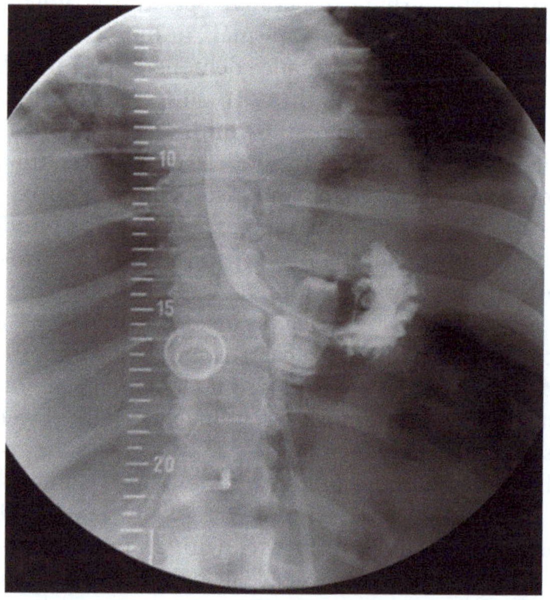

Fig. 13.11. A 31 year old woman with a BMI of 40 kg/m² 3 months after placement of the gastric band. To obtain better weight loss the lumen of the band was narrowed by injection of fluid into the port. Fluoroscopically, contrast material should pass the pouch without a persistent level of contrast material or delayed transit as shown here

agus by low patient compliance with overeating, may all lead to acute concentric pouch dilatation. Chronic concentric pouch dilatation is diagnosed, when a normal stomal width of 3–8 mm is combined with pouch dilatation. This is also due to volume overload. Pronounced posterior slippage

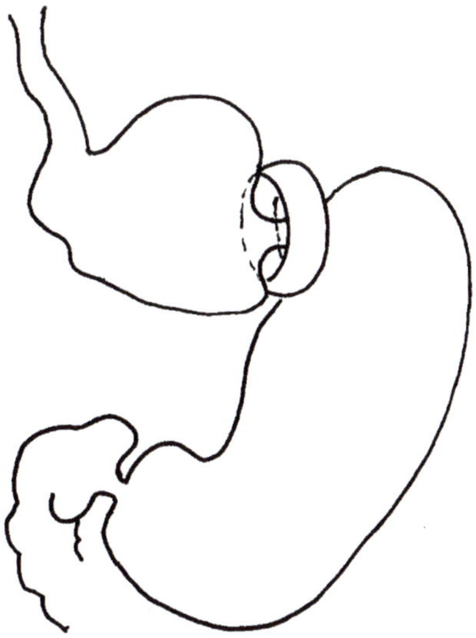

Fig. 13.12. Diagram showing the appearance of pouch dilatation due to slippage of the gastric band

due to older surgical techniques (before 2000) can lead to eccentric pouch dilatation, which seldom can be cured by emptying the system. Furthermore, system disconnections, transmural band penetration and infections around the port are all reported complications.

Biliopancreatic diversion is a malabsorptive procedure (Scopinaro et al. 2002), which represents a horizontal gastrectomy with an up to 250 cm long Roux-en-Y limb to create fat malabsorption. This may be combined with the restrictive gastric sleeve resection (Aggarwal et al. 2007) (Fig. 13.13). Biliopancreatic diversion is the most effective bariatric surgical method, as after 18 years, an average excessive weight loss of 78% was documented (Scopinaro et al. 2002). Morbidity ranges around 20%–25% and includes long term problems such as anaemia (5%–40%) and protein loss (10%) in these cases.

Neither restrictive nor malabsorption is the aim of gastric pacing systems. Laparascopically, a bipolar electrode is attached 3 cm distally to the oesophagogastric junction under endoscopic control. The electrode is connected to a pacemaker which constantly stimulates the fundus. The mechanism of effect remains unclear but a weight loss of 32%–22% is documented (Miller et al. 2002).

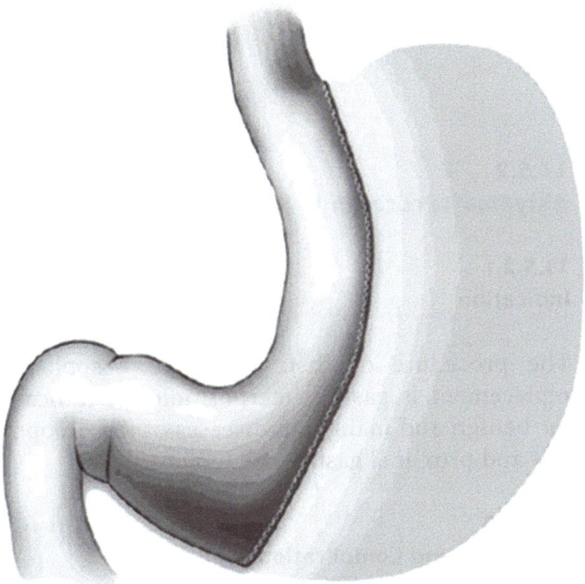

a

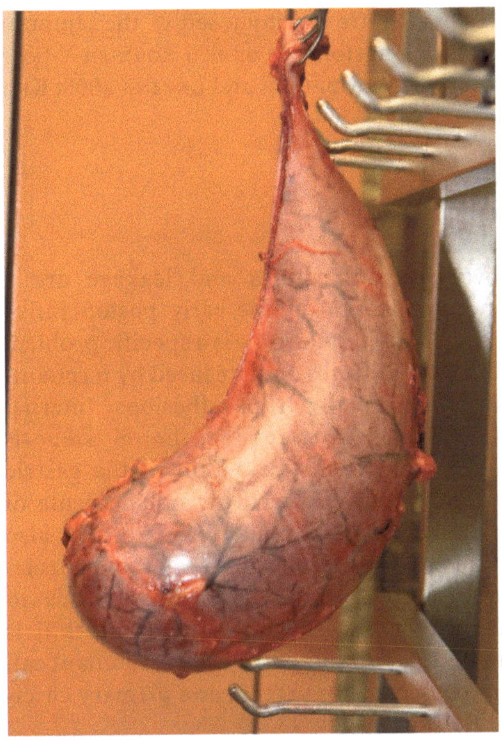

b

Fig. 13.13. a Diagram of a gastric sleeve procedure showing the creation of a narrow gastric tube using staplers against a bougie. The resected part of the stomach (right lateral part of the diagram) is also shown as a specimen in (**b**)

13.5 Gastric and Duodenal Resections

13.5.1 Partial Resections

13.5.1.1 Indication

Partial resections of the stomach and duodenum for peptic ulcer disease have disappeared over the past few decades because of the success of medical therapy. However these procedures remain an option for treatment of cancer in the distal stomach.

13.5.1.2 Procedures

Billroth I gastroduodenostomy, Billroth II gastrojejunostomy with a Roux-en-Y or loop-type gastrojejunostomy, and total gastrectomy with oesophagojejunostomy are the most common procedures. The Billroth I procedure consists of a partial gastrectomy with resection of the antrum. Continuity is performed by end- to end gastroduodenostomy. Billroth II procedures are much more common because of lesser complications of bile reflux. In Billroth II the entire or parts of the free edge of the resected stomach are anastomosed to the jejunum via end-to side anastomosis or as a Roux-en-Y type reconstruction (Woodfield and Levine 2005; Kim et al. 2002).

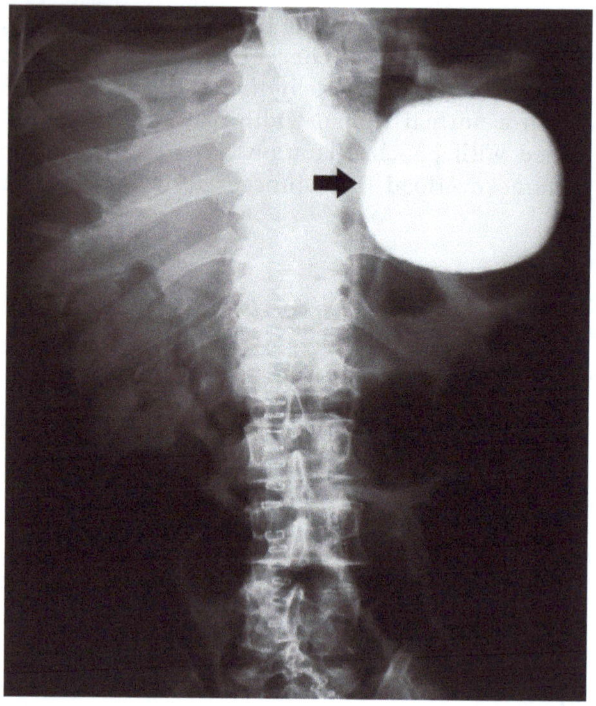

Fig. 13.14. A 76 year old male with persistent vomiting and 10 kg weight loss over the past 6 months. A Billroth II procedure had been performed 30 years ago and since then he had experienced multiple episodes of gastritis and ulcers, confirmed at endoscopic examinations. Upper GI series with water soluble contrast material revealed a round structure, measuring 8 cm, representing total obstruction of the gastric remnant at the level of the gastrojejunostomy. This was due to chronic ulcer stenosis and was followed by successful surgery

13.5.1.3 Complications

Breakdown of suture lines and leakage are a common complication of the early postoperative phase. Afferent loop syndrome is a specific problem of Billroth II procedures and is caused by mechanical obstruction usually from adhesions. Internal hernias, extrinsic compression, bowel stenosis may also occur. Bezoar formation in the gastric remnant, anastomotic ulcers, incisional hernia of the abdominal wall and hiatal hernia are all also potential complications. Stenosis of the gastrojejunostomy after Billroth II procedures leads to obstruction (Fig. 13.14). Fistula after Billroth II is rare (Fig. 13.15). Tumour of the gastric remnant can be due to recurrence or present as a primary carcinoma of the stump (Fig. 13.16).

13.5.2 Akiyama's Procedure

13.5.2.1 Indication

The procedure of first choice for oesophageal replacement is gastric interposition (1), indicated for benign and malignant diseases of the oesophagus and proximal gastric carcinomas.

13.5.2.2 Procedure and Complications

Gastric pull through procedures are successfully performed via the transthoracic and the transhiatal approach with a cervical or intrathoracic oesophagogastric anastomosis. Early postoperative leaks are

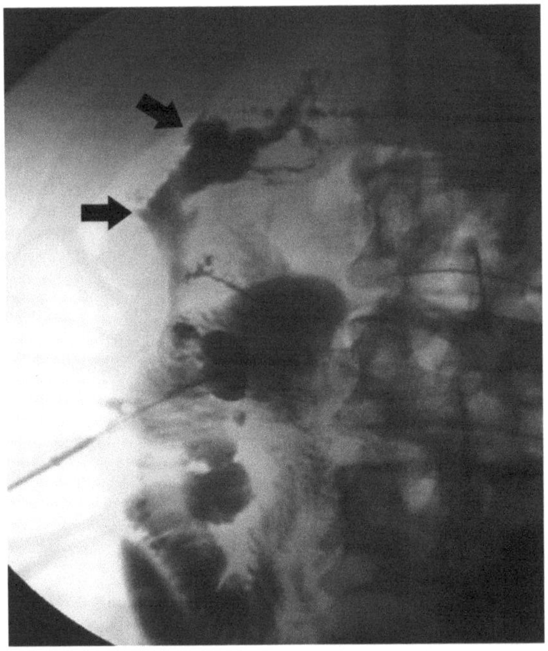

Fig. 13.15. A 67 year old male, suffering from a chronic enterocutaneous fistula after Billroth II procedure. Fistulography displays a large system of branched fistula within the abdominal wall and the peritoneal fat (*arrows*)

common (Urschel 1995). When the anastomosis is located at the level of the thoracic inlet, special techniques have to be incorporated into the examination. Only oblique projections allow sufficient evaluation of the anastomosis, with LPO and RPO projections, as well as additional frontal images. Furthermore, as the contrast material advances rapidly in this area, even in the horizontal position, recording is a great asset. Performed at 25 frames/s, it helps to define leaks, especially in these cases. Correlation with CT is recommended for doubtful cases, or if extraintestinal disease is suspected. Almost all leaks lead to strictures later on (Fig. 13.17). The intrathoracic stomach can be placed orthotopically or retrosternal (Fig. 13.18). If dysphagia is present, video fluoroscopy or oesophagrams are often the first diagnostic procedure, and subtle signs of complications should not be overlooked (Fig. 13.19).

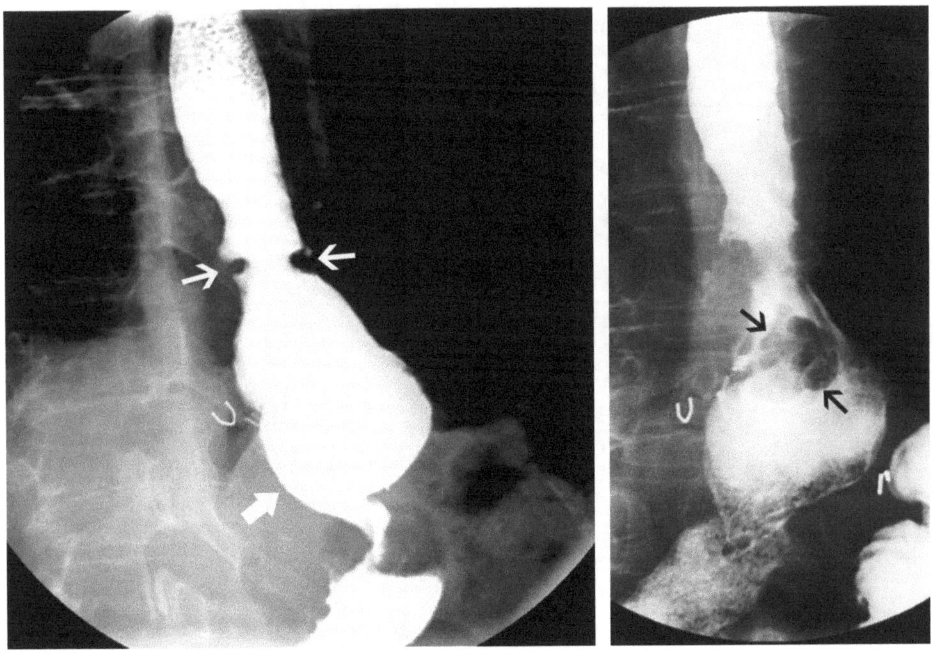

a b

Fig. 13.16a,b. An 81 year old man with weight loss and intermittent solid food dysphagia for 2 years, especially for meat and hard bread. A Billroth I procedure had been performed when the patient was 43 years old. **a** Upper GI series with barium. *Thin arrows* point to a typical Schatzki ring with a lumen about 10 mm. The gastric remnant following Billroth I is herniated axially (*thick arrow*), whilst the gastroduodenostomy is just below the diaphragmatic level, and appears slightly narrowed. **b** Later mono contrast image detects a lobulated polypoid mass in the gastric remnant, measuring about 3 cm (*arrows*) – Polypoid adenocarcinoma of the gastric remnant

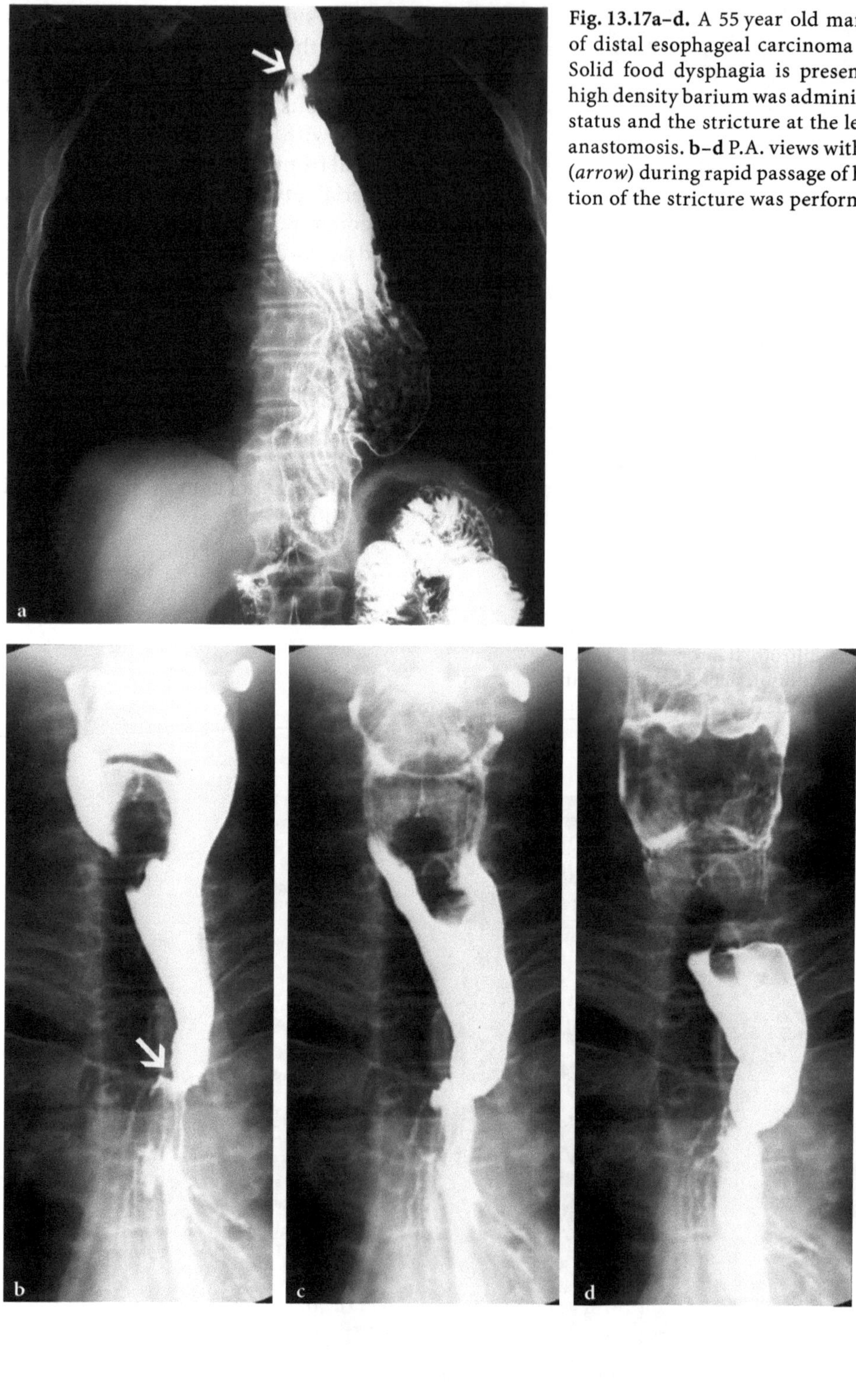

Fig. 13.17a–d. A 55 year old man, 9 months after treatment of distal esophageal carcinoma with Akyiama's procedure. Solid food dysphagia is present. **a** Overview images after high density barium was administered show the topographic status and the stricture at the level of the oesophagogastric anastomosis. **b–d** P.A. views with delineation of the stricture (*arrow*) during rapid passage of high density barium. Dilatation of the stricture was performed

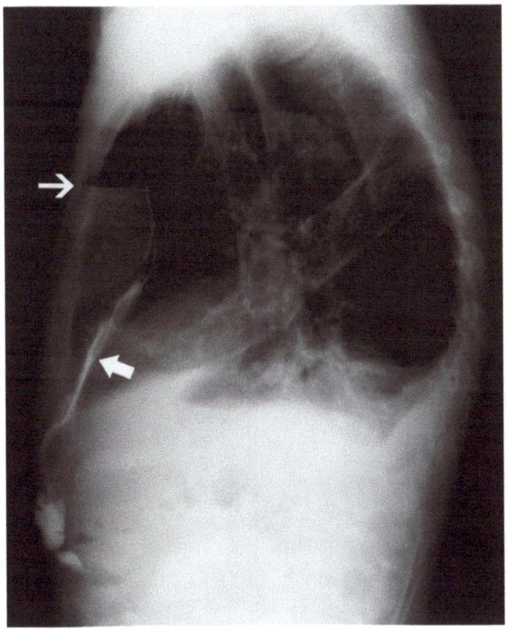

Fig. 13.18. A 52 year old man, 7 days after Akyiamas procedure for esophageal carcinoma. The patient was well and chest films had been performed as a routine. The stomach lies in a retrosternal position (*thick arrow*), there was no leak, but an air/fluid level in the mediastinum was visible (*thin arrow*). There were no clinical or laboratory findings to suggest infectious complication. The air and fluid had been resorbed one week later

13.5.3 Total Gastrectomy

13.5.3.1 Indication

The mainstay of treatment for gastric cancer is surgical excision with adequate margins on either side of the neoplasm and resection of locoregional lymph nodes. Extensive procedures with total gastrectomy and oesophagojejunostomy involve removal of the spleen and the pancreatic tail. Often total resections are palliative as at least one third of the patients are inoperable at the time of diagnosis. Gastric carcinoma does not respond to radiotherapy but regression can be achieved with combination chemotherapy.

13.5.3.2 Complications

After total resections, leaks are a common complication at the level of the oesophagojejunal anastomosis (Fig. 13.20). Less frequently leaks are found at the duodenal stump. Intraabdominal bleeding (Fig. 13.21), wound complications and abscesses may also be encountered (Fig. 13.22).

a 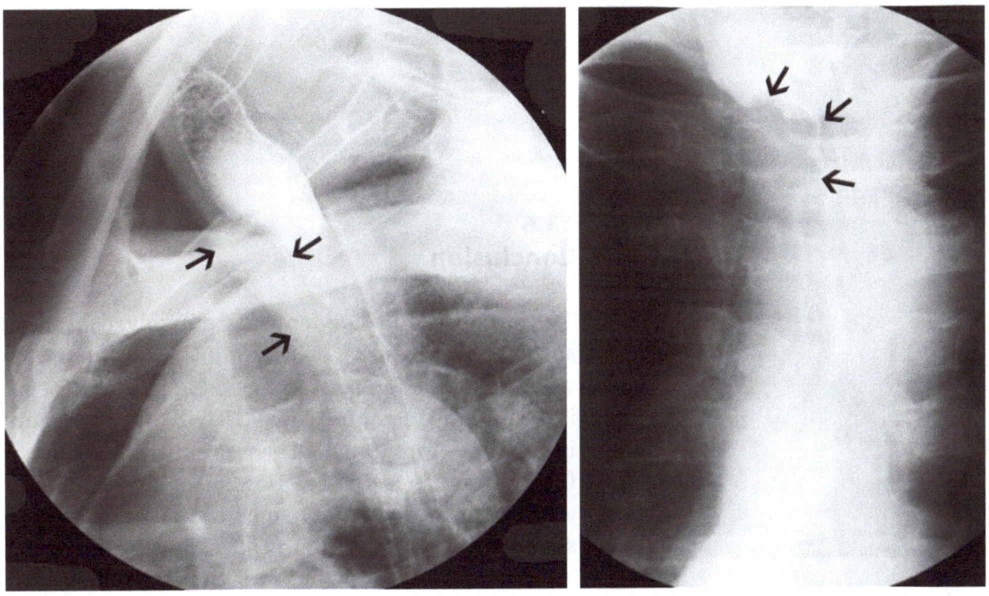 b

Fig. 13.19a,b. A 67 year old man, 6 months after Akyiama's procedure presents with dysphagia. Endoscopy was planned immediately after video fluoroscopy and so, water soluble contrast material was chosen. **a** RPO oblique projection shows a local enlargement of the retrotracheal space, the distance between the trachea and the cervical esophagus is widened (*arrows*). **b** A.P view revealed a lobulated mass with narrowing at the level of the anastomosis. Recurrent oesophageal tumour was diagnosed endoscopically

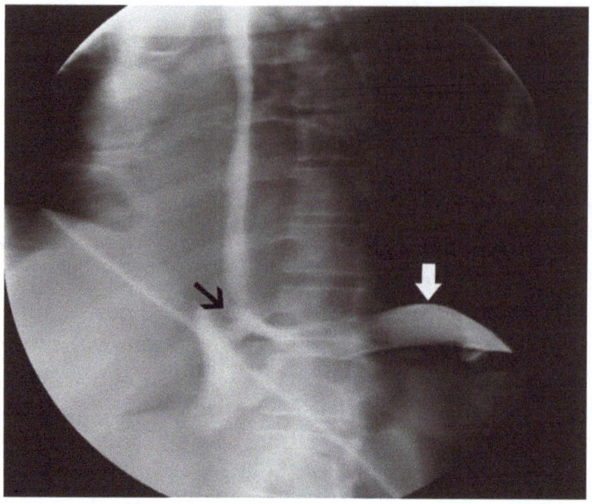

Fig. 13.20. A 67 year old man, 2 days after total gastrectomy. At the level of the oesophagojejunostomy (*black arrow*), an extensive extravasation develops in the left lateral direction and delineates the left dome of the diaphragm (*white arrow*). This was a typical leak and he was reoperated upon immediately as his clinical course was deteriorating rapidly

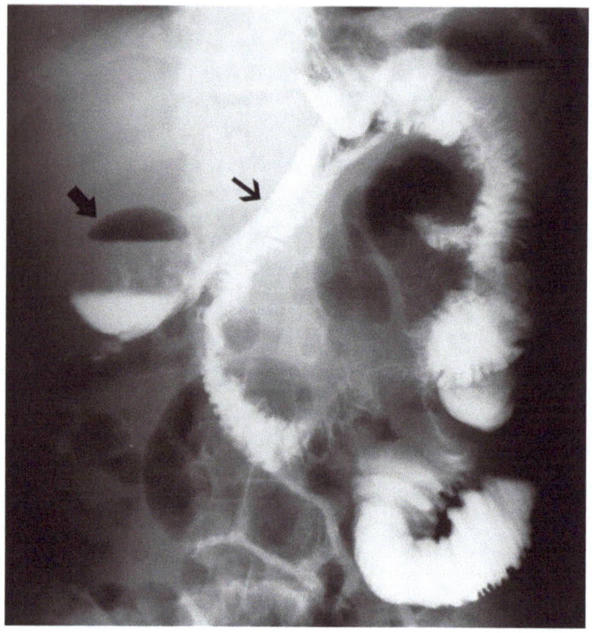

Fig. 13.22. A 62 year old man, 4 weeks after gastrectomy, presenting with fever, tachycardia and abdominal pain. Upper GI series revealed a leak of the oesophagojejunal anastomosis. The extravasation extends along the lower border of the left hepatic lobe (*thin arrow*) to a round structure measuring several centimeters (*thick arrow*). Within the structure, there is an air/fluid level and a level between the contrast material and secretions. CT and subsequent surgery confirmed a subhepatic abscess. The leak was oversewn

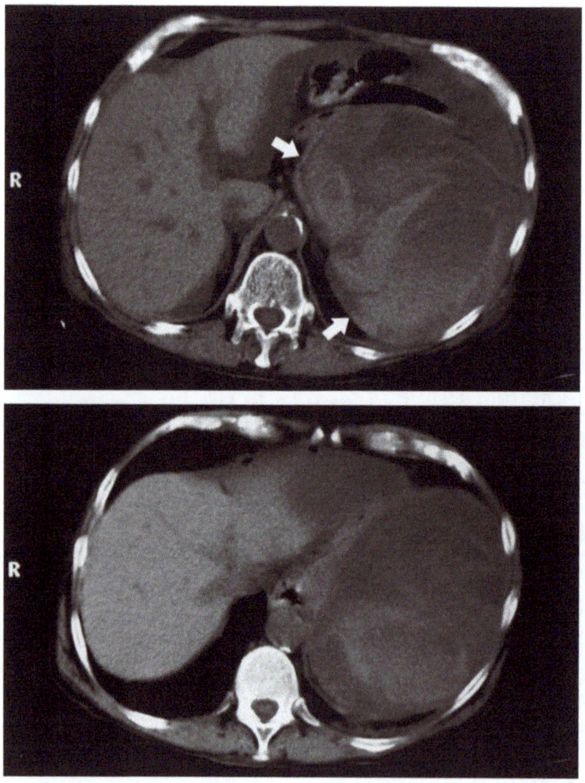

a

b

Fig. 13.21a,b. A 70 year old man, 8 h after gastrectomy. CT was performed for severe loss of hematocrit. **a** The spleen is massively enlarged (*arrows*) with an expansive global shape and shows irregular hypodense compartments. **b** Free fluid and air were present in the peritoneal cavity. Splenectomy was performed immediately after the CT

13.6 Conclusion

The stomach and duodenum are involved in many surgical procedures. The complementary use of video fluoroscopy spot images, CT and endoscopy is developing fast. Multislice CT will take over many indications for upper GI series, but the ability of fluoroscopy to visualize flow of contrast material within the bowel lumen means that it remains a strong tool to answer many specific questions.

Close inter-relation between the responsible radiologist and the surgeon is mandatory, and feed back can be achieved easily at clinical meetings. Radiology after GI surgery needs considerable experience and examinations have to be reviewed by the most experienced colleagues.

References

Aggarwal S, Kini SU, Herron DM (2007) Laparoscopic sleeve gastrectomy for morbid obesity: a review. Surg Obes Relat Dis 3:189–194

Angrisani L, Lorenzo M, Borrelli V (2007) Laparoscopic adjustable gastric banding versus Roux-en-Y gastric bypass: 5-year results of a prospective randomized trial. Surg Obes Relat Dis 3:127–133

Belachew M, Legrand M, Vincent V, Monami B, Jaquet N (1997) Láppr coelioscopique dans le traitment de la chirurgie de lóbesite morbide: technique et resultats. Ann Chi 51:165–172

Blachar A, Federle MP, Pealer KM et al. (2002) Gastrointestinal complications of laparoscopic Roux- en-Y gastric bypass surgery: clinical and imaging findings. Radiology 223(3):625–632

Bohdjalian A, Langer F, Hoda M, Felberbauer F, Silberhumer G, Zacherl J, Schindler K, Luger A, Ludvik B, Prager G (2004) Surgical treatment of obesity. Wien Med Wochenschr 154(13/14):329–333

Graziano K, Teitelbaum DH, McLean K et al. (2003) Recurrence after laparoscopic and open Nissen fundoplication: a comparison of the mechanisms of failure. Surg Endosc 17(5):704–707

Kahrilas PJ (2001) Management of GERD: Medical versus surgical. Semin Gastrointest Dis 12(1):3–15

Kim KA, Park CM, Park SW, Cha SH, Seol HY, Cha IH, Lee KY (2002) CT findings in the abdomen and pelvis after gastric carcinoma resection. AJR Am J Roentgenol 179:1037–1041

Kim TH, Daud A, Ude AO et al. (2006) U.S outcomes of laparoscopic gastric bypass versus laparascopic adjustable silicone gastric banding for morbid obesity. Surg Endosc 20:202–209

Kluthe R, Schubert A (1985) Obesity in Europe. Ann Intern Med 103:1037–1042

Mason EE, Ito C (1969) Gastric bypass. Ann Surg 170:329–339

Miller K, Holler E, Hell E (2002) Intragastric stimulation (IGS) for treatment of morbid obesity. Zentralbl Chir 127(12):1049–1054

National Institutes of Health Consensus Development Conference Statement (1992) Gastrointestinal surgery for severe obesity. Am J Clin Nutr 55 [Suppl2]:S615–S619

Rubino F, Forgione A, Cummings D et al. (2006) The mechanism of diabetes control after intestinal bypass surgery reveals a role of the proximal intestine in the pathophysiology of type 2 diabetes. Ann Surg 244:742–749

Rubino F, Marescaux J (2004) Efect of duodenal-jejunal exclusion in a non-obese animal model of type 2 diabetes: a new perspective for an old disease. Ann Surg 239:1–11

Sandrasegaran K, Rajesh A, Lall CH, Gomez GA, Lappas JC, Maglinte DD (2005) Gastrointestinal complications of bariatric Roux-en-Y gastric bypass surgery. Eur Radiol 15:254–262

Scopinaro N, Marinari GM, Camerini G (2002) Laparoscopic standard biliopancreatic diversion: technique and preliminary results. Obes Surg 12(2):241–244

Szucs RA, Turner MA, Kellum JM, De Maria EJ, Sugermann HJ (1998) Adjustable gastric band for the treatment of morbid obesity: radiologic evaluation. AJR Am J Roentgenol 170:993–996

Toppino M, Cesarani F, Comba A, Denegri F, Mistrangelo M, Gandini G, Morinno F (2001) The role of early radiological studies after gastric bariatric surgery. Obes Surg 11:447–454

Urschel JD (1995) Esophagogastrostomy anastomotic leaks complicating esophagectomy: a review. Am J Surg 169(6):634–640

Waring JP (1999) Postfundoplication complications. Prevention and management. Gastroenterol Clin North Am 28(4):1007–1019,viii–ix

Wiesner W, Hauser M, Schöb O, Weber M, Hauser R (2001) Spontaneous volume changes in gastric banding devices: complications of a semipermeable membrane. Eur Radiol 11:417–421

Woodfield CA, Levine MS (2005) The postoperative stomach. Eur J Radiol 53:341–352

Yu J, Turner MA, Cho S, Fulcher AS, DeMaria EJ, Kellum JM, Sugerman HJ (2004) Normal anatomy and complications after gastric bypass surgery: helical CT findings. Radiology 231:753–760

Angiography of the Stomach and Duodenum

14

Claire Cousins

CONTENTS

The indications for angiography of the stomach and duodenum have reduced with the development of improved endoscopic techniques and non-invasive vascular imaging. Angiography does, however, have a role particularly in the management of gastrointestinal bleeding refractory to other diagnostic and therapeutic options. Localization and possible embolization of the bleeding site are important in those patients who are at high risk for surgery. Interventional radiologists need to maintain their skills in upper gastrointestinal angiography as there are occasions when angiography and intervention are the only possible treatment option.

14.1 Anatomy

The arterial supply to the stomach and upper duodenum is from the coeliac axis. The superior mesenteric artery supplies the mid and distal duodenum. The coeliac axis arises from the aorta anteriorly at the level of the upper L1 vertebral body. Its main three branches are the left gastric, splenic and common hepatic arteries and these all give arterial supply to the stomach. The short gastric arteries arise from the splenic artery and the gastroduodenal artery (GDA) from the common hepatic artery. The right gastroepiploic artery is a terminal branch of the GDA and this courses around the greater curve of the stomach. The superior pancreaticoduodenal branches of the GDA supply the proximal duodenum.

The superior mesenteric artery (SMA) has its origin approximately 1 cm inferior to the coeliac axis on the anterior aspect of the aorta. Its inferior pancreaticoduodenal branches anastomose with the superior pancreaticoduodenal artery to supply the mid and distal duodenum.

14.2 Angiographic Technique

Selective digital subtraction angiography (DSA) is the standard technique to examine the coeliac axis and SMA. The radiographic detail obtained from an aortic injection is usually inadequate for diagnosis. The two main exceptions to this are when a lateral aortogram is necessary. These include the necessity to examine the origin of the vessels from the aorta in suspected mesenteric ischaemia, and, secondly if there is a suspected aortoduodenal fistula. The latter should be considered in any case of gastrointestinal bleeding with a history of previous aortic surgery.

Selective catheterisation of the coeliac axis may be performed using a sidewinder or femorovisceral (cobra) catheter. The former is often the catheter of choice as it allows greater catheter stability during a pump injection. A sheath is recommended if further selective angiography that requires catheter exchange is likely. Artefact from bowel peristalsis makes image interpretation difficult when using DSA and hence the bowel should be paralyzed with

C. Cousins, MB, BS, MRCP, FRCR
Department of Radiology, Addenbrooke's Hospital, Box 219, Hills Road, Cambridge, CB2 0QQ, UK

an anti-motility agent, e.g. hyoscine (Buscopan) 20–40 mg. This may be injected intra-arterially via the catheter before the angiographic run. An alternative agent is glucagon (GlucaGen) up to 1 mg.

The coeliac axis is usually opacified with 25–35 ml of contrast injected over 4–5 s using a pump injector; 30–35 ml contrast should be sufficient to opacify the SMA at a similar rate. Images are typically acquired at two frames/s and the radiographic sequence should be long enough to allow visualisation of the venous phase of the angiographic run. The patient should be asked to suspend respiration for the duration of the run but an adequate breath hold may be difficult or impossible when the patient is very sick. In this case it is better not to suspend respiration at all and acquire images with the patient breathing throughout. This requires the acquisition of several more masks and delaying the contrast injection by a few seconds. The frame rate may be reduced to one frame/s. This technique requires more detailed post processing to find an appropriate mask to match each image.

14.3 Indications

14.3.1 Gastrointestinal Bleeding

The commonest indication for performing angiography of the stomach or duodenum is gastrointestinal bleeding. Endoscopy is obviously the primary investigation and should always be performed prior to angiography. However, angiography is indicated when endoscopy has either failed to localise the site of bleeding or to successfully treat it (Fig. 14.1). Active bleeding is identified angiographically when contrast medium extravasates into the bowel lumen (Fig. 14.2). This finding may be absent if the bleeding is intermittent and other more indirect angiographic signs such as an aneurysm, early venous return, vascular irregularity or truncation should be sought.

For many years it has been accepted that the identification of a bleeding source requires a blood loss at a rate of 0.5 ml/min (Nusbaum and Baum 1963), but in general the chance of localising the site of bleeding is greater with a higher rate of blood loss. The timing of angiography is evidently critical and a good 'rule of thumb' is that the patient's pulse should be greater than 100 beats/min and the systolic blood pressure less than 100 mmHg, to maximise the chance of localisation. This may mean the patient is unstable at the time of the procedure and close collaboration with the clinical team is vital. The likelihood of success is obviously lower in a stable patient requiring little transfusion. It has been shown that patients who have been successfully embolized for upper gastrointestinal bleeding had a significantly higher transfusion rate and a higher rate of shock than those who were not embolized; largely

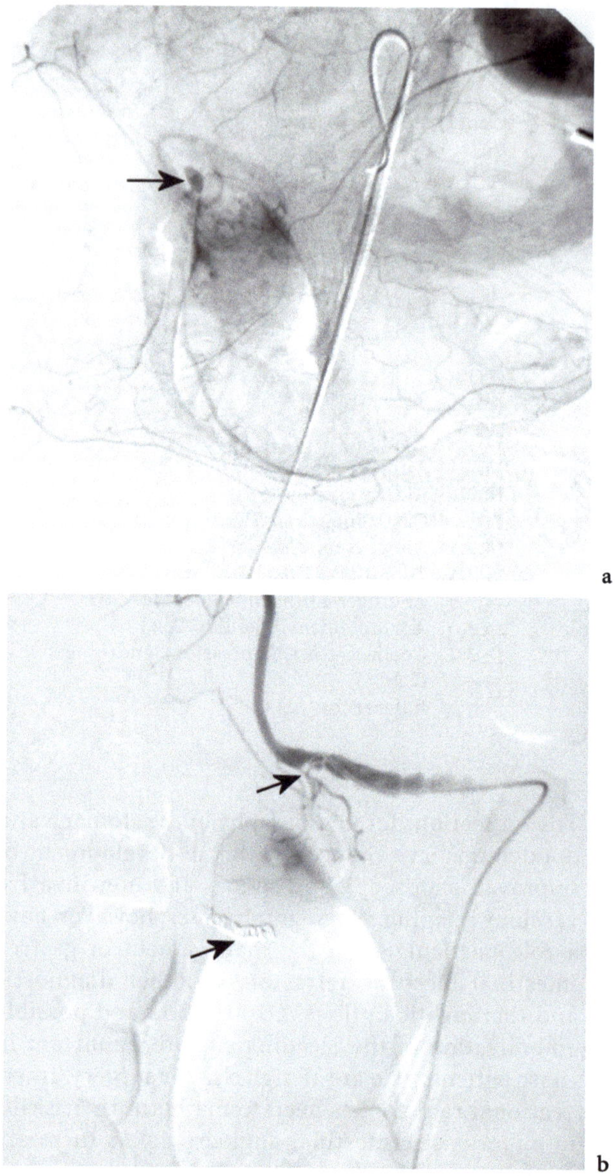

Fig. 14.1a,b. Duodenal ulcer. Coeliac axis arteriogram (**a**) demonstrates contrast medium pooling (*arrow*) in an ulcer in the duodenal bulb. Post-embolization arteriogram (**b**) after insertion of coils into the gastroduodenal artery (*arrows*)

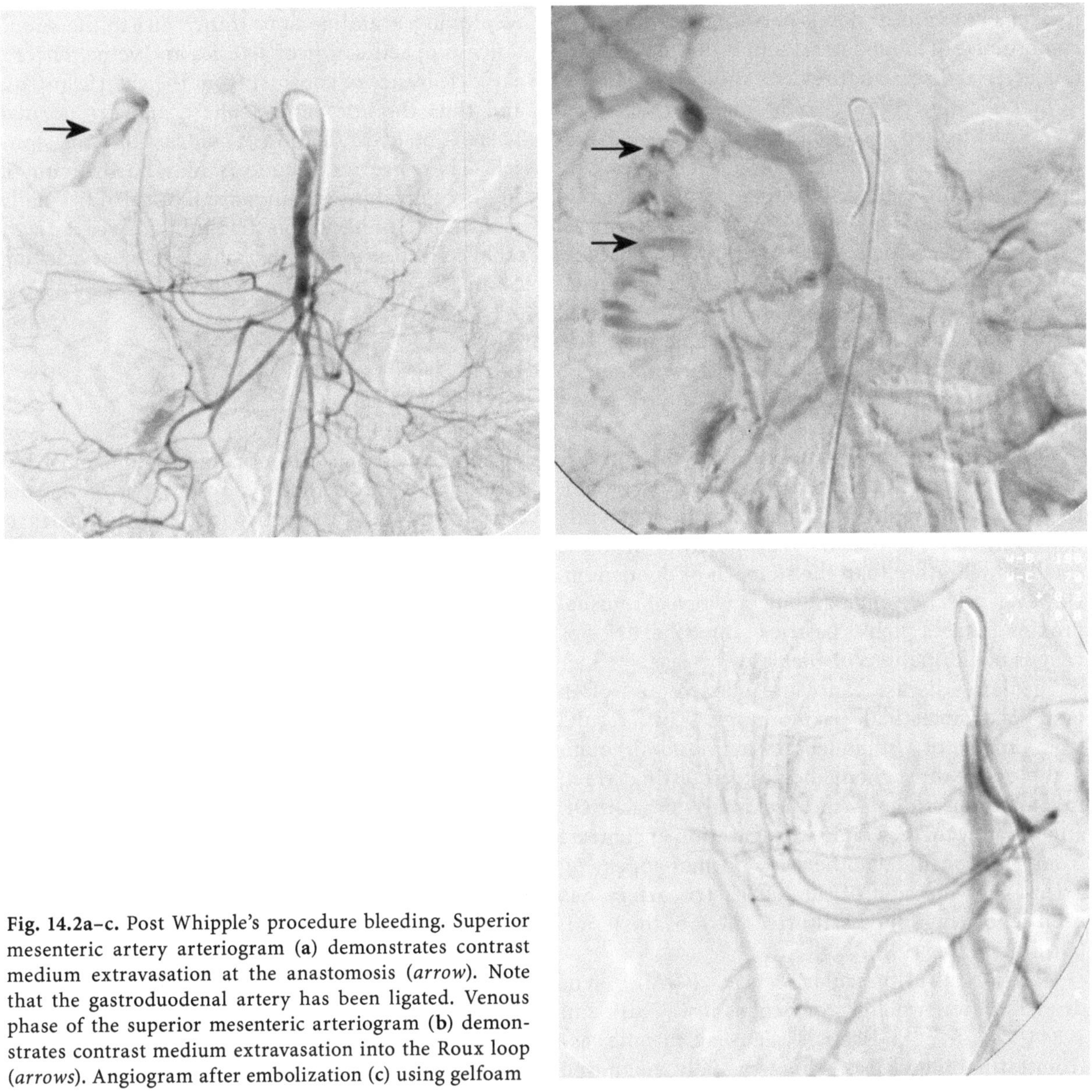

a b c

Fig. 14.2a–c. Post Whipple's procedure bleeding. Superior mesenteric artery arteriogram (**a**) demonstrates contrast medium extravasation at the anastomosis (*arrow*). Note that the gastroduodenal artery has been ligated. Venous phase of the superior mesenteric arteriogram (**b**) demonstrates contrast medium extravasation into the Roux loop (*arrows*). Angiogram after embolization (**c**) using gelfoam

because the latter group had no established aetiology (Defreyne et al. 2003).

The most frequent causes of gastric or duodenal bleeding are peptic ulcers, followed by iatrogenic causes, e.g. following biopsy or surgery, and most rarely aneurysms, particularly of the pancreaticoduodenal arteries. The role of angiography in the upper gastrointestinal tract is focussed more on therapy by embolization than purely diagnosis, particularly in elderly patients with high co-morbidity who are poor surgical candidates (Fig. 14.1). These are also the group in whom angiography may be more challenging.

The stomach and duodenum have a rich collateral blood supply and hence embolization of branches of the coeliac axis can be performed with a low risk of infarction of the viscera. Conversely, the extensive vascular supply may make embolization more difficult to achieve. Thus, in addition to coils, a small particulate embolic agent is often required for a more distal block. A co-axial catheter system is likely to be necessary for this. The method of embolization depends on the angiographic findings but occlusion of the artery needs to be performed on either side of the abnormality (eroded artery or aneurysm) to achieve haemostasis. Ischaemia may be provoked if extensive embolization is performed or if there is compromise of the collateral supply due to concomitant arterial disease or previous surgery.

Embolization of massively bleeding duodenal ulcers constituted 5% of endoscopically treated duodenal ulcers and as little as 0.6% of all cases with upper gastrointestinal bleeding who underwent emergency endoscopy in one large series. Contrast extravasation was demonstrated in only half of these cases. Embolization did however induce haemostasis in 90% of cases (Toyoda et al. 1995). 'Prophylactic' embolization of the GDA is sometimes performed with success (as in this series) even when no angiographic abnormality is demonstrated despite a proven endoscopic source of haemorrhage.

Patients with chronic gastrointestinal bleeding are often repeatedly investigated with numerous modalities and angiography is performed more frequently in this group. Of course this is primarily to study the small bowel rather than the stomach or duodenum. However, selective angiography may reveal unusual proximal causes such as gastric or duodenal arteriovenous malformations or Dieulafoy disease.

Dieulafoy disease can cause massive and often fatal gastrointestinal haemorrhage. This results from erosion of a submucosal artery and although it can occur throughout the gastrointestinal tract, the commonest site is the proximal stomach. On angiography there is rapid extravasation of contrast from an eroded but otherwise normal-appearing artery. Embolisation of the left gastric artery has been reported as successful treatment of the lesion (Durham et al. 1990).

Gastric antral vascular ectasia (GAVE) syndrome, or 'watermelon stomach' as it was called in 1984 (Jabbari et al. 1984), is a cause of chronic gastrointestinal blood loss. This is usually diagnosed at endoscopy but the angiographic features have also been described (Robertson et al. 1996). The syndrome is commoner in women and is associated with autoimmune diseases. Cirrhosis and portal hypertension is present in 30% of cases (Mesihovic et al. 2004). On endoscopy there are prominent longitudinal erythematous folds traversing the gastric antrum and hence the name 'watermelon'. However, many cases are not typical and there may be diffuse gastric reddening, which is impossible to distinguish from gastritis without biopsy. The angiographic features on selective coeliac axis, common hepatic or gastroduodenal angiography are hypervascularity restricted to the gastric antrum with a well defined demarcation between the normal and abnormal stomach and early arteriovenous shunting. This results in a tramline appearance due to the simultaneous opacification of arteries and veins. There is early clearance of contrast from the gastric antrum and thus the late venous phase appears normal. There is no extravasation of contrast into the stomach. Therefore the diagnosis may be difficult on angiography if the findings are subtle. Additionally, superimposition of the gastric antrum over the right renal collecting system may obscure hypervascularity and arteriovenous shunting.

14.3.3 Aneurysms

Visceral aneurysms are uncommon and most frequently involve the splenic artery. They may also arise from the pancreaticoduodenal branches of either the GDA or SMA and the left gastric artery (Fig. 14.3). Although an underlying cause may not be demonstrated, many of these are associated with acute or chronic pancreatitis or are secondary to atheromatous disease. Atheromatous stenosis of the coeliac axis or compression of the coeliac axis by the median arcuate ligament of the diaphragm results in hypertrophy of the pancreaticoduodenal arteries and is associated with aneurysm formation.

Some aneurysms are asymptomatic and found incidentally on computed tomography (CT) performed for other reasons. Other patients may have a history of chronic abdominal pain but if haemorrhage occurs the pain may be more severe and circulatory collapse can occur. Contrast enhanced CT is usually performed and this may reveal a haematoma and sometimes the aneurysm itself, which is a useful guide for subsequent angiography.

14.3.4 Tumours

The stomach and duodenum may be involved by primary tumours, by tumour in adjacent organs (e.g. pancreas, gallbladder) or by metastatic deposits (e.g. breast, melanoma). Angiography and embolization have little to offer in the management of these tumours. The tumours that are referred for embolization are inoperable primary leiomyosarcomas, which can cause severe bleeding, and large invading pancreatic neuroendocrine tumours. Angiography often reveals extensive neovascularity and therefore venous occlusion and embolization is limited to occluding tumour vessels in an attempt to reduce

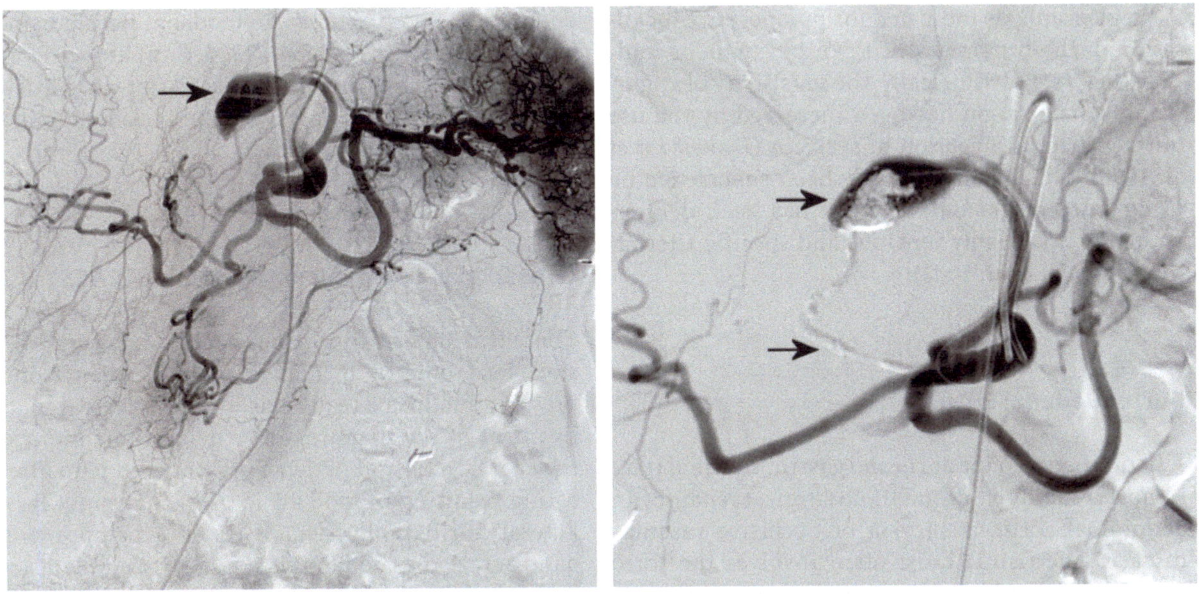

a b

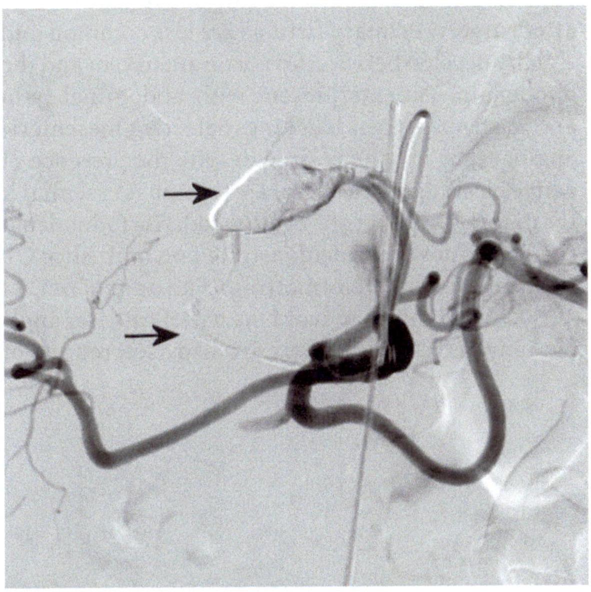

c

Fig. 14.3a–c. Left gastric aneurysm. Coeliac axis arteriogram (a) demonstrating a left gastric artery aneurysm (*arrow*). Post-embolisation images (b,c) show successful embolisation of the left gastric artery aneurysm using onyx (*arrows*)

perfusion pressure. The results are typically rather disappointing and short-lived.

14.3.5 Zollinger-Ellinson Syndrome

Zollinger-Ellinson syndrome is a severe form of peptic ulcer disease related to the presence of a gastrin secreting tumour. These tumours can develop from pancreatic islets or the endocrine cells of duodenal or gastric mucosa and therefore may form part of multiple endocrine neoplasia type I (MEN1) (Tonelli et al. 2005). The excess gastrin production causes gastric hypersecretion rich in hydrochloric acid. This results in multiple ulcerations of the oesophagus, stomach and duodenum. There is marked thickening and irregularity of the gastric rugae and duodenal folds. Multiple ulcers, which may be sizeable, are usual although a solitary ulcer can also occur. These findings on endoscopy or barium studies suggest the diagnosis, which is typically confirmed by elevation of blood gastrin levels. The majority of duodenal gastrinomas occur in the first or second part of the duodenum (83%) (Zogakis et al. 2003).

Angiography is indicated for preoperative localisation of the tumour, which can be single or multiple (Fig. 14.4). Historically, the sensitivity of angiographic localisation has been increased by the use of intra-arterial injection of secretin (Doppman et al. 1990). This has now largely been superseded by using calcium gluconate, which has been demonstrated to be a highly sensitive and specific alternative (Turner et al. 2002).

14.3.6 Aortoduodenal Fistula

A fistula between the aorta and gastrointestinal tract is most commonly secondary to surgical repair of an abdominal aortic aneurysm or occlusive vascular disease. The fistula most often involves the third part of the duodenum and can occur many years after surgery. Primary fistulas are less common and usually develop between an aortic aneurysm and the duodenum. Patients present with abdominal pain and gastrointestinal bleeding. Selective mesenteric angiography may be normal despite the presence of active bleeding and a lateral aortogram is essential if the diagnosis is not to be overlooked. Aortoduodenal fistula has now been demonstrated on multislice CT with multiplanar reformatting (Frauenfelder et al. 2004) and this may avoid the use of catheter angiography in the future. There are also a few reports of endovascular repair of aortoduodenal fistula using a stent-graft (Chuter et al. 2000; Schlensak et al. 2000). However, these have failed after only a few months and at present are advocated as a temporary measure to control bleeding.

14.3.7 Coeliac Axis Compression Syndrome (CACS)

There is debate as to whether coeliac axis compression syndrome or median arcuate ligament compression syndrome really exists. The median arcuate ligament of the diaphragm is thought to compress the coeliac axis and patients present with pain after eating resulting in food avoidance and weight loss. Lateral aortography demonstrates a compression band across the coeliac axis (Fig. 14.5) and there are reports of symptomatic improvement following surgical interruption of the ligament. It is possible that the syndrome can develop in patients with a poorly developed collateral circulation between the coeliac axis and SMA resulting in pain in the ischaemic stomach. However, coeliac axis stenosis has been demonstrated in 7.3% of asymptomatic individuals and this was due to median arcuate ligament compression in half of the cases (Park et al. 2001).

Theoretically angioplasty or stent insertion could be used as treatment but the median arcuate ligament is a very strong structure and it is unlikely that

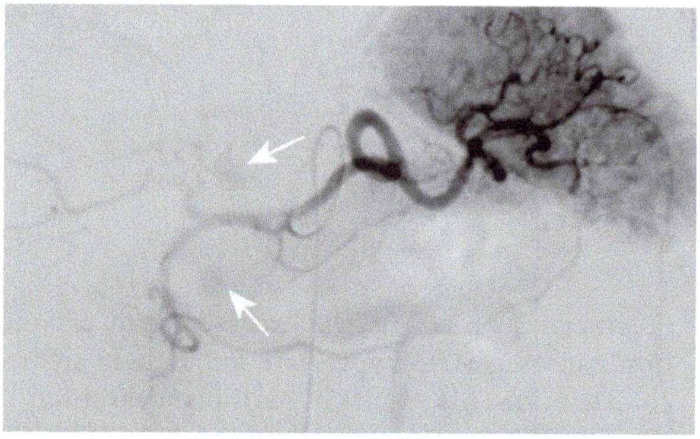

a

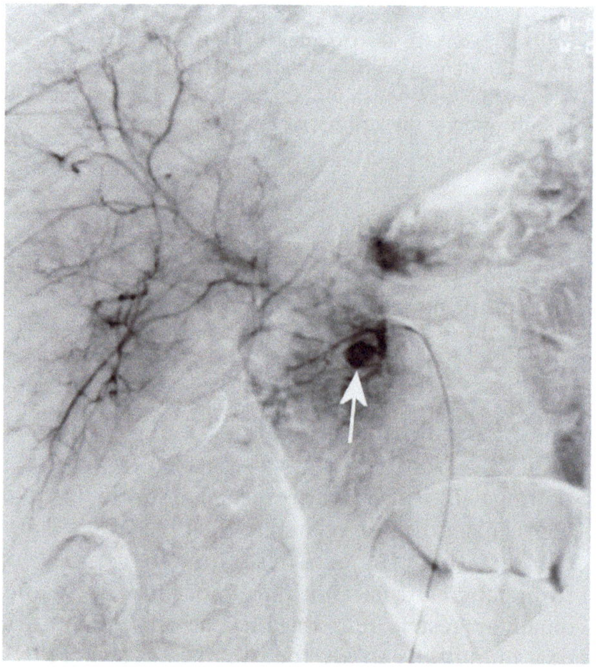

b

Fig. 14.4a,b. Zollinger-Ellison Syndrome. Selective celiac artery injection (**a**) demonstrates two faint focal areas of increased vascularity, one in the left lobe of the liver (*upper arrow*) and one in the second part of the duodenum (*lower arrow*). These represented two separate gastrinomas. Selective injection of the right hepatic artery (**b**) in a second case demonstrated an area of increased vascularity (*arrow*) in the second part of the duodenum. This corresponded to a positive octreotide scan and again represented a small gastrinoma

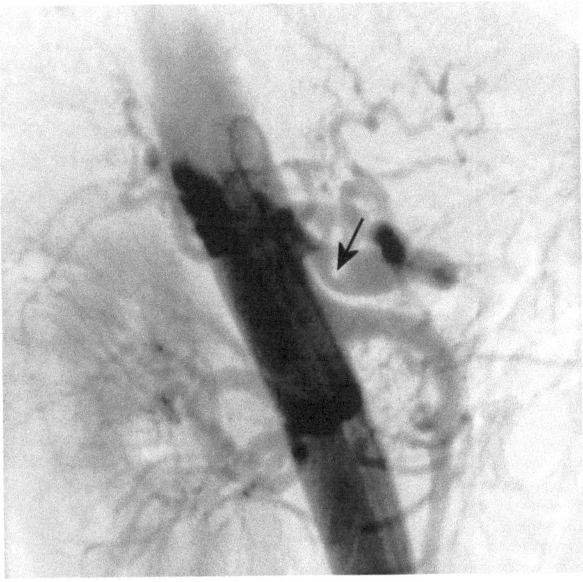

Fig. 14.5. Median arcuate ligament compression. Lateral abdominal aortogram showing compression of the celiac axis (*arrow*) by the median arcuate ligament of the diaphragm

either would achieve therapeutic benefit. Laparoscopic division of the ligament has been reported (Dordoni et al. 2002).

References

Chuter TA, Lukaszewicz GC, Reilly LM, Kerlan RK, Faruqi R, Sawhney R, Wall SD, Canto C, LaBerge JM, Gordon RL, Messina LM (2000) Endovascular repair of a presumed aortoenteric fistula: late failure due to recurrent infection. J Endovasc Ther 7:240–244

Defreyne L, Vanlangenhove P, Decruyenaere J, Van Maele G, De Vos M, Troisi R, Pattyn P (2003) Outcome of acute nonvariceal gastrointestinal haemorrhage after nontherapeutic arteriography compared with embolization. Eur Radiol 13:2604–2614

Doppman JL, Miller DL, Chang R, Maton PN, London JF, Gardner JD, Jensen RT, Norton JA (1990) Gastrinomas: localization by means of selective intraarterial injection of secretin. Radiology 174:25–29

Dordoni L, Tshomba Y, Giacomelli M, Jannello AM,Chiesa R (2002) Celiac artery compression syndrome: successful laparoscopic treatment – a case report. Vasc Endovascular Surg 36:317–321

Durham JD, Kumpe DA, Rothbarth LJ, Van Stiegmann G (1990) Dieulafoy disease: arteriographic findings and treatment. Radiology 174:937–941

Frauenfelder T, Wildermuth S, Marincek B, Boehm T (2004) Nontraumatic emergent abdominal vascular conditions: advantages of multi-detector row CT and three-dimensional imaging. Radiographics 24:481–496

Jabbari M, Cherry R, Lough JO, Daly DS, Kinnear DG, Goresky CA (1984) Gastric antral vascular ectasia: the watermelon stomach. Gastroenterology 87:1165–1170

Mesihovic R, Prohic D, Gribajcevic M, Vanis N, Gornjakovic S, Sarac A (2004) Portal hypertensive gastropathy (PHG). Med Arh 58:377–379

Nusbaum M, Baum S (1963) Radiographic demonstration of unknown sites of gastrointestinal bleeding. Surg Forum 14:374–375

Park CM, Chung JW, Kim HB, Shin SJ, Park JH (2001) Celiac axis stenosis: incidence and etiologies in asymptomatic individuals. Korean J Radiol 2:8–13

Robertson IR, Tait NP, Jackson JE (1996) Vascular ectasia of the gastric antrum: angiographic findings. AJR Am J Roentgenol 166:87–89

Schlensak C, Doenst T, Spillner G, Blum U, Geiger A, Beyersdorf F (2000) Palliative treatment of a secondary aortoduodenal fistula by stent-graft placement. Thorac Cardiovasc Surg 48:41–42

Tonelli F, Fratini G, Falchetti A, Nesi G, Brandi ML (2005) Surgery for gastroenteropancreatic tumours in multiple endocrine neoplasia type 1: review and personal experience. J Intern Med 257:38–49

Toyoda H, Nakano S, Takeda I, Kumada T, Sugiyama K, Osada T, Kiriyama S,Suga T (1995) Transcatheter arterial embolization for massive bleeding from duodenal ulcers not controlled by endoscopic hemostasis. Endoscopy 27:304–307

Turner JJ, Wren AM, Jackson JE, Thakker RV, Meeran K (2002) Localization of gastrinomas by selective intraarterial calcium injection. Clin Endocrinol (Oxf) 57:821–825

Zogakis TG, Gibril F, Libutti SK, Norton JA, White DE, Jensen RT, Alexander HR (2003) Management and outcome of patients with sporadic gastrinoma arising in the duodenum. Ann Surg 238:42–48

Subject Index

D

E

F

G

M

N

O

P

List of Contributors

Kottekattu Balan, BSc, MBBS, MD, FRCP
Consultant Physician in Nuclear Medicine
Department of Nuclear Medicine
Addenbrooke's Hospital
Box 170, Hills Road
Cambridge, CB2 2QQ
UK

Ahmed Ba-Ssalamah, MD
Department of Radiology
University of Vienna
Waehriner Guertel 18–20
1090 Vienna
Austria

Nicholas R. Carroll, MB, BS, MRCP, FRCR
Department of Radiology
Addenbrooke's Hospital
Box 219, Hills Road
Cambridge, CB2 2QQ
UK

Claire Cousins, MB, BS, MRCP, FRCR
Department of Radiology
Addenbrooke's Hospital
Box 219, Hills Road
Cambridge, CB2 2QQ
UK

Markus Dux, MD, PhD
Department of Diagnostic and Interventional Radiology
Krankenhaus Nordwest
Teaching Hospital of the
Johann Wolfgang Goethe University of Frankfurt
Steinbacher Hohl 2-26
60488 Frankfurt am Main
Germany

Frans-Thomas Fork, MD, PhD
Department of Diagnostic Radiology
Malmö University Hospital
20502 01 Malmö
Sweden

Alan H. Freeman, MB, BS, FRCR
Consultant Radiologist
Department of Radiology
Addenbrooke's Hospital
Box 219, Hills Road
Cambridge, CB2 2QQ
UK

Keith M. Harris, MB, BS, FRCS, FRCR
Department of Radiology
The General Infirmary
Great George Street
Leeds LS1 3EX
UK

Hans-Ulrich Laasch, MD, MRCP, FRCR
Consultant Radiologist
Christie Hospital NHS Trust
Wilmslow Road
Manchester M20 4BX
UK

Derrick Martin, FRCP, FRCR
Professor of GI-Radiology
Academic Dept. of GI-Radiology
South Manchester University Hospitals NHS Trust
Southmoor Road, Wythenshawe
Manchester M23 9LT
UK

Mazda Memarsadeghi, MD
Department of Radiology
University of Vienna
Waehriner Guertel 18–20
1090 Vienna
Austria

Peter Pokieser, MD
Medical Media Services of the
Core Unit of Medical Education
and
Department of Radiology
University of Vienna
Waehriner Guertel 18–20
1090 Vienna
Austria

Mathias Prokop, MD
Department of Radiology
University of Vienna
Waehriner Guertel 18–20
1090 Vienna
Austria

Jacques W. A. J. Reeders, MD, PhD
Consultant Radiologist
Department of Radiology
St. Elisabeth Hospital Willemstad
Breedestraat 193(O)
Curaçao
Netherlands Antilles

Evis Sala, MD, PhD
University Lecturer/Honorary Consultant
University Department of Radiology
Addenbrooke's Hospital
Box 219, Hills Road
Cambridge CB2 2QQ
UK

Teik C. See, MB, BS, MRCP, FRCR
Consultant Radiologist
Department of Radiology
Addenbrooke's Hospital
Box 219, Hills Road
Cambridge, CB2 2QQ
UK

Philip John Shorvon, MA, FRCP, FRCR
Consultant Radiologist
Department of Radiology
North West London Hospitals NHS Trust
Central Middlesex Hospital
Acton Lane
London NW10 7NS
UK

Martin Uffmann, MD
Department of Radiology
University of Vienna
Waehriner Guertel 18–20
1090 Vienna
Austria

Rivka Zissin, MD
Head of CT Unit
Department of Diagnostic Imaging
Meir General Hospital
Sapir Medical Center Kfar Saba
affiliated to the Sackler Faculty of Medicine
Tel-Aviv University
Tchernichovsky St., Kfar Saba 44281
Tel-Aviv
Israel

MEDICAL RADIOLOGY Diagnostic Imaging and Radiation Oncology

Titles in the series already published

DIAGNOSTIC IMAGING

Innovations in Diagnostic Imaging
Edited by J. H. Anderson

Radiology of the Upper Urinary Tract
Edited by E. K. Lang

The Thymus - Diagnostic Imaging, Functions, and Pathologic Anatomy
Edited by E. Walter, E. Willich, and W. R. Webb

Interventional Neuroradiology
Edited by A. Valavanis

Radiology of the Pancreas
Edited by A. L. Baert, co-edited by G. Delorme

Radiology of the Lower Urinary Tract
Edited by E. K. Lang

Magnetic Resonance Angiography
Edited by I. P. Arlart, G. M. Bongartz, and G. Marchal

Contrast-Enhanced MRI of the Breast
S. Heywang-Köbrunner and R. Beck

Spiral CT of the Chest
Edited by M. Rémy-Jardin and J. Rémy

Radiological Diagnosis of Breast Diseases
Edited by M. Friedrich and E.A. Sickles

Radiology of the Trauma
Edited by M. Heller and A. Fink

Biliary Tract Radiology
Edited by P. Rossi, co-edited by M. Brezi

Radiological Imaging of Sports Injuries
Edited by C. Masciocchi

Modern Imaging of the Alimentary Tube
Edited by A. R. Margulis

Diagnosis and Therapy of Spinal Tumors
Edited by P. R. Algra, J. Valk, and J. J. Heimans

Interventional Magnetic Resonance Imaging
Edited by J. F. Debatin and G. Adam

Abdominal and Pelvic MRI
Edited by A. Heuck and M. Reiser

Orthopedic Imaging
Techniques and Applications
Edited by A. M. Davies and H. Pettersson

Radiology of the Female Pelvic Organs
Edited by E. K.Lang

Magnetic Resonance of the Heart and Great Vessels
Clinical Applications
Edited by J. Bogaert, A.J. Duerinckx, and F. E. Rademakers

Modern Head and Neck Imaging
Edited by S. K. Mukherji and J. A. Castelijns

Radiological Imaging of Endocrine Diseases
Edited by J. N. Bruneton in collaboration with B. Padovani and M.-Y. Mourou

Trends in Contrast Media
Edited by H. S. Thomsen, R. N. Muller, and R. F. Mattrey

Functional MRI
Edited by C. T. W. Moonen and P. A. Bandettini

Radiology of the Pancreas
2nd Revised Edition
Edited by A. L. Baert. Co-edited by G. Delorme and L. Van Hoe

Emergency Pediatric Radiology
Edited by H. Carty

Spiral CT of the Abdomen
Edited by F. Terrier, M. Grossholz, and C. D. Becker

Liver Malignancies
Diagnostic and Interventional Radiology
Edited by C. Bartolozzi and R. Lencioni

Medical Imaging of the Spleen
Edited by A. M. De Schepper and F. Vanhoenacker

Radiology of Peripheral Vascular Diseases
Edited by E. Zeitler

Diagnostic Nuclear Medicine
Edited by C. Schiepers

Radiology of Blunt Trauma of the Chest
P. Schnyder and M. Wintermark

Portal Hypertension
Diagnostic Imaging-Guided Therapy
Edited by P. Rossi
Co-edited by P. Ricci and L. Broglia

Recent Advances in Diagnostic Neuroradiology
Edited by Ph. Demaerel

Virtual Endoscopy and Related 3D Techniques
Edited by P. Rogalla, J. Terwisscha Van Scheltinga, and B. Hamm

Multislice CT
Edited by M. F. Reiser, M. Takahashi, M. Modic, and R. Bruening

Pediatric Uroradiology
Edited by R. Fotter

Transfontanellar Doppler Imaging in Neonates
A. Couture and C. Veyrac

Radiology of AIDS
A Practical Approach
Edited by J.W.A.J. Reeders and P.C. Goodman

CT of the Peritoneum
Armando Rossi and Giorgio Rossi

Magnetic Resonance Angiography
2nd Revised Edition
Edited by I. P. Arlart, G. M. Bongratz, and G. Marchal

Pediatric Chest Imaging
Edited by Javier Lucaya and Janet L. Strife

Applications of Sonography in Head and Neck Pathology
Edited by J. N. Bruneton in collaboration with C. Raffaelli and O. Dassonville

Imaging of the Larynx
Edited by R. Hermans

3D Image Processing
Techniques and Clinical Applications
Edited by D. Caramella and C. Bartolozzi

Imaging of Orbital and Visual Pathway Pathology
Edited by W. S. Müller-Forell

Pediatric ENT Radiology
Edited by S. J. King and A. E. Boothroyd

Radiological Imaging of the Small Intestine
Edited by N. C. Gourtsoyiannis

Imaging of the Knee
Techniques and Applications
Edited by A. M. Davies and V. N. Cassar-Pullicino

Perinatal Imaging
From Ultrasound to MR Imaging
Edited by Fred E. Avni

Radiological Imaging of the Neonatal Chest
Edited by V. Donoghue

Diagnostic and Interventional Radiology in Liver Transplantation
Edited by E. Bücheler, V. Nicolas, C. E. Broelsch, X. Rogiers, and G. Krupski

Radiology of Osteoporosis
Edited by S. Grampp

Imaging Pelvic Floor Disorders
Edited by C. I. Bartram and J. O. L. DeLancey
Associate Editors: S. Halligan, F. M. Kelvin, and J. Stoker

Imaging of the Pancreas
Cystic and Rare Tumors
Edited by C. Procacci and A. J. Megibow

High Resolution Sonography of the Peripheral Nervous System
Edited by S. Peer and G. Bodner

Imaging of the Foot and Ankle
Techniques and Applications
Edited by A. M. Davies, R. W. Whitehouse, and J. P. R. Jenkins

Radiology Imaging of the Ureter
Edited by F. Joffre, Ph. Otal, and M. Soulie

Imaging of the Shoulder
Techniques and Applications
Edited by A. M. Davies and J. Hodler

Radiology of the Petrous Bone
Edited by M. Lemmerling and S. S. Kollias

Interventional Radiology in Cancer
Edited by A. Adam, R. F. Dondelinger, and P. R. Mueller

Duplex and Color Doppler Imaging of the Venous System
Edited by G. H. Mostbeck

Multidetector-Row CT of the Thorax
Edited by U. J. Schoepf

Functional Imaging of the Chest
Edited by H.-U. Kauczor

Radiology of the Pharynx and the Esophagus
Edited by O. Ekberg

Radiological Imaging in Hematological Malignancies
Edited by A. Guermazi

Imaging and Intervention in Abdominal Trauma
Edited by R. F. Dondelinger

Multislice CT
2nd Revised Edition
Edited by M. F. Reiser, M. Takahashi, M. Modic, and C. R. Becker

Intracranial Vascular Malformations and Aneurysms
From Diagnostic Work-Up to Endovascular Therapy
Edited by M. Forsting

Radiology and Imaging of the Colon
Edited by A. H. Chapman

Coronary Radiology
Edited by M. Oudkerk

Dynamic Contrast-Enhanced Magnetic Resonance Imaging in Oncology
Edited by A. Jackson, D. L. Buckley, and G. J. M. Parker

Imaging in Treatment Planning for Sinonasal Diseases
Edited by R. Maroldi and P. Nicolai

Clinical Cardiac MRI
With Interactive CD-ROM
Edited by J. Bogaert, S. Dymarkowski, and A. M. Taylor

Focal Liver Lesions
Detection, Characterization, Ablation
Edited by R. Lencioni, D. Cioni, and C. Bartolozzi

Multidetector-Row CT Angiography
Edited by C. Catalano and R. Passariello

Paediatric Musculoskeletal Diseases
With an Emphasis on Ultrasound
Edited by D. Wilson

Contrast Media in Ultrasonography
Basic Principles and Clinical Applications
Edited by Emilio Quaia

MR Imaging in White Matter Diseases of the Brain and Spinal Cord
Edited by M. Filippi, N. De Stefano, V. Dousset, and J. C. McGowan

Diagnostic Nuclear Medicine
2nd Revised Edition
Edited by C. Schiepers

Imaging of the Kidney Cancer
Edited by A. Guermazi

Magnetic Resonance Imaging in Ischemic Stroke
Edited by R. von Kummer and T. Back

Imaging of the Hip & Bony Pelvis
Techniques and Applications
Edited by A. M. Davies, K. J. Johnson, and R. W. Whitehouse

Imaging of Occupational and Environmental Disorders of the Chest
Edited by P. A. Gevenois and P. De Vuyst

Contrast Media
Safety Issues and ESUR Guidelines
Edited by H. S. Thomsen

Virtual Colonoscopy
A Practical Guide
Edited by P. Lefere and S. Gryspeerdt

Vascular Embolotherapy
A Comprehensive Approach
Volume 1: *General Principles, Chest, Abdomen, and Great Vessels*
Edited by J. Golzarian. Co-edited by S. Sun and M. J. Sharafuddin

Vascular Embolotherapy
A Comprehensive Approach
Volume 2: *Oncology, Trauma, Gene Therapy, Vascular Malformations, and Neck*
Edited by J. Golzarian. Co-edited by S. Sun and M. J. Sharafuddin

Head and Neck Cancer Imaging
Edited by R. Hermans

Vascular Interventional Radiology
Current Evidence in Endovascular Surgery
Edited by M. G. Cowling

Ultrasound of the Gastrointestinal Tract
Edited by G. Maconi and G. Bianchi Porro

Imaging of Orthopedic Sports Injuries
Edited by F. M. Vanhoenacker, M. Maas, J. L. M. A. Gielen

Parallel Imaging in Clinical MR Applications
Edited by S. O. Schoenberg, O. Dietrich, and M. F. Reiser

MRI and CT of the Female Pelvis
Edited by B. Hamm and R. Forstner

Ultrasound of the Musculoskeletal System
S. Bianchi and C. Martinoli

Spinal Imaging
Diagnostic Imaging of the Spine and Spinal Cord
Edited by J. W. M. Van Goethem, L. van den Hauwe, and P. M. Parizel

Radiation Dose from Adult and Pediatric Multidetector Computed Tomography
Edited by D. Tack and P. A. Gevenois

Computed Tomography of the Lung
A Pattern Approach
J. A. Verschakelen and W. De Wever

Clinical Functional MRI
Presurgical Functional Neuroimaging
Edited bei C. Stippich

Imaging in Transplantation
Edited by A. A. Bankier

Radiological Imaging of the Digestive System in Infants and Children
Edited by A. S. Devos and J. G. Blickman

Pediatric Chest Imaging
Chest Imaging in Infants and Children
2nd Revised Edition
Edited by J. Lucaya and J. L. Strife

Radiological Imaging of the Neonatal Chest
2nd Revised Edition
Edited by V. Donoghue

Radiology of the Stomach and Duodenum
Edited by A. H. Freeman and E. Sala

Imaging in Pediatric Skeletal Trauma
Techniques and Applications
Edited by K. J. Johnson and E. Bache

Percutaneous Tumor Ablation in Medical Radiology
Edited by T. J. Vogl, T. K. Helmberger, M. G. Mack, and M. F. Reiser

Screening and Preventive Diagnosis with Radiological Imaging
Edited by M. F. Reiser, G. van Kaick, C. Fink, and S. O. Schoenberg

Color Doppler US of the Penis
Edited by M. Bertolotto

Image Processing in Radiology
Current Applications
Edited by E. Neri, D. Caramella, and C. Bartolozzi

MIX
Papier aus verantwortungsvollen Quellen
Paper from responsible sources
FSC® C105338

If you have any concerns about our products,
you can contact us on
ProductSafety@springernature.com

In case Publisher is established outside the EU,
the EU authorized representative is:
Springer Nature Customer Service Center GmbH
Europaplatz 3, 69115 Heidelberg, Germany

Printed by Libri Plureos GmbH
in Hamburg, Germany